A CLINICAL GUIDE TO TREATING BEHAVIORAL ADDICTIONS

Amanda L. Giordano, PhD, LPC, is an associate professor in the counseling program at the University of Georgia. She specializes in addiction counseling with clinical, instructional, and scholarly experience related to both chemical and behavioral addictions. Giordano works to advance the counseling field with rigorous research and has published over 45 peer-reviewed articles and book chapters. She earned the Addictions/Offender Educator Excellence Award from the International Association of Addictions and Offender Counselors and has experience as an editorial board member for the *Journal of Addictions and Offender Counseling* and *Counseling & Values*. Giordano is dedicated to raising public awareness about addiction and frequently conducts conference presentations, webinars, and training related to addiction counseling.

A CLINICAL GUIDE TO TREATING BEHAVIORAL ADDICTIONS

Conceptualizations, Assessments, and Clinical Strategies

Amanda L. Giordano, PhD, LPC

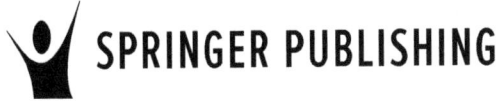

Copyright © 2022 Springer Publishing Company, LLC
All rights reserved.

No part of this publication may be reproduced, stored in a retrieval system, or transmitted in any form or by any means, electronic, mechanical, photocopying, recording, or otherwise, without the prior permission of Springer Publishing Company, LLC, or authorization through payment of the appropriate fees to the Copyright Clearance Center, Inc., 222 Rosewood Drive, Danvers, MA 01923, 978-750-8400, fax 978-646-8600, info@copyright.com or on the Web at www.copyright.com.

Springer Publishing Company, LLC
11 West 42nd Street, New York, NY 10036
www.springerpub.com
connect.springerpub.com/

Acquisitions Editor: Rhonda Dearborn
Compositor: Exeter Premedia Services Private Ltd.

ISBN: 978-0-8261-6316-5
ebook ISBN: 978-0-8261-6317-2
DOI: 10.1891/9780826163172

21 22 23 24 / 5 4 3 2 1

The author and the publisher of this work have made every effort to use sources believed to be reliable to provide information that is accurate and compatible with the standards generally accepted at the time of publication. The author and publisher shall not be liable for any special, consequential, or exemplary damages resulting, in whole or in part, from the readers' use of, or reliance on, the information contained in this book. The publisher has no responsibility for the persistence or accuracy of URLs for external or third-party Internet websites referred to in this publication and does not guarantee that any content on such websites is, or will remain, accurate or appropriate.

Library of Congress Cataloging-in-Publication Data

Names: Giordano, Amanda L., author.
Title: A clinical guide to treating behavioral addictions :
  conceptualizations, assessments, and clinical strategies / Amanda L.
  Giordano.
Description: First Springer Publishing edition. | New York, NY : Springer
  Publishing Company, LLC, 2021. | Includes bibliographical references and
  index.
Identifiers: LCCN 2021011266 (print) | LCCN 2021011267 (ebook) | ISBN
  9780826163165 (paperback) | ISBN 9780826163172 (ebook)
Subjects: MESH: Behavior, Addictive
Classification: LCC RC533 (print) | LCC RC533 (ebook) | NLM WM 176 | DDC
  616.86--dc23
LC record available at https://lccn.loc.gov/2021011266
LC ebook record available at https://lccn.loc.gov/2021011267

Contact sales@springerpub.com to receive discount rates on bulk purchases.

Publisher's Note: New and used products purchased from third-party sellers are not guaranteed for quality, authenticity, or access to any included digital components.

Printed in the United States of America.

*To my parents, Anthony and Diane Giordano.
Just two kids from Collingswood—who have given me every opportunity
I could have hoped for.*

*Not to us, Lord, not to us but to your name be the glory, because of your love
and faithfulness.*

PSALM 115:1

CONTENTS

Contributors   *xi*
Foreword   Zsolt Demetrovics   *xiii*
Preface   *xv*
Acknowledgments   *xix*

1. Introduction to Behavioral Addictions   1
   Why Read a Book About Behavioral Addictions?   1
   What Makes a Behavior an Addiction?   3
   Public Health Model of Behavioral Addiction   7
   Summary   12
   References   13

2. Neuroscience of Behavioral Addictions   17
   Why Is Neuroscience Important?   17
   Neurotransmission   18
   Reward Circuitry   19
   Genetic Predisposition to Behavioral Addictions   24
   Neuroadaptations Caused by Addictive Behaviors   26
   Interaction Between Genetic and Environmental Factors   28
   Summary   31
   References   31

3. Internet Gaming Addiction   35
   How Do I Conceptualize It?   35
   How Do I Identify It?   42
   How Do I Assess It?   44
   How Do I Treat It?   46
   Voices From the Field: Clinical Work With Internet Gaming Addiction   47
   How Can I Learn More?   50
   References   51

4. Social Media Addiction   55
   How Do I Conceptualize It?   55

How Do I Identify It? 63
How Do I Assess It? 65
How Do I Treat It? 67
Voices From the Field: Clinical Work With Social Media Addiction 68
How Can I Learn More? 72
References 72

5. Sex Addiction 77
How Do I Conceptualize It? 77
How Do I Identify It? 84
How Do I Assess It? 86
How Do I Treat It? 87
Voices From the Field: Clinical Work With Sex Addiction 88
How Can I Learn More? 93
References 94

6. Pornography and Cybersex Addiction 99
How Do I Conceptualize It? 99
How Do I Identify It? 107
How Do I Assess It? 108
How Do I Treat It? 110
Voices From the Field: Clinical Work With Porn Addiction 111
How Can I Learn More? 115
References 116

7. Love Addiction 121
How Do I Conceptualize It? 121
How Do I Identify It? 129
How Do I Assess It? 131
How Do I Treat It? 132
Voices From the Field: Clinical Work With Love Addiction 133
How Can I Learn More? 137
References 138

8. Gambling Addiction 143
How Do I Conceptualize It? 143
How Do I Identify it? 151
How Do I Assess It? 153
How Do I Treat It? 155
Voices From the Field: Clinical Work With Gambling Addiction 156
How Can I Learn More? 160
References 161

9. Nonsuicidal Self-Injury 165
How Do I Conceptualize It? 165
How Do I Identify It? 171
How Do I Assess It? 174
How Do I Treat It? 175

Voices From the Field: Clinical Work With NSSI 176
How Can I Learn More? 180
References 181

10. Food Addiction 185
How Do I Conceptualize It? 185
How Do I Identify It? 192
How Do I Assess It? 193
How Do I Treat It? 194
Voices From the Field: Clinical Work With Food Addiction 195
How Can I Learn More? 200
References 201

11. Exercise Addiction 205
How Do I Conceptualize It? 205
How Do I Identify It? 213
How Do I Assess It? 215
How Do I Treat It? 216
Voices From the Field: Clinical Work With Exercise Addiction 217
How Can I Learn More? 220
References 221

12. Work Addiction 225
How Do I Conceptualize It? 225
How Do I Identify It? 229
How Do I Assess It? 232
How Do I Treat It? 234
Voices From the Field: Clinical Work With Work Addiction 235
How Can I Learn More? 239
References 240

13. Shopping Addiction 245
How Do I Conceptualize It? 245
How Do I Identify It? 252
How Do I Assess It? 254
How Do I Treat It? 255
Voices From the Field: Clinical Work With Shopping Addiction 257
How Can I Learn More? 260
References 261

14. Advocating for Clients With Behavioral Addictions 265
What Is Advocacy? 265
Addiction Advocacy 266
Advocating for Those With Behavioral Addictions 268
Looking to the Future 275
References 276

Index 279

CONTRIBUTORS

Sarah Bridge, LCSW, LLC, Senior Clinical Advisor for The Meadows Behavioral Health, Scottsdale, Arizona

Hilarie Cash, PhD, LMHC, CSAT, WSGC, Founding Member, Chief Clinical Officer, Education Director; reSTART Life, PLLC, restartlife.com, Bellevue, Washington

Lauren Colston, PsyD, Licensed Clinical Psychologist, Registered Health Service Psychologist, Oxon Hill, Maryland

Pamela Dobbs, LCADC, CCS, SAC, MA, ICGC-II, Marlton Office Site Director, Genesis Counseling Centers, Marlton, New Jersey

Jon A. Parker, MAMFT, LPC, NCC, Counselor, Atlanta, Georgia

Tal Prince, MDiv, MA, NCC, LPC, CSAT, Director, Insights Counseling Center, Birmingham, Alabama

Kiersten Rapstine, LPC-S, CEDS-S, Counselor, Dallas, Texas

Bryan E. Robinson, PhD, Counselor, Asheville, North Carolina

Jennifer Rollin, MSW, LCSW-C, Therapist and Founder of The Eating Disorder Center, Rockville, Maryland

Thorn Winkler, MA, APC, AMFT, Stonegate Counseling Associates, Counselor, Watkinsville, Georgia

Taylor Zebrosky, MS, LPC, Owner/Therapist, Highland Village Counseling, PLLC, Highland Village, Texas

FOREWORD

Until very recently, addictions have been considered as disorders that are exclusively linked to psychoactive substance use. That was clearly reflected by the diagnostic systems as neither the section "Psychoactive Substance Use Disorders" in *Diagnostic and Statistical Manual of Mental Disorders,* Fourth Edition, nor the section "Mental and Behavioural Disorders Due to Psychoactive Substance Use" in *International Classification of Diseases,* 10th Revision, made it possible to include any nonsubstance-related disorders into these classes. Those disorders or problem behaviors that were often reflected as addictions had either been classified in other sections (e.g., pathological gambling as an impulse control disorder) or had not been recognized as disorders at all (e.g., work addiction, exercise addiction, shopping addiction).

Due to the research done in the past quarter of a century, this picture has changed substantially. Besides the increase in studying the "traditional" behavioral addictions such as gambling, compulsive buying, hypersexual behavior, and exercise addiction, the technological development of the past 25 years opened a new field for the study of internet-related addictive behaviors, with a special focus on video game use and problematic social media use. Not only the interest toward the understanding of technology-related addictive behaviors increased rapidly but also this stimulated further interest toward other nonsubstance-related addictive behaviors.

All this resulted in the strengthening of the concept of considering these behaviors as part of a larger class "behavioral addictions" or even, together with psychoactive substance use disorders as "addictive behaviors." Increasing numbers of studies examining genetic, neurobiological, and psychological factors confirmed the assumption that these behaviors are not only similar in their symptomatology, but they also share common etiologic roots. This recognition finally led to the opening of the addiction section both in the *Diagnostic and Statistical Manual of Mental Disorders,* Fifth Edition (*DSM-5;* "Substance-Related and Addictive Disorders") and in the *International Classification of Diseases,* 11th Revision (*ICD-11;* "Disorders Due to Substance Use or Addictive Behaviours"). While the main text of the new classification in *DSM-5* (in 2013) only included "Gambling Disorder," the *ICD-11* (in 2019) already included both "Gambling Disorder" and "Gaming Disorder."

The current book by Dr. Amanda Giordano reflects very much on these changes by summarizing the most recent literature on different behavioral addictions. The introduction of all these phenomena includes the detailed discussion of their symptomatology, etiologic factors, assessment issues as well as treatment possibilities. This book therefore could serve as a very useful handbook and comprehensive guide for all those who want to receive a general insight into the recent developments of the study of behavioral addictions, and especially for clinicians seeing patients with these disorders.

Zsolt Demetrovics
Chair, Centre of Excellence in Responsible Gaming, University of Gibraltar
Professor of Psychology, Institute of Psychology, Eötvös Loránd University,
Budapest, Hungary
Editor-in-Chief, Journal of Behavioral Addictions
President, International Society for the Study of Behavioral Addictions

PREFACE

Clinician, I had you in mind as I wrote each page of this book. I wanted you to have a practical, accessible resource to consult when your clients present with behavioral addictions. Therefore, I kept asking myself questions like, "What would help a school counselor who learns that her client has a problem with social media use?" or "What would a private practitioner want to know when his client discloses pornography addiction?" or "What information would a college counselor need to effectively address her client's internet gaming addiction?" or "What would help the clinician working with a client with a food addiction, or exercise addiction, or nonsuicidal self-injury, or sex addiction, or work addiction, or gambling addiction …." My goal was to create a clinical reference book that would meaningfully impact the work of mental health professionals in diverse settings.

The growing prevalence of behavioral addictions makes it clear that the majority of counselors (if not all) will work with clients with addictive behaviors. As such, I aspired to write a book that would aid in your conceptualization, assessment, and treatment of a variety of behavioral addictions. To accomplish this goal, I tried to consume as much information about behavioral addictions as I could find: reading mounds of published scholarship and books, listening to podcasts, watching documentaries, and conducting interviews with dozens of clinicians and members of 12-step programs. This book is the culmination of 18 months of investigation into the most current information related to behavioral addictions. In each chapter, I answered what I thought would be the most meaningful questions for clinical practice: *How do I conceptualize it?*, *How do I identify it?*, *How do I assess it?*, *How do I treat it?*, and *How do I learn more?*. Eleven behavioral addictions are covered in this text, including: internet gaming addiction, social media addiction, sex addiction, pornography and cybersex addiction, love addiction, gambling addiction, nonsuicidal self-injury, food addiction, exercise addiction, work addiction, and shopping addiction. Although not exhaustive, this list includes many of the most widely accepted behavioral addictions and those that the majority of you will encounter in your clinical practice.

Along with describing each behavioral addiction in detail, I also address important issues related to the addictive behaviors, such as distinguishing between gaming enthusiasts and those with internet gaming addiction, the association between social media addiction and cyberbullying, ethical considerations when clients disclose viewing illegal pornography, considerations related to adolescent sexting, the relationship between love addiction and codependence, the difference between sex addiction and sexual offending, the effects of legalized sports betting on gambling rates, distinguishing between nonsuicidal self-injury and a suicide attempt, the relationship between shopping addiction and hoarding disorder, the potential impact of neuromarketing, cultural considerations of work and study addiction, and conceptualizing exercise addiction with and without an eating disorder. Additionally, each chapter has a section devoted to the current state of neuroscience related to the behavioral addiction. The medical and mental health fields have made incredible gains with regard to understanding the neuroscience of addiction, and this information has the potential to dramatically impact our clinical work and advocacy efforts. I feel so strongly about the importance of increasing knowledge related to neuroscience that I also dedicated an entire chapter to the topic (Chapter 2).

Furthermore, in each chapter, I intentionally present a variety of treatment methods as potential strategies for clinical work with behavioral addictions. Although cognitive behavioral therapy or motivational interviewing may be effective for a number of behavioral addictions, I did not describe them in each chapter. Instead, I sought to present diverse treatment approaches to fit the widest range of clinical styles. Thus, in this book you will read about the application of dialectical behavior therapy, acceptance and commitment therapy, eye movement desensitization and reprocessing, mindfulness-based interventions, exposure and response prevention, internal family systems therapy, psychodrama, trauma-focused cognitive behavioral therapy, rational emotive behavioral therapy, positive psychology, meditation awareness, attachment work, group counseling, and more. I also address diagnostic considerations for each behavioral addiction, referencing both the *Diagnostic and Statistical Manual of Mental Disorders,* Fifth Edition, and the *International Classification of Diseases,* 11th Revision.

In addition to clinical strategies, I included an entire chapter dedicated to advocating for clients with behavioral addictions at the individual, community, and public levels (Chapter 14). Counselors are advocates, and our work occurs both inside and outside of our counseling rooms. There are numerous ways we can use our positions and influence to remove barriers faced by individuals with behavioral addictions (e.g., stigma, bias, misinformation, obstacles to treatment, lack of evidence-based treatment protocols, current laws and regulations related to addictive behaviors, lack of local treatment options). As you read this book and work with clients with behavioral addictions, I hope that you will feel moved to advocate, whether that means developing a clinical treatment manual for an addictive behavior to help educate novice counselors, providing accurate information about behavioral addictions to the public (e.g., podcasts, magazine articles, blogs, research papers), or initiating prevention programs related to protective factors for behavioral addictions (e.g., emotion regulation) in local schools. The possibilities for advocating for this population are endless.

Finally, one of the features of this book that I am most excited for you to read is the Voices From the Field sections. In these passages, clinicians who specialize in each of the 11 behavioral addictions share their thoughts related to their clinical work and describe what they want other counselors to know. Their insight and wisdom related to their personal experiences treating behavioral addictions is invaluable. Many counselors have been doing this important work for years, and it is imperative that we learn from each other.

In sum, my sincere hope is that this clinical reference book will help you provide compassionate, effective services to clients with a variety of behavioral addictions. As mental health professionals, we owe it to our clients to be informed about addictive behaviors and ready to join with them on their treatment and recovery journeys. For those of you who did not receive ample education related to behavioral addictions in your graduate training programs, I believe this comprehensive book will be a beneficial tool for self-study. Thank you for your desire to continue developing your clinical and advocacy skills related to behavioral addictions, and for choosing this book as a resource to that end.

Amanda L. Giordano

ACKNOWLEDGMENTS

I have an overwhelming sense of gratitude for the many clinicians and members of 12-step programs who shared their wisdom, insight, and experiences with me. My interviews with these men and women greatly shaped the content of this book and increased my understanding of the lived experiences of those with behavioral addictions. Each interviewee spoke candidly about their experiences, provided important resources and examples, and demonstrated a genuine passion to raise awareness about the nature of behavioral addictions. This book would not have come together without these individuals. I want to sincerely thank the members of 12-step programs who took the time to speak with me and share their stories. In addition, I am so grateful to the following clinicians, who are doing this very important work and generously imparted their wisdom to me.

Ms. Sarah Bridge, MSW, LCSW
Dr. Hilarie Cash, LMHC, CSAT, WSGC
Dr. Lauren Colston, LCP, HSP
Ms. Pamela Dobbs, LCADC, CCS, SAC, MA, ICGC-II
Mr. Aaron Hunt, MS, LPC, NCC, CSAT, LCDC-I
Ms. Lindsay Lundeen, MA, NCC
Dr. Raissa Miller, LPC
Mr. George Mladenetz, MEd, LCADC, ICGC-II
Mr. Jon Parker, MAMFT, LPC, NCC
Ms. Michelle Peteet, MA, LAPC
Mr. Tal Prince, MDiv, MA, NCC, LPC, CSAT
Ms. Kiersten Rapstine, LPC-S, CEDS-S
Ms. Megan Richardson, LMFT, NCC
Dr. Bryan Robinson, LMFT, LPC
Ms. Jennifer Rollin, MSW, LCSW-C
Mr. Thorn Winkler, MA, APC, AMFT
Ms. Taylor Zebrosky, MS, LPC

I am also so grateful to my community who encouraged me during this project—especially Jessica and Keith Abraham, Theresa and Seth Taylor, Elizabeth Prosek, Michael Schmit, and Erika Schmit. I could not have done this without you!

1

Introduction to Behavioral Addictions

WHY READ A BOOK ABOUT BEHAVIORAL ADDICTIONS?

All counselors, regardless of setting, will work with clients affected by addiction. Clients may struggle with addiction themselves, be in relationships with others with addiction (e.g., family members, romantic partners, friends, coworkers), or have childhood histories of living in homes where active addiction was present. Clinicians must be prepared to serve clients who struggle with a myriad of addictive behaviors—both those that involve substances (i.e., chemical addiction) and those that involve behaviors (i.e., behavioral addiction). This book focuses specifically on conceptualizing, assessing, and treating behavioral addictions in light of the growing prevalence rates of addictive behaviors and need for more training. Indeed, behavioral addictions are a widespread, global phenomenon. For example, scholars have posited that internationally, up to 5.5% of children and adolescents have internet gaming addiction (Paulus et al., 2018). With regard to problem gambling, researchers determined prevalence rates among adolescents in various countries ranging from 0.9% (Norway) to 7.9% (Finland; Floros, 2018). Moreover, a literature review of sex addiction studies uncovered prevalence rates ranging from 3% to 16.8% (Karila et al., 2014). Finally, researchers found that 12% of participants in Great Britain and 16% of participants in Taiwan had compulsive shopping (Lo & Harvey, 2014). It is clear that behavioral addictions affect individuals worldwide, and there are no signs that these addictions are subsiding. Instead, the availability and accessibility of potentially addictive behaviors continues to increase, particularly with the ubiquity of the internet and smartphones. Now, individuals can game, gamble, bet on fantasy sports, shop, access pornography, scroll social media, check work email, or use an app to find a sexual partner anytime, anywhere. Offline addictive behaviors also continue to be prevalent in light of the availability and affordability of highly palatable foods, social norms that promote and reward overworking, the popularity of electronic gambling machines, legalization of sports betting, frequent depictions of nonsuicidal self-injury in the media and on social networking sites, and societal approval of overexercising.

Although many people can engage in rewarding behaviors without experiencing significant issues, for a small portion of people, these behaviors can become compulsive and lead to a host of negative consequences. Thus, whether counselors work in schools, colleges, private practices, hospitals, or community mental health settings, all clinicians will undoubtedly encounter clients who struggle with addictive behaviors. It is therefore imperative that *all* counselors become familiar with behavioral addictions and able to recognize the signs and symptoms in their clinical work, assess appropriately, craft holistic conceptualizations, and implement effective treatment plans. Rather than considering clinical work with behavioral addictions as a niche or counseling specialty, all counselors must be prepared to serve clients with addictive behaviors. Hence, the aim of this book is to help mental health professionals become informed about behavioral addictions and develop the competence to work effectively with clients who present with a variety of addictive behaviors.

THE EVOLVING DEFINITION OF ADDICTION

Historically, the concept of *addiction* was marked by the loss of control over one's use of alcohol or another drug of abuse. However, with advances in neuroscience and empirical research, it is now known that addiction can manifest with or without the ingestion of psychoactive chemicals. Indeed, the most recent definition provided by the American Society of Addiction Medicine (ASAM, 2019) clearly describes addiction as a medical disease involving the compulsive use of substances, or compulsive engagement in behaviors, which continue despite negative consequences (ASAM, 2019). Furthermore, the latest version of the *Diagnostic and Statistical Manual of Mental Disorders* (5th ed.; *DSM-5*; American Psychiatric Association [APA], 2013) has a chapter titled, "Substance-Related and Addictive Disorders," reflecting both chemical and behavioral addictions. The inclusion of gambling disorder within this chapter was an important step toward the widespread recognition of behavioral addictions. Additionally, although not included in the *DSM-5* proper, internet gaming disorder and nonsuicidal self-injury disorder were listed as conditions for further study in Section III, suggesting that other potentially addictive behaviors likely will be added to the *DSM* in the future (APA, 2013). In addition to these changes in the *DSM*, the most recent revision of the *International Classification of Diseases, 11th Revision* (*ICD-11*; World Health Organization, 2018) contains a section titled "Disorders Due to Addictive Behaviours," which includes both gambling disorder and gaming disorder. The *ICD-11* also includes compulsive sexual behavior disorder in the section for impulse control disorders.

Furthermore, recent standards of a prominent accrediting body for counseling and related programs (i.e., Council for Accreditation of Counseling and Related Educational Programs [CACREP]) now require counseling students to have knowledge pertaining to both "addictions and addictive behaviors" (Section 2, F.3.d., CACREP, 2016). Moreover, internationally known clinicians, like Claudia Black (known for her family systems work with addictions) and William Miller (one of the developers of motivational interviewing), have been raising awareness about behavioral addictions for decades. Specifically, Black (2001) wrote, "Addictive obsession can exist in whatever generates significant mood alterations, whether it is the self-nurturing of food, the excitement of gambling, or the intoxication of alcohol or other drugs" (p. 3). Miller et al. (2019) noted in their clinical guide for treating addiction that the word "addiction" is used "as the most generic term for SUDs [substance use disorders] as well as other addictive behaviors, encompassing a broad range of severity" (p. 13). Thus, prominent medical societies, diagnostic manuals, classifications of diseases, accrediting bodies, and renowned clinicians all endorse the fact that addiction entails both chemicals and behaviors. The question is no longer "Can behaviors be addictive?" but rather, "How can clinicians best serve clients with behavioral addictions?" This book aims to answer that question.

WHAT MAKES A BEHAVIOR AN ADDICTION?

The fact that certain behaviors can become addictive for some individuals is widely recognized, yet it is important to delineate between enthusiastic engagement in a behavior and a behavioral addiction. Specifically, the amount of time engaging in an activity is not a sufficient determinant of whether or not a behavioral addiction exists. Kardefelt-Winther et al. (2017) warned that without a uniform definition of behavioral addictions, clinicians are at risk of pathologizing nonaddictive, albeit excessive, behaviors. To decrease this risk, the scholars proposed two necessary criteria of behavioral additions: (a) engagement in the behavior must persist over time; and (b) engagement in the behavior must yield distress, impaired functioning, and/or harm to the individual. Furthermore, the scholars posited that if the behavior is a manifestation of a mental disorder, if it is willfully chosen, if it is a temporary coping strategy, or if it does not lead to impairment, the behavior should not be considered an addiction (Billieux et al., 2017; Kardefelt-Winther et al., 2017). From this perspective, a professional eSport player who willfully chooses when and how long to game, and does not experience any distress or impairment from the activity, is unlikely to have a behavioral addiction. On the other hand, an adolescent who games for 8 to 10 hours at a time, misses school, foregoes sleep, has poor personal hygiene, has lost control over his gaming, and experiences significant conflict due to the prominence of gaming in his life should be assessed for a behavioral addiction. Thus, the presence of impaired functioning, negative consequences, and/or distress resulting from prolonged engagement in a behavior can serve as an initial indicator that a behavioral addiction may be present.

CLINICAL NOTE 1.1

In his seminal piece describing the components model of addiction, Griffiths (2005) stated, "the difference between an excessive healthy enthusiasm and an addiction is that healthy enthusiasm adds to life whereas addiction takes away from it" (p. 195). As counselors gain information about clients' engagement in rewarding behaviors, they can pay attention to the consequences of the behavior on various realms of clients' lives.

COMPONENTS MODEL OF ADDICTION

In addition to the two-criterion definition posited by Kardefelt-Winther et al. (2017), researchers have identified specific components necessary for a behavior to be considered an addiction. Adapted from a model suggested by Brown (1993), Griffiths (1996, 2005, 2019) proposed a *components model of addiction* identifying six components necessary for a behavior to be considered an addiction: (a) salience (the behavior becomes central to the individual's life), (b) mood modification (the behavior alters the individual's emotional experience), (c) tolerance (the individual must engage in more of the behavior to achieve the desired effect, such as more time, more frequency, or more intensity), (d) withdrawal (upon cessation of the behavior, the individual experiences unpleasant physical or psychological effects), (e) conflict (as a result of engagement in the behavior, the individual experiences discord with others or discord within themselves), and (f) relapse (despite efforts to refrain from engaging in the behavior, the individual returns to previous patterns of engagement after a period of abstinence). According to Griffiths (2005), each of the six components must be present in order for the behavior to be deemed an addiction. To better understand the components model, consider the following hypothetical case example.

Asher is a 25-year-old, heterosexual, biracial graduate student who presents to counseling due to feelings of anxiety. After several sessions in which a strong therapeutic alliance is built, Asher discloses that he believes the root cause of his anxiety is his relationship with internet pornography. He began using pornography after he was first exposed to it by a neighborhood friend at the age of 12. Since then, he has used pornography regularly, beginning with a few times a month, advancing to a few times a week, and now he uses it daily (tolerance). Not only has his frequency increased over time, he uses pornography for longer durations (often for 2–3 hours per night), and is viewing types of pornography he never thought he would view (e.g., violent porn). Asher discloses that even when he is not using pornography, he is thinking about it and recalling the images and videos he last viewed (salience). It is difficult for him to be attentive in class because his mind almost always is on pornography. Additionally, Asher reports that he has found himself gradually becoming more depressed over the past year. The only thing that gives him any sense of happiness or pleasure anymore is using pornography (mood modification), and when he does not have access to it (e.g., during class), he feels agitated, angry, and restless (withdrawal). Asher said that over the years, he has discontinued the activities he used to enjoy (e.g., going out with friends, playing sports, attending church services) because he does not have an interest in them anymore. Additionally, his romantic relationship recently ended because his girlfriend was frustrated with his seeming obsession with pornography (conflict). When she first threatened to end the relationship, Asher committed to end his pornography use and was successful for 3 weeks. However, despite his genuine desire to stop, he began using again in secret until his girlfriend caught him (relapse). Asher noted that he feels like his life has spiraled completely out of control and he does not know what to do. Viewing and thinking about pornography to the exclusion of other people and activities is not congruent with his personal values (conflict), yet he does not know how, or if, he can make a change.

In this example, the six components of addiction are clearly present, demonstrating the addictive nature of the behavior. Although this case involved pornography, the components model can be applied to a variety of potentially addictive behaviors including gaming, gambling, eating, shopping, social media use, exercise, and others. When counselors become aware of these components in their clients' experiences, they can begin to accurately conceptualize, assess, and treat behavioral addictions.

THE FOUR Cs OF ADDICTION

Along with the components model of addiction, it may be helpful for counselors to apply an even shorter screening tool in their clinical work to help recognize potential behavioral addictions. For example, there may be times in which a counselor is working with a client in early addiction and tolerance has not yet developed. Or, consider a situation in which a counselor is unable to determine whether a client is experiencing actual withdrawal symptoms, or just irritability from not being able to continue an activity that they enjoy (e.g., when parents require an adolescent to log off social media; Griffiths et al., 2016; Kuss et al., 2017). Thus, a simple way to assess whether engagement in an activity may be a behavioral addiction is to consider the *four Cs*:

- Is the behavior compulsive?
- Is there a loss of control over the behavior?
- Does the individual continue the behavior despite negative consequences?
- Does the individual experience cravings or demonstrate mental preoccupation with the behavior?

The four Cs represent features of prominent definitions of addiction (ASAM, 2019; Kardefelt-Winther, 2017; S. Sussman & A. N. Sussman, 2011) and the components model of addiction (Griffiths, 2005); yet as a simple screener, it may be an easy way to alert counselors to the potential of behavioral addictions in their clinical work. If a counselor recognizes that a client's behavior is compulsive, out of control, leads to negative consequences, and the client craves or is mentally preoccupied with the behavior, it can prompt the clinician to engage in further assessment related to behavioral addictions. For example, consider the case of Gretchen.

Gretchen, a Caucasian woman in her early 60s, reports that she has a problem with online shopping. She spends hours scrolling through retail websites ordering gifts for herself, friends, and members of her family. Whenever she has a spare moment, Gretchen feels compelled to pick up her smartphone and hunt for the best deals. Whether sitting at a red light when driving, waiting at the doctor's office, or in bed at night, it is hard for her to resist the urge to shop online (compulsivity). Her daughter has expressed concern over the quantity of her purchases; so Gretchen has tried setting limits for herself (e.g., no online shopping after 9 p.m., not spending more than 1 hour at a time online shopping, not spending more than $100 in one sitting), but she continues to break her own rules (loss of control). She finds herself shopping more frequently and purchasing more items than she intended. As a result, Gretchen's credit card bills have become unmanageable (negative consequences). She has more debt than she has ever had, and this has caused conflicts with her siblings (who have repeatedly loaned her money) and her daughter (negative consequences). Although she is aware of the problems it is causing, Gretchen finds herself thinking about online shopping most of the time and unable to resist the desire to search for deals and make purchases (craving). Scrolling through the retail sites gives her a sense of excitement that she does not feel at other times and helps her forget her problems.

A counselor would be able to identify the four Cs of addiction in Gretchen's case and begin considering the potential of shopping addiction. The clinician may then choose to utilize a formal shopping addiction assessment, such as the Bergen Shopping Addiction Scale (Andreassen et al., 2015) to further investigate the potential of a behavioral addiction. Thus, the four Cs screening tool is a useful, preliminary way to identify signs of behavioral addictions.

CLINICAL NOTE 1.2

A client comes to your office reporting that he thinks he may be addicted to skydiving. What would you want to assess in order to determine whether the client is indeed engaging in an addictive behavior or if it is another issue?

PUBLIC HEALTH MODEL OF BEHAVIORAL ADDICTION

In addition to being able to identify behavioral addictions, it is important for counselors to have a framework for conceptualizing the complex, multifaceted nature of addictive behaviors. For example, not all individuals have the same degree of susceptibility to addiction, not all behaviors have the same addiction potential, and not all cultures and societies have the same availability, accessibility, and environmental conditions necessary to promote specific behaviors. Consider the fact that although many people can play internet games socially, with control, and without negative consequences, there are some individuals who engage compulsively, lose control, experience many negative consequences, and crave gaming when it is unavailable. Thus, different people respond to potentially addictive behaviors in different ways. Moreover, although gambling, sex, nonsuicidal self-injury, and shopping can be addictive for some individuals, activities such as folding laundry, baking cookies, or going to the dentist are not addictive. Thus, the nature of specific activities seems important to the development of addiction. Finally, some behavioral addictions are more prominent among some cultural groups or in particular countries compared to others. How is one to make sense of all of these distinctions?

Taking a *public health perspective*, particularly utilizing the epidemiologic triad, can help mental health professionals, clients, and communities better understand behavioral addiction (Ahrens et al., 2014; Centers for Disease Control and Prevention [CDC], 2012). This model postulates that infectious diseases involve three factors: the agent (i.e., disease or pathogen), the host (i.e., susceptible individual), and the environment (i.e., setting, context, culture; Ahrens et al., 2014; CDC, 2012). Some scholars also include a fourth factor, namely, the vector, which refers to mechanisms that connect agents and hosts (e.g., mosquitoes, ticks; Wilson et al., 2017). Scholars have applied this public health model to the disease of addiction as a means of conceptualizing the nature of the disorder (Compton & Jones, 2019; Giovino, 2002; Miller et al., 2019; Rasmussen, 2000). With regard to behavioral addictions specifically, counselors, clients, and communities can benefit from considering the public health perspective, including agents, hosts, environments, and vectors.

AGENT

Human beings engage in innumerable behaviors, yet only a few emerge as potentially addictive (*agents*). The potential for a behavior to be addictive depends on the nature of the activity and the effects of the behavior on the individual. Specifically, addictive behaviors are rewarding, meaning they activate reward circuitry in the brain (described in detail in Chapter 2) and are both positively and negatively reinforcing (Goodman, 2001; Parylak et al., 2011; Wise & Koob, 2014). Consider eating a piece of highly palatable food, like chocolate cake. The experience of ingesting this high-energy, high-sugar food activates the reward centers in the brain creating positive, gratifying sensations (Leigh & Morris, 2018). The activation of reward circuitry and resulting emotional state is a form of positive reinforcement, which increases the probability that the behavior will be repeated. Thus, addictive behaviors initially have appetitive effects (Sussman & Sussman, 2011). Additionally, when an individual is stressed, anxious, or irritated, eating highly palatable foods also can serve to reduce negative emotions (consider the colloquial terms "comfort food" or "stress eating;" Parylak et al., 2011). Therefore, eating chocolate cake can provide temporary relief from aversive mood states, which constitutes negative reinforcement (i.e., removing or reducing an undesirable stimulus or condition). Negative reinforcement also increases the probability that a behavior will be repeated. Thus, behaviors that have the potential to be addictive (i.e., agents) are both positively and negatively reinforcing.

Importantly, the positively and negatively reinforcing properties of addictive behaviors make them effective mechanisms of emotion regulation or mood modification (Griffiths, 2005). For example, if an individual is feeling depressed, they may engage in a sexual act to experience both positive reinforcement (e.g., rewarding sensations) and negative reinforcement (e.g., escape from feelings of depression). However, due to neurological changes resulting from the chronic overstimulation of reward circuitry (i.e., neuroadaptations, described in Chapter 2), the initial appetitive effects of addictive behaviors eventually wane, while aversive emotional states in response to the absence of the behavior emerge (Koob, 2009; Wise & Koob, 2014). This pattern is reflected in the addiction cycle, which is composed of (a) preoccupation/anticipation, (b) binge/intoxication, and (c) withdrawal/negative affect (Koob & Le Moal, 2008). Thus, as addiction progresses, there is a shift from the prominence of positive reinforcement (engaging in an addictive behavior to feel good) to the prominence of negative reinforcement (engaging in an addictive behavior to avoid feeling bad; Koob & Le Moal, 2008; Parylak et al., 2011; Wise & Koob, 2014). In sum, potentially addictive behaviors activate neurological reward systems, are both positively and negatively reinforcing, and initially fulfill appetitive effects while subsequently transitioning to function primarily as a means to relieve withdrawal distress (Koob & Le Moal, 2008). Although not an exhaustive list, this book explores the potential addictive nature of several behaviors including internet gaming, social media, sex, pornography and cybersex, love, gambling, nonsuicidal self-injury, food, exercise, work, and shopping.

HOST

There is no single factor that determines whether an individual will develop a behavioral addiction over the course of their life. Instead, susceptible individuals (i.e., *hosts*) must be conceptualized from a *biopsychosocial model* of addiction (Marlatt & Baer, 1988). Specifically, the individual's genetic makeup and biological characteristics (e.g., heredity, epigenetics, mesolimbic dopaminergic system functioning), psychological traits (e.g., temperament, self-esteem, degree of sensation-seeking, impulsivity, anxiety, depression), and personal experiences (e.g., trauma, neglect, abandonment, early exposure to addictive behaviors) all contribute to their degree of susceptibility to addiction. Due to unique neurobiological characteristics, rewarding behaviors feel subjectively different to different people. For example, one individual might be introduced to gambling and find it moderately entertaining, while another person may find it extremely rewarding and, subsequently, difficult to resist. Additionally, given that addictive behaviors serve the function of emotion regulation (Griffiths, 2005), unique personal experiences (e.g., early trauma) may prime some individuals to seek and respond to the mood modifying effects of addictive behaviors more intensely than others. For example, a woman with a history of childhood emotional abuse who never developed effective coping strategies may have a very different response to feelings of being in love than another individual with a different childhood history. Indeed, individual characteristics affect the attractiveness, desirability, and level of reward associated with potentially addictive behaviors. Thus, a person's susceptibility to behavioral addictions is influenced by neurobiological and psychological factors, as well as the individual's past experiences and the nature and effectiveness of coping and emotion regulation strategies.

ENVIRONMENT

The *environment* plays a critical role in behavioral addictions as it determines what behaviors are available, the ease of accessibility, legality of particular activities, the extent to which behaviors are modeled, marketed, and visible, the extent of social approval of behaviors, and cultural norms related to engagement in various activities. Specifically, Sussman et al. (2011) noted, "acquisition of some specific addictions versus others also involves exposure to unique social environmental experience" (p. 3402). For example, there are some environments in which technology is available and easily accessible, making internet-based addictive behaviors (e.g., gaming, social media, shopping, pornography, cybersex, gambling) more prevalent than environments without reliable internet access (i.e., a consequence of the digital divide). Additionally, some populations may be disproportionately targeted with advertising, promotional material, and access to particular behaviors, such as gambling advertisements and electronic gaming machines in impoverished or low-income communities (Tse et al., 2012). Moreover, some societies celebrate, reward, or expect certain behaviors, such as overworking, while other societies are more disapproving (Cheung et al., 2018; Hoffman & Unger, 2020).

Sussman et al. (2011) proposed a model to help explain *addiction specificity*, or why some individuals engage in one addictive behavior over another. This model, titled PACE, is composed of four elements, all of which are linked to the environment: (a) pragmatics (access to the behavior, availability, exposure), (b) attraction (social acceptance of the behavior, reinforcing consequences of engagement), (c) communication (exposure to language associated with addictive behavior, in-group vocabulary), and (d) expectations (anticipated outcomes of behavioral engagement, media portrayals, social learning; Sussman et al., 2011). With these four processes in mind, it is easy to understand differing rates of addictive behaviors among various cultural groups and societies. For example, in the study of university students in four Middle Eastern countries, researchers found higher prevalence of smartphone addiction in countries in which smartphones and the internet were more widely available (59.8% of the Jordan sample had smartphone addiction) compared to students in countries without reliable internet or affordable smartphones (8.6% of the Yemen sample had smartphone addiction; Albursan et al., 2019). Additionally, researchers noted higher rates of problem gambling among English adolescents (4.8%) compared to Portuguese adolescents (2.6%), noting differences in gambling laws, legislation, and opportunities between England and Portugal (Calado et al., 2020). Moreover, in their study of German and Polish university students, Martyniuk and Briken (2016) found more high pornography users among the German sample, which had more liberal views of sex and lower rates of religious identities (61% Christian) compared to the Polish sample, which had more conservative views of sex and higher rates of religious identities (93% Christian; Martyniuk & Briken, 2016). It is clear, therefore, that the environment plays a critical role in the development and perpetuation of behavioral addictions. Cultural norms, environmental contexts, and location-specific laws and regulations all contribute to the availability, affordability, access, social modeling, and social acceptance of potentially addictive behaviors.

Another environmental feature relevant to the understanding of behavioral addictions is systemic privilege and oppression. Members of marginalized cultural groups (e.g., race, ethnicity, religion/spirituality, ability status, socioeconomic status, sexual orientation, gender, age) face higher rates of injustice and oppression than members of privileged groups (Johnson, 2018). These experiences of systemic oppression and discrimination can be traumatic (Bryant-Davis, 2007; Carter, 2007), which may make members of marginalized groups, specifically those without effective coping strategies, more vulnerable to the mood-modifying properties of addictive behaviors. For example, Currie et al. (2013) studied the relationship between racial discrimination and problem gambling among a sample of Aboriginal or First Nation adults in Canada. The researchers found that as experiences of racial discrimination increased, so too did problem gambling scores among participants. The data suggested that Aboriginal adults who experience racial discrimination may use gambling as a means to escape the negative emotions triggered by acts of racism (Currie et al., 2013). In addition, researchers examined food addiction symptoms among a sample of 154 lesbian, gay, or bisexual (LGB) participants and 202 heterosexual participants (Rainey et al., 2018). Not only did the researchers find that LGB participants endorsed more food addiction symptoms than heterosexual participants, they also determined that as experiences of harassment and discrimination increased among LGB individuals, so too did their food addiction symptomology. The authors noted that food addiction symptoms may be influenced by the stress associated with discrimination related to participants' sexual orientation (Rainey et al., 2018).

Thus, in addition to the rewarding nature of specific behaviors and biological and psychological vulnerabilities of certain individuals, counselors should consider clients' cultural identities and cultural contexts when conceptualizing behavioral addictions. Specifically, counselors can best serve clients by being informed regarding cultural norms, systems of privilege and oppression, and the impact of their own cultural identities on their clinical work. The *Multicultural and Social Justice Counseling Competencies* (MSJCC; Ratts et al., 2016) endorsed by the American Counseling Association can be extremely helpful as counselors strive to increase their multicultural competence when addressing behavioral addictions (find the MSJCC at www.counseling.org/docs/default-source/competencies/multicultural-and-social-justice-counseling-competencies.pdf?sfvrsn=8573422c_20).

CLINICAL NOTE 1.3

Racial discrimination currently is not listed as an example of trauma in the *DSM-5* (APA, 2013). However, researchers have found empirical support for the relationship between race-based traumatic stress and trauma symptoms. Specifically, among 155 participants who experienced race-based traumatic stress, researchers found significant relationships between race-based traumatic stress symptoms and trauma symptoms, indicating that the two constructs are strongly related (Carter et al., 2020). As counselors consider clients' histories of trauma (which may increase the risk of coping through addictive behaviors), they should explore experiences of racism and oppression.

VECTOR

In the public health model, vectors refer to stimuli that transmit agents to hosts (CDC, 2012). In the case of infectious diseases, vectors could be mosquitoes or ticks (Wilson et al., 2017). In the case of chemical addiction, vectors could be individuals who sell drugs of abuse, prescribe drugs that can be abused (e.g., prescription opioids, benzodiazepines, stimulants), or pharmaceutical companies that produce and market these drugs (Compton & Jones, 2019). With regard to behavioral addictions, vectors can include the people, organizations, or companies that connect individuals to potentially addictive behaviors, such as casinos, the pornography industry, social media platforms, daily fantasy sports betting servers, anonymous sex or hook-up app developers, internet gaming distributors and streaming services, food processing companies, or stockholders of these businesses. The influence of vectors on the maintenance of behavioral addictions is substantial. As these companies and organizations multiply and the number of mediums through which individuals can access addictive behaviors grows (e.g., increasing number of pornography websites, virtual reality pornography), vectors may use compelling strategies to accrue more hosts. When describing the addictive potential of internet-based activities, Alter (2017) wrote,

> The people who create and refine tech, games, and interactive experiences are very good at what they do. They run thousands of tests with millions of users to learn which tweaks work and which ones don't—which background colors, fonts, and audio tones maximize engagement and minimize frustration. (p. 5)

Therefore, it is important for clinicians to consider the effects of various strategies, operations, goals, marketing tactics, and regulations used by companies and organizations related to potentially addictive behaviors. Specifically, it is important for counselors to inquire: (a) How are the companies/organizations seeking to attract users?, (b) What strategies are the companies/organizations using to capture users' attention and encourage continued engagement in the behavior?, (c) Are there particular populations targeted by certain companies/organizations?, and (d) What are the policies or legislation that serve to regulate the industries related to addictive behaviors?. As counselors become aware of the role of vectors in behavioral addictions, they may discover opportunities to advocate for individuals with behavioral addictions and their local communities (e.g., age restrictions for engagement in particular potentially addictive behaviors, funding for awareness campaigns in schools or communities, or marketing regulations to reduce targeting specific cultural groups; see Chapter 14 for more information on advocacy).

SUMMARY

It is clear that addiction includes the compulsive use of alcohol or other drugs as well as the compulsive engagement in rewarding behaviors. Despite the variance of addictive behaviors, there are some common features that can help counselors recognize behavioral addictions in their work. The components model of addiction (Brown, 1993; Griffiths, 1996, 2005, 2019) identifies six aspects of addiction, namely, salience, mood modification, tolerance, withdrawal, conflict, and relapse. Many popular assessment instruments for behavioral addictions are based on these six components and can be useful methods of identifying addictive behaviors. Additionally, the four Cs of addiction (the behavior is compulsive, there is a loss of control over the behavior, continued engagement in the behavior despite negative consequences, and the experience of cravings or mental preoccupation with the behavior) is a helpful screening tool for the initial recognition of behavioral addictions among clients.

Given the complexity of behavioral addictions, it is important for counselors to consider the nature of the rewarding behavior (agents), unique susceptibility among individuals (hosts), the influence of culture and society (environment), and the role of companies, organizations, and individuals who connect people with potentially addictive behaviors (vectors). A public health perspective of behavioral addictions allows mental health professionals to take a holistic view of the condition and discover opportunities for advocacy. Thus, the models and frameworks outlined in this chapter are a good starting place to help counselors and clients identify and conceptualize behavioral addictions.

REFERENCES

Ahrens, W., Krickeberg, K., & Pigeot, I. (2014). An introduction to epidemiology. In W. Ahrens & I. Pigeot (Eds.), *Handbook of epidemiology* (2nd ed., pp. 3–41). Springer Publishing Company.

Albursan, I. S., Al Qudah, M. F., Dutton, E., Hassan, E. M. A. H., Bakhiet, S. F. A., Alfnan, A. A., Aljomaa, S. S., & Hammad, H. I. (2019). National, sex and academic discipline differences in smartphone addiction: A study of students in Jordan, Saudi Arabia, Yemen, and Sudan. *Community Mental Health Journal, 55*, 825–830. https://doi.org/10.1007/s10597-019-00368-x

Alter, A. (2017). *Irresistible: The rise of addictive technology and the business of keeping us hooked*. Penguin Books.

American Psychiatric Association. (2013). *Diagnostic and statistical manual of mental disorders* (5th ed.). Author.

American Society of Addiction Medicine. (2019). *Definition of addiction*. https://www.asam.org/docs/default-source/quality-science/asam's-2019-definition-of-addiction-(1).pdf?sfvrsn=b8b64fc2_2

Andreassen, C. S., Griffiths, M. D., Pallesen, S., Bilder, R. M., Torsheim, T., & Aboujaoude, E. (2015). The Bergen shopping addiction scale: Reliability and validity of a brief screening test. *Frontiers in Psychology, 6*, 1374. https://doi.org/10.3389/fpsyg.2015.01374

Billieux, J., van Rooij, A. J., Heeren, A., Schimmenti, A., Maurage, P., Edman, J., Blaszczynski, A., Khazaal, Y., & Kardefelt-Winther, D. (2017). Behavioural addiction 2.0- using open science framework for collaborative and transparent theoretical development. *Addiction, 112*, 1723–1724. https://doi.org/10.1111/add.13938

Black, C. (2001). *It will never happen to me: Growing up with addiction as youngsters, adolescents, adults* (2nd ed). Hazelden.

Brown, R. I. F. (1993). Some contributions of the study of gambling to the study of other addictions. In W. R. Eadington, & J. A. Cornelius (Eds.), *Gambling behaviour and problem gambling* (pp. 341–272). University of Nevada Press.

Bryant-Davis, T. (2007). Healing requires recognition: The case for race-based traumatic stress. *The Counseling Psychologist, 35*, 135–143. https://doi.org/10.1177/0011000006295152

Calado, F., Alexandre, J., & Griffiths, M. D. (2020). Gambling among adolescents and emerging adults: A cross-cultural study between Portuguese and English youth. *International Journal of Mental Health and Addiction, 18*, 737–753. https://doi.org/10.1007/s11469-018-9980-y

Carter, R. T. (2007). Racism and psychological and emotional injury: recognizing and assessing race-based traumatic stress. *The Counseling Psychologist, 35*, 13–105. https://doi.org/10.1177/0011000006292033

Carter, R. T., Kirkinis, K., & Johnson, V. E. (2020). Relationships between trauma symptoms and race-based traumatic stress. *Traumatology, 26*, 11–18. https://doi.org/10.1037/trm0000217

Centers for Disease Control and Prevention. (2012). *Principles of epidemiology in public health practice* (3rd ed). Author.

Cheung, F., Tang, C. S. K., Lim, M. S. M., & Koh, J. M. (2018). Workaholism on job burnout: A comparison between American and Chinese employees. *Frontiers in Psychology, 9*, 2546. https://doi.org/10.3389/fpsyg.2018.02546

Compton, W. M., & Jones, C. M. (2019). Epidemiology of the U.S. opioid crisis: The importance of the vector. *Annals of the New York Academy of Sciences, 1451*, 130–143. https://doi.org/10.1111/nyas.14209

Council for Accreditation of Counseling and Related Educational Programs. (2016). *2016 CACREP standards*. www.cacrep.org

Currie, C., Wild, T., Schopflocher, D., Laing, L., Veugelers, P., & Parlee, B. (2013). Racial discrimination, post traumatic stress, and gambling problems among urban Aboriginal adults in Canada. *Journal of Gambling Studies, 29*, 393–415. https://doi.org/10.1007/s10899-012-9323-z

Floros, G. D. (2018). Gambling disorder in adolescents: Prevalence, new developments, and treatment challenges. *Adolescent Health, Medicine and Therapeutics, 9*, 43–51. https://doi.org/10.2147/AHMT.S135423

Giovino, G. A. (2002). Epidemiology of tobacco use in the United States. *Oncogene, 21*, 7326–7340. https://doi.org/10.1038/sj.onc.1205808

Goodman, A. (2001). What's in a name? Terminology for designating a syndrome of driven sexual behavior. *Sexual Addiction & Compulsivity, 8*, 191–213. https://doi.org/10.1080/107201601753459919

Griffiths, M. (1996). Behavioral addiction: An issue for everybody? *Employee Counselling Today, 8*, 19–25. https://doi.org/101108/13665629610116872

Griffiths, M. (2005). A 'components' model of addiction within a biopsychosocial framework. *Journal of Substance Use, 10*, 191–197. https://doi.org/10.1080/14659890500114359

Griffiths, M. D. (2019). The evolution of the 'components model of addiction' and the need for a confirmatory approach in conceptualizing behavioral addictions. *Dusunen Adam The Journal of Psychiatry and Neurological Sciences, 32*, 179–184. https://doi.org/10.14744/DAJPNS.2019.00027

Griffiths, M. D., Rooij, A. J., Kardefelt-Winther, D., Starcevic, V., Kiraly, O., Pallesen, S., Müller, K., Dreier, M., Carras, M., Prause, N., King, D. l., Aboujaoude, E., Kuss, D. J., Pontes, H. M., Fernandez, O. L., Nagygyorgy, K., Achab, S., Billieux, J., Quandt, T., & Carbonell, X. (2016). Working towards an international consensus on criteria for assessing internet gaming disorder: A critical commentary on Petry et al. (2014). *Addiction, 111*, 167–175. https://doi.org/10.111/add.13057

Hoffman, B. R., & Unger, J. B. (2020). The role of culture in addiction. In S. Sussman (Ed.), *The Cambridge handbook of substance and behavioral addictions* (pp. 171–181). Cambridge University Press.

Johnson, A. G. (2018). *Privilege, power, and difference* (3rd ed.). McGraw-Hill Education.

Kardefelt-Winther, D., Heeren, A., Schimmenti, A., van Rooij, A., Maurage, P., Carras, M., Edman, J., Blaszczynski, A., Khazaal, Y., & Billieux, J. (2017). How can we conceptualize behavioral addiction without pathologizing common behaviors? *Addiction, 112,* 1709–1715. https://doi.org/10.1111/add.13763

Karila, L., Wery, A., Weinstein, A., Cottencin, O., Petit, A., Reynaud, M., & Billieux, J. (2014). Sexual addiction or hypersexual disorder: Different terms for the same problem? A review of the literature. *Current Pharmaceutical Design, 20,* 4012–4020. https://doi.org/10.2174/13816128113199990619

Koob, G. F. (2009). Dynamics of neuronal circuits in addiction: Reward, antireward, and emotional memory. *Pharmacopsychiatry, 42,* 532–541. https://doi.org/10.1055/s-0029-1216356

Koob, G. F., & Le Moal, M. (2008). Addiction and the brain antireward system. *Annual Review of Psychology, 59,* 29–53. https://doi.org/10.1146/annurev.psych.59.103006.093548

Kuss, D. J., Griffiths, M. D., & Pontes, H. M. (2017). Chaos and confusion in DSM-5 diagnosis of internet gaming disorder: Issues, concerns, and recommendations for clarity in the field. *Journal of Behavioral Addictions, 6,* 103–109. https://doi.org/10.1556/2006.5.2016.062

Leigh, S. J., & Morris, M. J. (2018). The role of reward circuitry and food addiction in the obesity epidemic: An update. *Biological Psychology, 131,* 31–42. https://doi.org/10.1016/j.biopsycho.2016.12.013

Lo, H. Y., & Harvey, N. (2014). Compulsive buying: Obsessive acquisition, collecting or hoarding? *International Journal of Mental Health and Addiction, 12,* 453–469. https://doi.org/10.1007/s11469-014-94772

Marlatt, G. A., & Baer, J. S. (1988). Addictive behaviors: Etiology and treatment. *Annual Review of Psychology, 39,* 223–252. https://doi.org/10.1146/annurev.ps.39.020188.001255

Martyniuk, U., & Briken, P. (2016). Pornography use and sexual behavior among Polish and German university students. *Journal of Sex and Marital Therapy, 42,* 494–514. https://doi.org/10.1080/0092623x.2015.1072119

Miller, W. R., Forcehimes, A. A., & Zweben, A. (2019). *Treating addiction: A guide for professionals* (2nd ed.). The Guilford Press.

Parylak, S. L., Koob, G. F., & Zorrilla, E. P. (2011). The dark side of food addiction. *Physiology and Behavior, 104,* 149–156. https://doi.org/10.1016/j.physbeh.2011.04.063

Paulus, F. W., Ohmann, S., Von Gontard, A., & Popow, C. (2018). Internet gaming disorder in children and adolescents: A systematic review. *Developmental Medicine & Child Neurology, 60,* 645–659. https://doi.org/10.111/dmcn.13754

Rainey, J. C., Furman, C. R., & Gearhardt, A. N. (2018). Food addiction among sexual minorities. *Appetite, 120,* 16–22. https://doi.org/10.1016/j.appet.2-17.08.019

Rasmussen, S. (2000). *Addiction treatment: Theory and practice*. Sage Publishing.

Ratts, M. J., Singh, A. A., Nassar-McMillan, S., Butler, S. K., & McCullough, J. R. (2016). Multicultural and social justice counseling competencies: Guidelines for the counseling profession. *Journal of Multicultural Counseling and Development, 44,* 28–48. https://doi.org/10.1002/jmcd.12035

Sussman, S., Leventhal, A., Bluthentahal, R. N., Freimuth, M., Foster, M., & Ames, S. L. (2011). A framework for the specificity of addictions. *International Journal of Environmental Research and Public Health, 8,* 3399–3415. https://doi.org/10.3390/ijerph8083399

Sussman, S., & Sussman, A. N. (2011). Considering the definition of addiction. *International Journal of Environmental Research and Public Health, 8*, 4025–4038. https://doi.org/10.3390/ijerph8104025

Tse, S., Dyall, L., Clarke, D., Abbott, M., Townsend, S., & Kingi, P. (2012). Why people gamble: A qualitative study of four New Zealand ethnic groups. *International Journal of Mental Health and Addiction, 10*, 849–861. https://doi.org/10.1007/s11469-012-9380-7

Wilson, A. J., Morgan, E. R., Booth, M., Norman, R., Perkins, S. E., Hauffe, H. C., Mideo, N., Antonovics, J., McCallum, H., & Fenton, A. (2017). What is a vector? *Philosophical Transactions of the Royal Society B: Biological Science, 372*, 20160085. https://doi.org/10.1098/rstb.2016.0085

Wise, R. A., & Koob, G. F. (2014). The development and maintenance of drug addiction. *Neuropsychopharmacology, 39*, 254–262. https://doi.org/10.1038/npp.2013.261

World Health Organization. (2018). *International statistical classification of diseases and related health problems* (11th Rev.). https://icd.who.int/browse11/l-m/en

2

Neuroscience of Behavioral Addictions

WHY IS NEUROSCIENCE IMPORTANT?

Counselors must be equipped with basic knowledge of brain functioning in order to accurately conceptualize their clients with behavioral addictions. The American Society of Addiction Medicine (ASAM, 2019) emphasized that addiction is a disease directly linked to brain circuitry in addition to one's personal experiences and genetic predispositions. Although only part of the larger picture of addiction, understanding brain circuitry is essential for providing effective, appropriate treatment for clients with addiction. This chapter focuses on specific aspects of brain functioning, but should be understood within the context of the *biopsychosocial model* of addiction, which emphasizes the interactions between an individual's genetic composition, psychological experiences, social context, and unique cultural identities on the development and progression of addiction.

There have been substantial advances in the field of neuroscience over the past few decades, particularly as technology and neuroimaging capabilities become more sophisticated. However, brain circuitry is complex and although more information is being garnered, there remain unanswered questions and hypotheses that require further confirmatory studies. For example, much of what is known about the neuroscience of behavioral addictions is an extension of the neuroscience of chemical addiction; and much of the research related to chemical addiction stems from animal studies (Blum et al., 2020; Gardner, 2011; Leeman & Potenza, 2013). Thus, more research specific to addictive behaviors (e.g., gambling, gaming, sex, shopping), using human participants, is needed to clarify and confirm the neuroscience in this area. Yet, it is clear that both behavioral and chemical addictions affect many of the same brain regions, notably those implicated in the experience and processing of rewards (Berridge & Kringelbach, 2015; Karim & Chaudhri, 2012; Wise & Robble, 2020). Furthermore, it appears that both conditions are at least partially explained by genetic factors, specifically those regulating the functioning of the reward system in the brain (Gold et al., 2014; Grant et al., 2006; Leeman & Potenza, 2013). Indeed, Blum, Werner, et al. (2012) noted, "malfunctioning of the brain's reward center is increasingly understood to underlie all addictive behaviors" (p. 41). Thus, the purpose of this chapter is to provide a concise overview of relevant neuroscience to help prepare counselors for their work with clients with behavioral addictions.

CLINICAL NOTE 2.1

It is important for counselors to be aware of the potential for chemical and behavioral addictions to co-occur. In a sample of 95 clients in treatment for alcohol use disorders, researchers found that 28.4% had at least one co-occurring behavioral addiction, compared to 15% of a healthy control group (which was a statistically significant difference; Di Nicola et al., 2015).

NEUROTRANSMISSION

The brain is composed of billions of specialized nerve cells called *neurons*, which are responsible for processing information (Erickson, 2007; C. A. Simpkins & A. M. Simpkins, 2012). Neurons are not physically connected to each other; instead, small gaps called *synapses* exist between them. In order for one neuron to communicate with another, an electrical impulse within the cell stimulates the release of chemicals that travel across the synapse and bind to a neighboring neuron. These chemical messengers, which are ejected from one neuron and received by another, are called *neurotransmitters*. Well-known neurotransmitters include dopamine, serotonin, endorphins, glutamate, and gamma-aminobutyric acid (GABA), yet more than 100 distinct neurotransmitters have been identified. Neurotransmitters can have excitatory functions (i.e., activate a response) or inhibitory functions (i.e., suppress a response), and these neurochemicals affect all that humans feel, think, and do (Erickson, 2007; Simpkins & Simpkins, 2013).

The process of communication between nerve cells is called *neurotransmission* (Erickson, 2007). The basic steps of neurotransmission include the release of neurotransmitters from the end (*axon*) of a neuron, the traversing of neurotransmitters across the synapse by way of transporter molecules, and the binding of those neurotransmitters to specific, corresponding receptors on the branch-like endings (*dendrites*) of an adjacent neuron (Siegel, 2012).

Understanding neurotransmission is vital to addiction counseling given that drugs of abuse mimic, interfere with, or alter the effects of neurotransmitters (Erickson, 2007). For example, cocaine interferes with the transporter molecules that remove dopamine (one of the primary neurotransmitters implicated in reward) from the synapse (Nestler, 2005; Wise & Robble, 2020). Rather than being reabsorbed into the neuron and thereby deactivated, cocaine blocks the process of dopamine reuptake, causing dopamine to remain active (in addition to other neurotransmitters such as norepinephrine and serotonin; Wise & Robble, 2020). This accumulation of dopamine in the synapse (in concert with other neurotransmitters) is implicated in the experience of reward. Thus, by blocking dopamine reuptake, cocaine interferes with the process of neurotransmission, creating powerfully rewarding effects (Nestler, 2005; Wise & Robble, 2020). In various ways, all drugs of abuse (e.g., alcohol, marijuana, cocaine, heroin) act upon neurotransmitters and affect the process of neurotransmission. Most abused substances act as *agonists*, meaning they activate receptors on neurons to cause reactions similar to those of natural neurotransmitters (e.g., heroin activates opioid receptors; Gardner, 2011). These drugs differ from chemicals that act as *antagonists*, which block receptor activation (e.g., medications such as haloperidol [used to treat schizophrenia] is a dopamine antagonist that blocks activation of dopamine receptors; Li et al., 2016).

Along with chemical addiction, the process of neurotransmission also is relevant to behavioral addictions. Rather than ingesting *exogenous* chemicals, which originate outside the body (e.g., drugs of abuse), certain behaviors can stimulate *endogenous* chemical release (e.g., neurotransmitters), which are naturally produced within the body (Sinacola et al., 2020). Specifically, engagement in certain behaviors can trigger the release of neurotransmitters, which, in turn, affect mood, motivation, and learning. The natural relationship between behaviors and endogenous neurotransmitter activation is adaptive and useful, yet in some instances, chronic engagement in highly rewarding behaviors can overstimulate neurotransmitter release and lead to changes in the brain (i.e., *neuroplasticity*; Doidge, 2007). Indeed, according to Sinacola et al. (2020), "the behavioral activities themselves can produce chemical changes in the brain similar to those produced by any exogenous drug" (p. 109). Thus, both chemical and behavioral addictions affect neurotransmission. The influence of addictive behaviors on neurotransmitters occurs in specific areas of the brain known as the *reward system*.

REWARD CIRCUITRY

To understand behavioral addictions, one must understand the neurological experience of reward. The idea that specific brain regions regulate rewards emerged from animal studies in the 1950s (Olds & Milner, 1954). Specifically, researchers found that by implanting electrodes on specific areas of the brain (i.e., the septal area), rats would repeatedly press a lever to self-stimulate with electrical shocks. The behavior of these rats seemed to indicate that the electrical stimulation of the septal area produced a pleasurable effect. Thus, the researchers concluded, "we have perhaps located a system within the brain whose peculiar function is to produce a rewarding effect on behavior" (Olds & Milner, 1954).

Over decades of research, much more is now known about the brain's reward circuitry, although many questions and hypotheses still remain. The brain is a complex organ, and the experience of reward involves several processes such as motivation ("wanting" a reward), pleasure ("liking" a reward), and learning (associating the experience of reward with particular stimuli; Berridge & Kringelbach, 2015). "Wanting," or desiring a reward, is presumably the appetitive phase of the reward cycle, while the experience of pleasure, or "liking," is the consummatory phase. When individuals experience rewards, those stimuli become salient as the brain learns how to anticipate and predict rewarding outcomes. In addition, multiple neurotransmitters are involved in the experience of reward (Blum et al., 2020) as well as various processes beyond the subjective experience of pleasure, such as focused attention, cognitive appraisal, memory formation, and decision-making (Berridge & Kringelbach, 2015).

Most scholars agree that the experience of reward involves the neural pathways of *dopamine*, although the exact role of the neurotransmitter continues to be debated. Previously, it was assumed that dopamine was the primary "pleasure neurotransmitter," responsible for producing hedonic reactions to rewards (Berridge & Kringelbach, 2015; Berridge & Robinson, 2016). However, recent studies have implicated dopamine in the desire or "wanting" aspect of reward, rather than the hedonic "liking" component. Although "wanting" and "liking" frequently co-occur, there are instances in which these aspects of the reward cycle act independently (e.g., wanting something without necessarily liking it; Berridge & Kringelbach, 2015; Berridge & Robinson, 2016). Thus, the dysregulation of the dopamine system underlying addiction may be more linked to desire, motivation, and seeking (i.e., "wanting") rather than experiences of pleasure (i.e., "liking"; Berridge & Robinson, 2016). When working with clients with behavioral addictions, it is important for counselors to consider the multifaceted nature of the reward cycle, which extends beyond subjective experiences of pleasure and includes aspects of desire, learning, attention, memory, expectancies, and incentive motivation (Blum, Gardner, et al., 2012).

Along with motivation, dopamine is involved in important functions such as movement, memory, and stress (Arias-Carrion et al., 2010; Blum et al., 2014; Erikson, 2007). There are two distinct dopaminergic pathways in the brain: mesolimbic and mesocortical. The *mesolimbic dopaminergic pathway* is implicated in the processing of rewards and appears central to the understanding of addiction. This pathway originates with dopamine in the ventral tegmental area, which is then released into the nucleus accumbens and travels to various brain regions including the olfactory tubercle, amygdala, and prefrontal cortex (Koob et al., 1998; Gardner, 2011; Simpkins & Simpkins, 2013). Activation of the mesolimbic dopaminergic pathway appears to serve the important evolutionary function of reinforcing behaviors necessary for survival (e.g., eating, drinking, sexual activity), thereby promoting the propagation of the species (Arias-Carrion et al., 2010). Specifically, "humans are biologically predisposed to drink, eat, reproduce, and desire pleasurable experiences" (Blum et al., 2013, p. 2). For example, when an individual is hungry and takes a bite of highly palatable food, specific neurotransmitters are released in their reward system that stimulate both the appetitive and consummatory function of reward, thereby reinforcing the behavior (i.e., eating) and increasing the probability that it will be repeated in the future.

Although dopamine is a primary neurotransmitter of the reward system (Blum et al., 2013), it does not work in isolation. It is hypothesized that dopamine is prominent in the desire or "wanting" phase of reward (anticipation), while the opioid system and, potentially, endocannabinoids, are responsible for the "liking" or hedonic phase of reward (satisfaction; Berridge & Kringelbach, 2015; Comings & Blum, 2000). Indeed, Blum et al. (2020) hypothesized that at least six neurotransmitter pathways are involved in the experience of reward including serotonin, cannabinoids, opioids, GABA, glutamate, and dopamine. Thus, the experience of reward is linked to several neurotransmitters and neuromodulators in complex, interrelated circuitry (Berridge & Kringelbach, 2015; Blum et al., 2014; Blum et al., 2020; Koob et al., 1998; Volkow & Boyle, 2018). Ingesting exogenous drugs of abuse, or stimulating endogenous neurotransmitter release via addictive behaviors, can affect multiple neurotransmitter systems leading to diverse responses among individuals.

REWARDS AND LEARNING

As described in Chapter 1, not all behaviors activate the brain's reward circuitry. Those that do are known as *rewards*. Rewards are any stimuli that produce positive effects (i.e., positive emotions or behaviors) or foster "wanting" and approach behaviors, and thus, are subjectively assigned value (Schultz, 2015). Examples of rewards include eating, drinking, sexual activity, enjoyable social interactions, listening to music, winning a football game, accruing likes on social media, hitting the jackpot on an electronic gambling machine, leveling up in a video game, or getting a promotion at work. Some rewards are natural, meaning they are biologically reinforced with neurochemicals to promote survival (e.g., eating food, drinking water, engaging in sexual activity; Comings & Brum, 2000). Other rewards are not natural, yet have been assigned value and thus become *learned* rewards (e.g., gambling, winning a bet, shopping, getting likes on social media, drinking alcohol, using marijuana; Comings & Brum, 2000). In this way, the reward circuitry is directly involved in the process of learning. When an individual experiences a positive effect ("wanting" or "liking") from a stimulus, the brain identifies the source of the reward, assigns value to the object or activity, and remembers the association between the particular stimulus and the experience of reward

(Arias-Carrion et al., 2010; Schultz, 2015). The amygdala and hippocampus are implicated in the formation and storage of these emotional memories and recalling stimuli that have been linked to rewards (Ashwell, 2019; Koob, 2009; Simpkins & Simpkins, 2013). Once the brain learns what stimuli are rewarding, individuals subsequently are motivated to seek out those rewards. Arias-Carrion et al. (2010) noted, "For the most part, one's motivation is to return to the rewards experienced in the past and to the cues that mark the way to such rewards" (p. 3).

Importantly, not all rewards have the same effect on the learning process. Specifically, "rewards with stronger effects on dopamine neurons are likely to have more impact on learning and choices" (Schultz, 2015, p. 937). Both chemical and nonchemical rewards exist on a spectrum and affect the dopamine system to varying extents (Wise & Rubble, 2020). It remains unclear as to why some individuals prefer one addictive behavior (e.g., gambling) over another (e.g., alcohol), yet it is possible that social contexts, availability, cultural norms, and individual preferences may mediate the pursuit of particular rewards (see Chapter 1 for more details). Although more research is needed in this area, it is clear that the "wanting," "liking," and learning processes of the reward cycle increase the salience of the reward (chemical or behavioral) in the individual's life (Berridge & Robinson, 2016). This increased salience is why clients may pursue addictive substances or behaviors to the neglect of family, romantic partners, job responsibilities, hobbies, friendships, or other previously valued rewards. The individual with addiction experiences strong, urgent desires for the addictive behavior that supersede desires for other rewarding stimuli. This information can be extremely helpful to clients and their family members as a means of understanding the client's seemingly illogical behavior (e.g., pursuing an addictive behavior at the expense of an important relationship). As they learn about the effects of rewarding behaviors in the brain, clients and their families can move away from a moral model conceptualization of addiction (i.e., addiction is the result of bad decisions and personal moral failings) to a biopsychosocial model of addiction (i.e., addiction is the result of biological, psychological, and environmental factors).

ADOLESCENT BRAIN DEVELOPMENT

A final consideration of the brain's response to rewards is the developmental period in which rewards are experienced. A large percentage of addictive behaviors begin during the adolescent years (Gladwin et al., 2011), and there are many factors that contribute to this occurrence (such as the influence of peers, which scholars have found to impact the subjective value of immediate rewards among adolescents; Albert et al., 2013). From a biopsychosocial model of addiction, adolescents have varying levels of risk for addiction as a result of genetic predispositions (e.g., functioning of reward circuitry), psychological traits (e.g., impulsivity, sensation-seeking, mental health symptomology), social networks (e.g., peer groups), environment (e.g., access, availability), and cultural norms (e.g., expectancies, beliefs, values). The following section discusses one component of the neurobiology of adolescence, namely, *myelination*, which should be considered in light of the holistic framework of an adolescent's biopsychosocial experience.

The process of neuronal myelination is a component of brain development that typically transpires during adolescence and young adulthood. As young brains mature, a fatty layer called a *myelin sheath* wraps around the axons of neurons, making the act of transmitting impulses much faster (Ashwell, 2019). The process of myelination begins at the base of the brain (e.g., brainstem) and progresses toward the front (e.g., prefrontal cortex). Thus, the limbic region in the midbrain (which is responsible for emotional and reward processing) experiences myelination and greater connectivity to other brain regions *prior* to the prefrontal cortex (which is responsible for executive functioning, decision-making, and self-regulation). In other words, in the developing brain, the emotional system is myelinated and more connected to other brain regions before the rational, control system. Adolescent brains are still in the process of maturing, so the emotional regions of the midbrain are connected and working quickly, while the rational regions at the front of the brain remain less connected and slower. Specifically, adolescence is "characterized by a tension between early emerging 'bottom-up' systems that express exaggerated reactivity to motivational stimuli and later maturing 'top-down' cognitive control regions" (Casey & Jones, 2010, p. 1197). This means that among adolescents, emotional responses occur more quickly and are much stronger than reasoned, goal-directed responses (Ashwell, 2019; Gladwin et al., 2011).

The process of brain maturation and myelination has important implications for adolescent engagement in addictive behaviors. Given that emotional and motivational circuitry develops prior to self-regulatory circuitry, adolescents are prone to act more impulsively and without as much control as adults with fully myelinated brains (Volkow & Boyle, 2018). Indeed, "during adolescence, the striatal reward/motivation and limbic-emotional circuits are hyperactive, leading to greater emotional reactivity and reward-seeking behaviors" (Volkow & Boyle, 2018, p. 730). It is not surprising, then, that adolescents are more sensitive to rewarding experiences and thereby more motivated to seek them out or return to them once exposed. These rewarding experiences can include using drugs of abuse or engaging in thrilling or hedonic behaviors such as gaming, gambling, social media, or sexual activity. When exposed to a rewarding stimulus (e.g., a social media notification), adolescents likely feel stronger approach behaviors and weaker inhibitory or control behaviors due to the state of their developing brain (Gladwin et al., 2011). The disproportionate strength of the limbic region coupled with the salience of social rewards among adolescents (Albert et al., 2013) provides at least a partial explanation for why addictive behaviors likely emerge during this developmental period. Counselors should be careful to assess for behavioral addictions with clients of all ages, yet mental health professionals working with adolescents should be particularly equipped to recognize, assess, and treat addictive behaviors.

GENETIC PREDISPOSITION TO BEHAVIORAL ADDICTIONS

Genetics is but one component of the broader conceptualization of addiction, yet remains an important consideration (ASAM, 2019). Clinicians should be careful to consider the effects of a client's genetic makeup within the constellation of other attributes such as personality traits, psychological states, environmental conditions, lived experiences, social contexts, and cultural norms. Genes, however, do play a role in the unique functioning of an individual's mesolimbic reward pathway (Blum et al., 2014). Variations in genes, or polymorphisms, related to the production, function, transportation, metabolism, or absorption of neurotransmitters have been proposed to cause impairments in the reward pathway leading to *hypodopaminergic functioning* (i.e., underactive dopamine system in the brain's reward center). This condition has been labeled *reward deficiency syndrome* (RDS; Blum et al., 1996; Blum et al., 2014; Comings & Blum, 2000) and is believed to result in a "biochemical inability to derive reward from ordinary, everyday activities" (Blum et al., 1996, p. 132). Specifically, proponents of the reward deficiency hypothesis believe that due to hypodopaminergic functioning, individuals with RDS experience constant cravings in response to their "reward deficient state" (Febo et al., 2017, p. 669). These cravings may be temporarily satisfied by engaging in behaviors that stimulate dopamine release, such as using drugs of abuse, gambling, gaming, or sexual activity. Specifically, it has been postulated that "an individual with low dopamine function will seek out substances and/or behaviors known to boost dopamine function" (Blum, Chen, et al., 2012).

Thus, from this perspective, individuals with RDS are predisposed to engage in addictive behaviors as a means of self-medication for underactive reward pathways (Blum et al., 2014; Comings & Blum, 2000). For example, an individual with an optimally functioning dopaminergic system (i.e., without RDS) is presumed to have the neurochemical composition necessary to experience rewards within their environments (e.g., coos from an infant, conversation with a close friend, taste of a good meal, beauty of a sunrise, smell of perfume, sight of a romantic partner). An individual with RDS who experiences underactive dopaminergic brain functioning, however, may lack the ability to experience rewards from these naturally occurring phenomena (Blum, Gardner, et al., 2012). Yet, if this individual comes upon a highly rewarding stimulus (e.g., internet pornography, internet gaming, high-sugar food, electronic gambling machine), they may experience an enhanced mood or a state of well-being previously unknown. Once the individual feels the enhanced emotional state, they are likely to return to the activity to once again stimulate reward circuitry of the brain and curb the cravings caused by RDS. Therefore, individuals with RDS are presumably predisposed to seek out their own means of stimulating their dopaminergic reward systems, which may include using drugs of abuse or chronically engaging in highly rewarding activities (Blum et al., 2014; Gold et al., 2014).

It is important to note that the reward pathway is a complex system. As more information regarding the multifaceted nature of reward emerged (i.e., "wanting" systems and "liking" systems; Berridge & Kringelbach, 2015; Berridge & Robinson, 2016), the reward deficiency hypothesis has become more nuanced (Blum et al., 2020). Indeed, scholars purport that dopamine deficiency is but one subtype of RDS along with others such as endorphinergic deficiency syndrome and opioid deficiency syndrome (Blum et al., 2020). Although dopamine is one of the primary neurochemicals of reward, it is affected by and affects several other neurotransmitters (Comings & Blum, 2000; Blum et al., 1996). Therefore, it has been proposed that aberrations in any component of the reward pathway can lead to RDS (Comings & Blum, 2000). It thereby behooves counselors to acknowledge that genetic vulnerabilities to behavioral addictions can involve multiple neurotransmitters and brain regions. For example, low serotonin levels are implicated in impaired control and impulsivity, and serotonergic deficiencies have been associated with addictive behaviors, including gambling (Bellegarde & Potenza, 2010). Additionally, variations in endogenous opioids, which are implicated in feelings of euphoria, also have been linked to addictive behaviors. Specifically, "Individuals with altered opioidergic systems may feel a more intense euphoria after engaging in rewarding behaviors and, thus, have greater difficulty controlling desires to continue the addictive behavior" (Grant et al., 2006, p. 926).

An important recognition for counselors is that a client's response to a rewarding behavior and level of felt euphoria varies depending, in part, on their genetic makeup (Schultz, 2015). Thus, one client's experience of reward while playing an internet game can be very different from the experience of other clients. The recognition of these differences can help increase empathy for clients who find particular behaviors very rewarding and thereby challenging to limit or control. Continued empirical investigation is needed to fully understand the neurochemical experience of reward, yet most scholars agree that genetic polymorphisms contribute, at least in part, to the predisposition to addiction.

CLINICAL NOTE 2.2

Some clients may have heard that addiction is a disease, but it is likely that many clients and their family members are unfamiliar with the details supporting that claim. One helpful way to engage in psychoeducation related to genetic factors and individual vulnerabilities is to have clients create an *addiction genogram* in which they depict at least three generations of their family system and identify all known addictions (both behavioral and chemical). These addiction genograms depicting addictive behaviors across generations can help facilitate a discussion about genetic vulnerabilities that can contribute, in part, to the development of addiction.

NEUROADAPTATIONS CAUSED BY ADDICTIVE BEHAVIORS

The preceding section described genetic predispositions that can contribute to an individual's vulnerability toward behavioral addictions. However, even among individuals without a genetic predisposition, the repeated, long-term engagement in addictive behaviors is believed to cause changes in the brain. As a reminder, all drugs of abuse and rewarding activities (e.g., shopping, eating, gaming, gambling, sex) are posited to affect the brain's mesolimbic dopamine system (Blum, Chen, et al., 2012). If neurotransmitter levels are too high due to chronic overstimulation (e.g., hours of continuous internet gaming, gambling, or pornography use), the brain may adjust in response to these heightened levels to restore equilibrium (Leeman & Potenza, 2013). These adjustments, or *neuroadaptations*, are the brain's way of reinstating homeostasis (Blum, Chen, et al., 2012; Koob, 2009). Rather than a hardwired, fixed machine, the brain is plastic and continually adapts and changes with experience (i.e., neuroplasticity; Doidge, 2007). For example, in response to the chronic overstimulation of dopamine in an individual's reward circuitry (e.g., years of gambling at casinos), they may experience the downregulation of the dopamine system. This downregulation occurs by reducing dopamine transporters, reducing dopamine receptors, or decreasing dopamine release to lessen the effect of the neurochemical in the reward system (Blum et al., 2014; Leeman & Potenza, 2013; Wise & Robble, 2020). With regard to chemical addiction, Blume, Chen, et al. (2012) summarized:

> Independent of one's genetic makeup, if one keeps taking drugs, the brain adjusts to the overwhelming surge in dopamine and other neurotransmitters causing a breakdown in the natural process of brain reward by producing less dopamine or by reducing the number of dopamine (D2) receptors. (p. 140)

Like drugs of abuse, it is hypothesized that the chronic engagement in highly rewarding behaviors also can lead to neuroadaptations, such as the downregulation of the dopamine system, regardless of an individual's genetic composition (Barrett, 2010; Hilton, 2013; Love et al., 2015; Parylak et al., 2011). Specifically, the use or consumption of objects known as *supernormal stimuli*, which are artificial, exaggerated versions of natural instincts (e.g., internet pornography; processed, high-sugar foods; electronic gambling machines) can cause heightened stimulation of reward circuitry, thereby triggering neuroadaptations. These supernormal stimuli are more enhanced and potent than natural stimuli (consider the processed sugar in a piece of hard candy compared to the natural sweetness of a strawberry) and can cause spikes in endogenous neurotransmitter release (especially dopamine) leading to neuroadaptations, much like those that follow the chronic use of drugs of abuse (Barrett, 2010; Hilton, 2013; Love et al., 2015; Parylak et al., 2011). Additionally, researchers have discovered that *novel stimuli* trigger greater releases of dopamine in the reward pathway (Menegas et al., 2017). This consideration is particularly relevant for behavioral addictions given the novelty inherent in many addictive behaviors. For instance, there is always another social media post to read, another aspect of a virtual world to explore in an internet game, and another pornographic image or video to view online. The novelty inherent in these behaviors may serve to stimulate more dopamine release, thereby triggering neuroadaptations as a result of chronic engagement.

As a consequence of the downregulation of the dopaminergic system, individuals may become less sensitive to naturally occurring rewards (Wise & Robble, 2020; Volkow & Boyle, 2018). For example, an individual who chronically engages in online gambling and experiences neuroadaptations may no longer experience reward from naturally occurring stimuli (e.g., beautiful weather, enjoyable music, pleasant social interactions, high score on an exam). Thus, for individuals with and without a genetic predisposition to addiction, overstimulation of the mesolimbic dopamine system may lead to decreased dopamine functioning (such as a decrease in dopamine [D2] receptors; Parylak et al., 2011; Wise & Robble, 2020) and, in turn, may lead to baseline feelings of dysphoria or anhedonia (i.e., the reduced capacity to feel pleasure; Koob et al., 1998; Leeman & Potenza, 2013; Simpkins & Simpkins, 2013; Volkow & Boyle, 2018). Known as the "dark side of addiction" (Koob & Le Moal, 2008, p. 38), the downregulation of the reward system in response to chronic overactivation is presumed to lead to negative emotional states marked by malaise, loss of motivation, stress, and irritability.

To provide another example, consider an adolescent who chronically activates his reward system via internet gaming for several hours each night. The downregulation of his dopaminergic functioning in response to excessive dopamine release from gaming may lead him to feel dysphoric or irritable when he is not gaming, even in response to otherwise pleasurable activities. The adolescent's parents may describe him as becoming increasingly moody or agitated, regularly unhappy, and report that he has lost interest in activities other than gaming. Thus, the cycle of addiction appears to apply to both drug use and behavioral addictions: (a) preoccupation/anticipation (craving), (b) binge/intoxication (pleasure and euphoria), and (c) withdrawal/negative affect (antireward or adverse mood states; Koob & Le Moal, 2008). Once these neuroadaptations have occurred, individuals may become dependent on engaging in the rewarding behavior (i.e., internet gaming) just to feel "normal" and ward off withdrawal symptoms (thus, drugs of abuse and addictive behaviors are both positively and negatively reinforcing; Goodman, 2001; Koob, 2009; Koob & Le Moal, 2008). For example, the adolescent described earlier may find that the only way he knows how to feel positive emotions is by gaming; so he plays for longer periods of time, more frequently, and may increase the intensity of gaming, just to reach his desired state (i.e., tolerance). The increased frequency and intensity of gaming continues to cause neuroadaptations, leading to dysphoric mood states when he is not playing. Thus, although he initially engaged in gaming due to its rewarding effects (i.e., positive reinforcement), he now engages to diminish his dysphoria (i.e., negative reinforcement), and the cycle continues.

It is important for counselors to understand, and perhaps explain to clients and their family members, that chronic engagement in highly rewarding behaviors (particularly the use or consumption of supernormal stimuli) can lead to neuroadaptations that are hypothesized to downregulate dopaminergic functioning. This downregulation may substantially impact clients' daily emotional experiences, such as the ability to seek and experience natural rewards. It may be helpful to ask clients and their families to provide a history of the clients' positive and negative emotional experiences, beginning with emotional experiences prior to the initiation of the addictive behavior (e.g., how often the client typically experienced positive and negative affect, descriptions of the client's baseline emotional experience, intensity of positive and negative emotions), during the first few engagements of the addictive behavior (e.g., how euphoric the behavior made the client feel, emotional response when the behavior stopped), and up until the present day (e.g., how does engagement in the behavior feel for the client now, current daily emotional experiences, baseline affect). For example, the client may report that it used to be extremely pleasurable to play internet games, yet now the client plays for hours and does not experience the same degree of pleasure. Moreover, the client and client's family may report that the client demonstrates more overall irritation, anger, and negative mood states than they did during the years prior to gaming. This information can help counselors and clients understand the impact of addictive behaviors on brain functioning and emotional responses.

INTERACTION BETWEEN GENETIC AND ENVIRONMENTAL FACTORS

As previously mentioned, genetics is but one component of the development and course of addiction. The *environment* and unique individual *experiences* also play critical roles, and the bidirectional interaction between genetics and environmental factors is well known. Genes are largely responsible for an individual's traits and temperaments, which impact the ways in which they engage with the world (Siegel, 2012), yet, at the same time, experience can change an individual's neural pathways (i.e., neuroplasticity; Doidge, 2007) and gene expression (i.e., epigenetics; Siegel, 2012). Specifically, "by altering both the activity and the structure of the connections between neurons, experience directly shapes the circuits responsible for such processes as memory, emotion, and self-awareness" (Siegel, 2012, p. 4). Thus, along with genetic vulnerabilities, environmental factors can affect neurobiological systems and increase one's risk of addiction (Blum, Chen, et al., 2012). Specifically, neglect and deprivation during infancy (Volkow & Boyle, 2018) or trauma and stress during childhood (Felitti et al., 1998) can heighten one's susceptibility for addiction later in life.

> **CLINICAL NOTE 2.3**
>
> Deans and Maggert (2015) defined epigenetics as "the study of phenomena and mechanisms that cause chromosome-bound, heritable changes to gene expression that are not dependent on changes to DNA sequence" (p. 892). Thus, experience (e.g., stress) does not change the structure of genes, but can change gene expression. Those changes in genetic expression can be passed from one generation to the next (van der Kolk, 2014). Epigenetics is a burgeoning field, yet more research may reveal links between epigenetics and the heredity of behavioral addictions.

TRAUMA AND ADDICTION

In their groundbreaking study, Felitti et al. (1998) investigated the relationship between childhood trauma (known as *adverse childhood experiences* [ACEs]) and an array of physical and behavioral outcomes among adults. The researchers examined the prevalence of several categories of ACEs including physical, sexual, and psychological abuse, mental illness or substance abuse in the home, exposure to the violent treatment of one's caregiver, and criminal behavior in the home. The results of the study clearly demonstrated a dose–response relationship between the number of ACE categories experienced in the first 18 years of life and the risk of numerous detrimental outcomes in adulthood. Specifically, as ACE scores increased, so too did the prevalence of smoking, alcohol use, and illicit drug use, among other physical and mental health problems. With particular relevance to behavioral addictions, the researchers also found that higher ACE scores predicted more severe obesity and an increased likelihood of having 50 or more sexual partners. Specifically, among respondents with ACE scores of 4 or more, 12% had severe obesity compared to 5.4% with no ACEs, and 6.8% had 50 or more sexual partners compared to 3.0% with no ACEs (Felitti et al., 1998), suggesting possible associations between ACEs and food and sex addiction. Along with additional studies connecting ACEs and alcohol use (Dube et al., 2002) and illicit drug use (Dube et al., 2003), ACEs also have been linked to problem gambling (Poole et al., 2017) and early sexual intercourse (at or before 15 years of age) and increased number of sex partners (30 or more) among women (Hillis et al., 2001).

What is the association between early trauma and addictive behaviors? It is hypothesized that the answer lies in the dysregulation of the body's stress response system (Nakazawa, 2015; van der Kolk, 2014). The stress response system involves an important cascade of hormones and neurochemicals to help human beings respond to danger. Consider a situation in which a woman thinks she is alone in the office, yet she notices a shadow move. Sensing danger, her stress response system is immediately activated.

The stress hormones *cortisol* and *adrenaline* are released, which prepare her to run or fight (van der Kolk, 2014). In that moment, she is highly focused, her heart beats faster, her blood pressure increases, and she breathes rapidly (Nakazawa, 2015; Siegel, 2012). As she looks in the direction of the shadow, she realizes that a window was left open and the movement she noticed was only a curtain blowing in the wind. With the resolution of the threat, her stress response is deactivated, stress hormone levels return to baseline, and she regains a sense of calm. This example demonstrates the adaptive functioning of a regulated stress response system (Burke Harris, 2018; Nakazawa, 2015).

A stress response system can become dysregulated, however, due to early trauma or ACEs, particularly in the absence of an attuned, buffering adult (Burke Harris, 2018; Nakazawa, 2015). Rather than normative or tolerable stress, which can be adaptive, stress that is chronic and unpredictable (known as *toxic stress*; Burke Harris, 2018; Nakazawa, 2015) can lead to alterations in a child's stress response system. For children in situations in which a threat persists over time (e.g., physical abuse from a caregiver, a parent with untreated mental illness, prolonged criminal activity within the home, active addiction in the home), coupled with the absence of a supportive caregiver, the stress response system can become chronically activated (consider the features of an activated stress response described in the example of the woman in her office that never "switch off" or return to baseline). Specifically, in the event of toxic stress, the hypothalamic–pituitary–adrenal (HPA) axis is continually stimulated, triggering the release of cortisol, while the sympathoadrenomedullary axis triggers the release of adrenaline (Burke Harris, 2018; Nakazawa, 2015; Volkow & Boyle, 2018). Chronic activation of the stress response system can result in high levels of stress hormones in the body, which can lead to insomnia, increased blood sugar, inflammation, cardiovascular disease, and a compromised immune system (Guilliams & Edwards, 2010; Nakazawa, 2015). Moreover, Nakazawa (2015) noted, "if we had early trauma, our adult HPA stress axis can't distinguish between real danger and perceived stress" (p. 38). Thus, ACEs can alter the functioning of a child's stress response, which can persist into adulthood.

The dysregulated stress response system can lead to a host of emotional and physical challenges, including difficulties in emotion regulation. The link between ACEs and emotion regulation difficulties is particularly relevant to addiction treatment, given that drugs of abuse and rewarding behaviors may be used as a means of mood modification by activating reward circuitry (Griffiths, 2005). Indeed, individuals with dysregulated stress responses due to early trauma may seek to regulate their heightened emotional states (e.g., hyperarousal, vigilance, fear, anxiety) by engaging in addictive behaviors. Specifically, Felitti et al. (1998) noted, "the linking mechanisms appear to center on behaviors such as smoking, alcohol or drug abuse, overeating, or sexual behaviors that may be consciously or unconsciously used because they have immediate pharmacological or psychological benefits as coping devices" (p. 253). For example, among a sample of individuals with gambling experience, researchers found that increases in ACE scores predicted more emotion dysregulation, which, in turn, predicted higher levels of gambling severity (Poole et al., 2017). Therefore, as a result of past trauma and current dysregulated stress response systems, individuals may rely on addictive behaviors or drugs of abuse as their primary means of modulating their emotional states. Although detrimental, addictive behaviors likely are the best way clients know how to manage their emotions.

In sum, ACEs can disrupt the functioning of the body's stress response system and, subsequently, create difficulties in emotion regulation, specifically in the absence of a supportive, attuned caregiver. In light of a dysregulated stress response system, certain individuals may be at higher risk of regulating their emotional states through addictive behaviors. Therefore, counselors may best serve clients with behavioral addictions by assessing for childhood trauma and, when appropriate, engaging in trauma-informed interventions and emotion regulation enhancement strategies.

SUMMARY

Counselors should be knowledgeable about neuroscience and its direct application to their work with behavioral addictions. The understanding of neurotransmission, the experience of reward, genetic vulnerabilities, neuroadaptations, and environmental risk factors such as childhood trauma can greatly enhance treatment for addictive behaviors. Additionally, clients often believe that their behavioral addictions are the result of moral failings and insufficient willpower, and, as a result, harbor immense amounts of shame and self-stigma. As counselors provide psychoeducation related to the neuroscience of behavioral addictions, their clients (and their clients' friends and family members) can feel empowered, optimistic, and hopeful as they work with, rather than against, their neurobiological systems.

REFERENCES

Albert, D., Chein, J., & Steinberg, L. (2013). The teenage brain: Peer influences on adolescent decision making. *Current Directions in Psychological Science, 22,* 114–120. https://doi.org/10.1177/0963721412471347

American Society of Addiction Medicine. (2019). *Definition of addiction.* https://www.asam.org/docs/default-source/quality-science/asam's-2019-definition-of-addiction-(1).pdf?sfvrsn=b8b64fc2_2

Arias-Carrion, O., Stamelou, M., Murillo-Rodriguez, E., Menendez-Gonzalez, M., & Poppel, E. (2010). Dopaminergic reward system: A short integrative review. *International Archives of Medicine, 3,* 24. https://doi.org/10.1186/1755-7682-3-24

Ashwell, K. (2019). *The brain book: Development, function, disorder, health* (2nd ed.). Firefly Books.

Barrett, D. (2010). *Supernormal stimuli: How primal urges overran their evolutionary purpose.* W. W. Norton & Company.

Bellegarde, J. D., & Potenza, M. N. (2010). Neurobiology of pathological gambling. In D. Ross, H. Kincaid, D. Spurrett, & P. Collins (Eds.), *What is addiction?* (pp. 27–52). The MIT Press.

Berridge, K. C., & Kringelbach, M. L. (2015). Pleasure systems in the brain. *Neuron, 86*, 646–664. https://doi.org/10.1016/j.neuron.2015.02.018

Berridge, K. C., & Robinson, T. E. (2016). Liking, wanting and the incentive-sensitization theory of addiction. *The American Psychologist, 71*, 670–679. https://doi.org/10.1037/amp0000059

Blum, K., Baron, D., McLaughlin, T., & Gold, M. S. (2020). Molecular neurological correlates of endorphinergic/dopaminergic mechanisms in reward circuitry linked to endorphinergic deficiency syndrome (EDS). *Journal of Neurological Sciences, 411*, 116733. https://doi.org/10.1016-j.jns.2020.116733

Blum, K., Chen, A. L. C., Giordano, J., Borsten, J., Chen, T. J. H., Hauser, M., Simpatico, T., Femino, J., Braverman, E. R., & Barh, D. (2012). The addictive brain: All roads lead to dopamine. *Journal of Psychoactive Drugs, 44*, 134–143. https://doi.org/10.1080/02791072.2012.685407

Blum, K., Cull, J. G., Braverman, E. R., & Comings, D. E. (1996). Reward deficiency syndrome. *American Scientist, 84*, 132–146.

Blum, K., Femino, J., Teitelbaum, S., Giordano, J., Oscar-Berman, M., & Gold, M. (2013). Introduction. In K. Blum, J. Femino, S. Teitelbaum, J. Giordano, M. Oscar-Berman, & M. Gold (Eds.), *Molecular neurobiology of addiction recovery: The 12 steps program and fellowship* (pp. 1–10). Springer Publishing.

Blum, K., Gardner, E., Oscar-Berman, M., & Gold, M. (2012). "Liking" and "wanting" linked to reward deficiency syndrome (RDS): Hypothesizing differential responsivity in brain reward circuitry. *Current Pharmaceutical Design, 18*, 113–118. https://doi.org/10.2174/1381612127989191100

Blum, K., Oscar-Berman, M., Demetrovics, Z., Barh, D., & Gold, M. S. (2014). Genetic addiction risk score (GARS): Molecular neurogenetic evidence for predisposition to reward deficiency syndrome (RDS). *Molecular Neurobiology, 50*, 765–796. https://doi.org/10.1007/s12035-014-8726-5

Blum, K., Werner, T., Carnes, S., Carnes, P., Bowirrat, A. Giordano, J., Oscar-Berman, M., & Gold, M. (2012). Sex, drugs, and rock 'n' roll: Hypothesizing common mesolimbic activation as a function of reward gene polymorphisms. *Journal of Psychoactive Drugs, 44*, 38–55. https://doi.org/10.1080/02791072.2012.662112

Burke Harris, N. (2018). *The deepest well: Healing the long-term effects of childhood adversity*. Bluebird.

Casey, B. J., & Jones, R. M. (2010). Neurobiology of the adolescent brain and behavior: Implications for substance use disorders. *Journal of the American Academy of Child and Adolescent Psychiatry, 49*, 1189–1201. https://doi.org/10.1016/j.jaac.2010.08.017

Comings, D. E., & Blum, K. (2000). Reward deficiency syndrome: Genetic aspects of behavioral disorders. *Progress in Brain Research, 126*, 325–341.

Deans, C., & Maggert, K. A. (2015). What do you mean, "epigenetic"? *Genetics, 199*, 887–896. https://doi.org/10.1534/genetics.114.173492

Di Nicola, M., Tedeschi, D., De Risio, L., Pettorruso, M., Martinotti, G., Ruggeri, F., Swierkosz-Lenart, K., Guglielmo, R., Callea, A., Ruggeri, G., Pozzi, G., Di Giannantonio, M., & Janiri, L. (2015). Co-occurrence of alcohol use disorder and behavioral addictions: Relevance of impulsivity and craving. *Drug and Alcohol Dependence, 148*, 118–125. https://doi.org/10.1016/j.drugalcdep.2014.12.028

Doidge, N. (2007). *The brain that changes itself: Stories of personal triumph from the frontiers of brain science*. Penguin Group.

Dube, S. R., Anda, R. F., Felitti, V. J., Edwards, V. J., & Croft, J. B. (2002). Adverse childhood experiences and personal alcohol abuse as an adult. *Addictive Behaviors, 27,* 713–725. https://doi.org/10.1016/s0306-4603(01)00204-0

Dube, S. R., Dong, M., Chapman, D. P., Giles, W. H., Anda, R. F., & Felitti, V. J. (2003). Childhood abuse, neglect, and household dysfunction and the risk of illicit drug use: The adverse childhood experiences study. *Pediatrics, 111,* 564–572. https://doi.org/10.1542/peds.111.3.564

Erickson, C. K. (2007). *The science of addiction: From neurobiology to treatment.* W. W. Norton & Company.

Febo, M., Blum, K., Badgaiyan, R. D., Baron, D., Thanos, P. K., Colon-Perez, L. M., Demotrovics, Z., & Gold, M. S. (2017). Dopamine homeostasis: Brain functional connectivity in reward deficiency syndrome. *Frontiers in Bioscience, 22,* 669–691. https://doi.org/10.2741/4509

Felitti, V. J., Anda, R. F., Nordenberg, D., Williamson, D. F., Spitz, A. M., Edwards, V., Koss, M. P., & Marks, J. S. (1998). Relationship of childhood abuse and household dysfunction to many of the leading causes of death in adults: The adverse childhood experiences (ACE) study. *American Journal of Preventive Medicine, 14,* 245–258. https://doi.org/10.1016/s0749-3797(98)00017-8

Gardner, E. L. (2011). Addiction and brain reward and antireward pathways. *Advances in Psychosomatic Medicine, 30,* 22–60. https://doi.org/10.1159/000324065

Gladwin, T. E., Figner, B., Crone, E. A., & Wiers, R. W. (2011). Addiction, adolescence, and the integration of control and motivation. *Developmental Cognitive Neuroscience, 1,* 364–376. https://doi.org/10.1016/j.dcn.2011.06.008

Gold, M. S., Blum, K., Febo, M., McLaughlin, T., Cronje, F. J., & Han, D. (2014). Hatching the behavioral addiction egg: Reward deficiency solution system (RDSS) as a function of dopaminergic neurogenetics and brain functional connectivity linking all addictions under a common rubric. *Journal of Behavioral Addictions, 3,* 149–156. https://doi.org/10.556/JBA.3.2014.019

Goodman, A. (2001). What's in a name? Terminology for designating a syndrome of driven sexual behavior. *Sexual Addiction and Compulsivity, 8,* 191–213. https://doi.org/10.1080/107201601753459919

Grant, J. E., Brewer, J. A., & Potenza, M. N. (2006). The neurobiology of substance and behavioral addictions. *CNS Spectrums, 11,* 924–930. https://doi.org/10.1017/S109285290001511X

Griffiths, M. (2005). A 'components' model of addiction within a biopsychosocial framework. *Journal of Substance Use, 10,* 191–197. https://doi.org/10.1080/14659890500114359

Guilliams, T. G., & Edwards, L. (2010). Chronic stress and the HPA axis: Clinical assessment and therapeutic considerations. *The Standard, 9,* 1–12.

Hillis, S. D., Anda, R. F., Felitti, V. J., & Marchbanks, P. A. (2001). Adverse childhood experiences and sexual risk behaviors in women: A retrospective cohort study. *Family Planning Perspectives, 33,* 206–212. https://doi.org/10-2307/2673783

Hilton, D. L. (2013). Pornography addiction- A supranormal stimulus considered in the context of neuroplasticity. *Socioaffective Neuroscience and Psychology, 3,* 20767. https://doi.org/10.3402/snp.v3i0.20767

Karim, R., & Chaudhri, P. (2012). Behavioral addictions: An overview. *Journal of Psychoactive Drugs, 44,* 5–17. https://doi.org/10.1080/02796072.2012.662589

Koob, G. F. (2009). Dynamics of neuronal circuits in addiction: Reward, antireward, and emotional memory. *Pharmacopsychiatry, 42,* 532–541. https://doi.org/10.1055/s-0029-1216356

Koob, G. F., & Le Moal, M. (2008). Addiction and the brain antireward system. *Annual Review of Psychology, 59,* 29–53. https://doi.org/10.1146/annurev.psych.59.103006.093548

Koob. G., F., Sanna, P. P., & Bloom, F. E. (1998). Neuroscience of addiction. *Neuron, 21,* 467–476. https://doi.org/10.1016/s0896-6273(00)80557-7

Leeman, R. T., & Potenza, M. N. (2013). A targeted review of the neurobiology and genetics of behavioral addictions: An emerging area of research. *Canadian Journal of Psychiatry, 58,* 260–273. https://doi.org/10.1177/070674371305800503

Li, P., Snyder, G. L., & Vanover, K. E. (2016). Dopamine targeting drugs for the treatment of schizophrenia: Past, present and future. *Current Topics in Medicinal Chemistry, 16,* 3385–3403. https://doi.org/10.2174/1568026616666160608084834

Love, T., Laier, C., Brand, M., Hatch, L., & Hajela, R. (2015). Neuroscience of internet pornography addiction: A review and update. *Behavioral Sciences, 5,* 388–433. https://doi.org/10.3390/bs5030388

Menegas, W., Babayan, B. M., Uchida, N., & Watabe-Uchida, M. (2017). Opposite initialization to novel cues in dopamine signaling in ventral and posterior striatum in mice. *eLife, 6,* e21886. https://doi.org/10.7554/eLife.21886

Nakazawa, D. J. (2015). *Childhood disrupted: How your biography becomes your biology, and how you can heal.* Atria.

Nestler, E. J., (2005). The neurobiology of cocaine addiction. *Science and Practice Perspectives, 3,* 4–10. https://doi.org/10.1151/spp05314

Olds, J., & Milner, P. (1954). Positive reinforcement produced by electrical stimulation of septal area and other regions of rat brain. *Journal of Comparative Psychology, 47,* 419–427. https://doi.org/10.1037/h0058775

Parylak, S. L., Koob, G. F., & Zorrilla, E. P. (2011). The dark side of food addiction. *Physiology and Behavior, 104,* 149–156. https://doi.org/10.1016/j.physbeh.2011.04.063

Poole, J. C., Kim, H. S., Dobson, K. S., & Hodgins, D. C. (2017). Adverse childhood experiences and disordered gambling: Assessing the mediating role of emotion dysregulation. *Journal of Gambling Studies, 33,* 1187–1200. https://doi.org/10.1007/s10899-017-9680-8

Schultz, W. (2015). Neuronal reward and decision signals: From theories to data. *Physiological Reviews, 95,* 853–951. https://doi.org/10.1152/physrev.0023.2014

Siegel, D. J. (2012). *The developing mind: How relationships and the brain interact to shape who we are* (2nd ed.). Guilford Press.

Simpkins, C. A., & Simpkins, A. M. (2013). *Neuroscience for clinicians: Evidence, models, and practice.* Springer Publishing.

Sinacola, R. S., Peters-Strickland, T., & Wyner, J. D. (2020). *Basic psychopharmacology for mental health professionals* (3rd ed.). Pearson.

van der Kolk, B. A. (2014). *The body keeps the score: Brain, mind, and body in the healing of trauma.* Penguin Books.

Volkow, N. D., & Boyle, M. (2018). Neuroscience of addiction: Relevance to prevention and treatment. *The American Journal of Psychiatry, 175,* 729–740. https://doi.org/10.1176/appi.ajp.2018.17101174

Wise, R. A., & Robble, M. A. (2020). Dopamine and addiction. *Annual Review of Psychology, 71,* 79–106. https://doi.org/10.1146/annurev-psych-010418-103337

3

Internet Gaming Addiction

HOW DO I CONCEPTUALIZE IT?

In the late 1970s, Multi-User Dungeons (MUDs) emerged as the first text-based, virtual, role-playing games for multiple players. These games did not have graphics, yet allowed gamers to chat via text with each other as they journeyed through narrated adventures (Sanchez, 2009). TinyMUDs were introduced in the late 1980s, which permitted small groups of users to socialize with one another and create objects within the game. Although the objects could not be used by players, TinyMUDs allowed gamers to add to their virtual worlds. In the 1990s, Multi-User Dungeon, object oriented (MOO) emerged, in which users could create objects to be utilized in the game by employing a programming language. MOO gamers were directly involved in the development of their virtual worlds, which they could share with other gamers. In the mid-to-late 1990s, a new genre of multiuser games, called *massively multiplayer online* (MMO) games, took over the gaming entertainment sphere. Within MMOs, gamers typically assume a character (in the form of an *avatar*) to socialize, create, compete, and perform tasks with thousands of other gamers within a virtual world (Sanchez, 2009). Today, a variety of MMOs exist, including first-person shooter (FPS), real-time strategy (RTS), role-playing games (RPGs), and multiplayer online battle arena (MOBA). Along with MMOs, individuals can engage in other forms of online games such as simulations (virtual depictions of real-world activities such as dancing, playing sports, or socializing), action games (requiring movement and physical activity), casual skill-based games (matching tasks or puzzles), casino or arcade games, and educational games. As a multibillion-dollar industry yielding an estimated 152.1 billion dollar revenue in 2019 (Newzoo, 2019a), it is clear that online gaming has become a substantial component of modern entertainment.

Like all rewarding behaviors, gaming exists on a continuum ranging from healthy to disordered play. Moderate online gaming has been linked to positive outcomes such as increasing response time (Gorman et al., 2018), decreasing loneliness and social anxiety (Martoncik & Loksa, 2016), and fostering skills such as communication and collaboration (Sourmelis et al., 2017). However, for a small portion of gamers, internet gaming can become compulsive, out of control, lead to negative consequences, and induce cravings or mental preoccupation with gaming. Gamers who exhibit these characteristics should be assessed for internet gaming addiction.

INTERNET ADDICTION VERSUS INTERNET GAMING ADDICTION

Dr. Kimberly Young is credited with introducing the concept of internet addiction after observing individuals who lost control over their internet usage (Young, 1998). These individuals would lose track of time while online, forego important responsibilities to spend time in chat rooms, and give up long-term relationships for sexual partners they met online. Although no substances were ingested, those with compulsive, out-of-control internet usage displayed the classic characteristics of addiction. Young (1998) noted, "In behavior-oriented addictions, those who get hooked are addicted to what they *do* and the *feelings* they experience when they're doing it" (p. 17).

Rather than the amount of time spent online, Young identified the desire to *escape* as the primary feature of internet addiction. She created the Internet Addiction Test (IAT), modeled after the criteria for pathological gambling, to assess all forms of online activities (Young, 1998). Since its inception, the concept of internet addiction and the IAT have been widely employed in research and clinical settings, yet given the multitude of available online activities, scholars began questioning whether individuals were actually addicted to the internet or to *specific activities that took place online*. For example, the experience of online gaming addiction is categorically different than cybersex addiction, yet both utilize the internet. Moreover, those who lose control over online gambling may require different treatment approaches than those who lose control over their social media use. Therefore, it seemed reasonable to forego the notion of internet addiction and, instead, conceptualize activities as specific behavioral addictions that may occur on- or offline (e.g., shopping addiction). Conversely, scholars in support of internet addiction noted that there is something distinct about engaging in behaviors online, and many online activities overlap. For example, sexually arousing content exists within internet games and on social media. Should clinicians consider sex addiction, gaming addiction, or social media addiction with their clients? Additionally, it has been argued that using real-world currency to pay to unlock virtual rewards in games (e.g., loot boxes, described later in this chapter) is a form of gambling (Macey & Hamari, 2019). Should a counselor investigate gaming addiction, gambling addiction, or both? Thus, some researchers question whether we can truly separate distinct types of addictive internet behaviors.

> **CLINICAL NOTE 3.1**
>
> Consider the argument for internet addiction versus the argument for specific behavioral addictions that take place online. In light of your experience, which conceptualization seems more fitting? How might this influence your practice?

Ultimately, many scholars contend that specific internet content (e.g., gambling, gaming, cybersex, pornography, shopping, social networking) is the addictive stimulus and the internet is merely the medium to access that stimulus (Saunders et al., 2017). In support of this view, researchers have noted that clients do not typically show signs of being addicted to all activities on the internet. Rather, clients seem to lose control over some online behaviors (e.g., pornography) but not others (e.g., gambling). For example, Kiraly et al. (2014) studied internet addiction and online gaming addiction among adolescents and found that only 6.7% of the sample met criteria for both. Almost 9% of the sample was classified as problematic internet users but not problematic gamers, and 4.3% was classified as problematic gamers but not problematic internet users (Kiraly et al., 2014). Thus, counselors may best understand their clients by inquiring about exact uses of the internet to identify the specific addictive stimulus.

THE NATURE OF GAMING

It is important for counselors to recognize that gaming is not a homogeneous activity. Games can be played on smartphones, tablets, personal computers, or consoles. They can be free-to-play or pay-to-play (which require a paid subscription or one-time payment) games. Gamers can play independently, with others online, with others in person, or with others online and in person. Additionally, gaming genres vary considerably and include independent puzzle and skill games, sports games, educational games, social games (often played on social networking sites), virtual simulations of real-world experiences, action games, and massively multiplayer competitions in fantasy worlds. When it comes to gaming addiction, any genre of gaming can be problematic for vulnerable users, yet researchers have found that MMOs (such as MMORPGs) are most strongly linked to internet gaming addiction (Bonnaire & Phan, 2017; Bonnaire & Baptista, 2019).

Online gaming, particularly MMOs, offers an all-encompassing immersive experience. Gamers enter a highly detailed virtual world and are able to socialize with other gamers through text or voice communication. Players can form guilds or clans and collectively work to advance in the game, developing strong attachments with one another along the way. The games also are perpetually adapting and updating (through patches), providing gamers with an endless supply of new adventures and experiences (and recall from Chapter 2 that novelty is linked to greater dopamine release in the reward pathway; Menegas et al., 2017). Several genres of online games do not have an end and persist even after the gamer has logged off. Thus, gaming can be a long-term investment spanning many years.

Internet games, such as simulations and MMOs, allow gamers to create virtual representations of themselves in online worlds. Through avatars, characters, and champions, gamers can experiment with different depictions of themselves and explore various aspects of their personalities (Young, 2009). Gamers can choose to portray themselves as a different race, different gender, different physical size, or different species. This online self-representation is important, as researchers have found that greater identification between gamers and their avatars is linked to greater degrees of gaming addiction (Burleigh et al., 2017). Counselors working with clients who game should have a genuine interest in their clients' gaming experience and inquire about the genre of game they play, what they like about that specific genre, the nature of their relationships with other gamers, how they represent themselves virtually, and the nature of their relationship with their avatar. This kind of dialogue can help build rapport (as the counselor shows genuine interest in something important to the client) and can help counselors understand the role of gaming in the client's life.

PREVALENCE OF INTERNET GAMING ADDICTION

Internet gaming addiction is a worldwide phenomenon, and several countries including Thailand, Vietnam, South Korea, and China have enforced regulations to limit gaming (Kiraly et al., 2018). With regard to frequency, researchers reviewed 252 articles examining internet gaming addiction among children and adolescents across the globe and found a median prevalence rate of up to 5.5% (Paulus et al., 2018). Prevalence rates, however, are difficult to obtain due to differences in samples (naturalistic populations versus gamers), geographic locations, and assessment instruments. For example, Mihara and Higuchi (2017) examined 37 research articles pertaining to internet gaming addiction and determined a wide variance of prevalence rates ranging from .7% to 27.5%. Although frequencies vary, reviews of internet gaming literature consistently conclude that gaming addiction rates are higher among males (Paulus et al., 2018) and younger populations (Mihara & Higuchi, 2017). Scholars believe that males are more afflicted with internet gaming addiction due to the fact that internet games often are designed for males (e.g., depicting masculine ideals, sexualization of women, competition) and many game designers are themselves male (Chen et al., 2018; King & Delfabbro, 2018). However, it is important for counselors to recognize that the number of female gamers continues to increase with recent statistics indicating that 46% of all gamers are female (Entertainment Software Association, 2019).

MOTIVES FOR GAMING

There are numerous reasons why individuals use internet games. Many motives are healthy and developmentally appropriate; yet some motives are more directly linked to internet gaming addiction. Possible motives for internet gaming include achievement (i.e., advancing in the game; demonstrating mastery), sociability (i.e., interacting with other gamers), and immersion (i.e., escaping into the game to avoid negative emotional states; Chen et al., 2018; Yee, 2006). While some researchers have found that the motive of immersion was most linked to gaming addiction (Chen et al., 2018; Yee, 2006), others identified achievement as the strongest predictor (Carlisle et al., 2019). Kiraly et al. (2015) seemed to link both motivations to addiction as they found motives of escape and competition to have the largest effect sizes in their relationship with problematic online gaming. Additionally, researchers examining psychiatric distress, gaming motivation, and problem gaming found that the motives to escape (i.e., avoid reality) and fantasy (i.e., take on a new identity) significantly mediated the relationship between psychiatric symptoms and problem gaming (Ballabio et al., 2017). Therefore, it is imperative that counselors explore clients' reasons for gaming. Asking questions such as, "What does gaming do for you?" or "When do you feel the strongest desire to game?" can help counselors and clients identify motives for gaming. Those individuals who turn to gaming as a means of escaping difficult feelings, assuming a new identity, or cultivating a sense of achievement may be more at risk for internet gaming addiction than those who game for other reasons (e.g., socialization, recreation, skill development).

CLINICAL NOTE 3.2

The concept of *teleology* from Adlerian theory posits that all behavior serves a function. How might you conceptualize a female adolescent client who says she games "to support her clan, the only people who really care about her." What might be the function of her gaming? How might you conceptualize a Black college student who says he games so that he can "spend time as his avatar (a mythical creature) who does not have to worry about racism." What might be the function of his gaming?

NEUROSCIENCE RELATED TO INTERNET GAMING ADDICTION

Internet games are designed to be highly rewarding and to keep gamers engaged. With visual stimulation, high graphic resolution, sounds and music, opportunities for team play, social reinforcement, unlimited opportunities for advancement, instant gratification, and a complete immersion experience, gaming can offer more rewards than many offline experiences. Indeed, positron emission tomography (PET) confirms that dopamine (the primary neurotransmitter implicated in desire and reward) is released while gaming (Kuss et al., 2018). Despite the rewarding nature of games, many individuals are able to play without demonstrating the characteristics of addiction. Like other addictive behaviors, it is the interaction between a highly rewarding behavior (e.g., gaming) and a vulnerable individual that contributes to the development of addiction (see the public health model in Chapter 1 describing the roles of agents, hosts, environments, and vectors in the development of addiction; Centers for Disease Control and Prevention, 2012). Indeed, King and Delfabbro (2018) stated, "Some individuals are susceptible—due to factors including psychological predisposition, stress, risky environments, and the availability of gaming opportunities—to developing a habitual and self-destructive pattern of gaming" (p. 2). Thus, it is the rewarding nature of gaming coupled with individual susceptibility that creates the risk of gaming addiction (King & Delfabbro, 2018).

One aspect of internet games that makes them so compelling, particularly among those predisposed to addiction, is the use of *variable ratio reinforcement schedules* (King & Delfabbro, 2018; Kiraly et al., 2018). Unlike fixed reinforcement schedules, in which a reward occurs each time an individual engages in a particular behavior (consider an elementary school student who receives a gold sticker each time they spell a word correctly), variable ratio reinforcement schedules are unpredictable and rewards are dispensed in an irregular fashion (consider playing a slot machine—the player knows a reward will come, but does not know when). The anticipation of irregularly dispensed rewards is a powerful reinforcer and one of the most difficult to extinguish (for more information about operant conditioning and reinforcement schedules, see the work of behaviorist B. F. Skinner [1969, 1976]). Variable ratio reinforcement schedules characterize much of online gaming as particular gaming behaviors are sometimes, but not always, accompanied by rewards. For example, loot boxes (i.e., virtual containers often unlocked with real-world currency) can contain very advantageous virtual items (producing a high degree of reward) or items that are not very valuable. Additionally, the beginning levels of games often can be completed fairly quickly and the gamer experiences the reward of leveling up. Subsequent levels in the game, however, may require long periods of grinding (i.e., performing repetitive behaviors) to complete; thus the reward of leveling up becomes more unpredictable. In sum, the rewards in internet games occur frequently enough to keep the gamer engaged, but not often enough to create a predictable pattern. Game designers utilize variable ratio reinforcement scheduling, the most powerful form of reinforcement, to keep gamers playing in anticipation of the next reward.

With regard to neurobiological studies, internet gaming addiction shares characteristics of both substance use disorders and gambling disorder (Weinstein et al., 2017). Neuroscientific investigations indicate differences in brain structure and neurotransmission among those with internet gaming addiction compared to healthy controls (Kuss et al., 2018). For example, researchers found decreased levels of glutamate, an excitatory neurotransmitter implicated in learning and memory (Simpkins & Simpkins, 2013), among those with internet gaming addiction compared to controls (Paik et al., 2018). Additionally, Yao et al. (2017) found lower gray matter volume in key brain structures related to emotion regulation and decision-making, including the anterior cingulate cortex and dorsolateral prefrontal cortex, among those with internet gaming addiction compared to controls. Moreover, researchers have identified changes in the brain's reward system (specifically, dopamine reductions) among those with internet gaming addiction, indicating that neuroadaptations (i.e., changes in the brain in response to experience) occur in some gamers as the result of excessive gaming (Weinstein et al., 2017). Finally, in a review of neurological literature related to internet gaming addiction, Kuss et al. (2018) summarized that those with internet gaming disorder (IGD) have demonstrated impaired cognitive control, impaired executive functioning, greater impulsivity, poorer emotion regulation, and deficiencies in the reward system in the brain. Therefore, although more research is needed, it is clear that neurobiological differences exist among those with internet gaming addiction.

eSPORTS

In order for counselors to have an accurate conceptualization of clients who game, they must be familiar with competitive electronic gaming or eSports, which continue to increase in popularity. Tournaments between teams of gamers from around the world, often competing in MOBAs (Banyai et al., 2019) or FPS games (King & Delfabbro, 2018), draw thousands of in-person and online viewers. In fact, in 2018, eSports had a global viewership of 395 million people, which is expected to rise to 495 million in 2020 (Newzoo, 2019b). Moreover, in 2019, over 5,000 eSport tournaments were held globally with total prize money exceeding $230 million (eSports Earnings, 2019). Professional gamers reach international stardom, and fans can watch them game via online streaming services such as Twitch and YouTube. Additionally, eSports are becoming institutionalized at the collegiate level as over 170 colleges are members of the National Association of Collegiate Esports (2019) with some offering competitive eSport scholarships. The popularity of eSports and potential aspiration to become a professional gamer can be compelling motivations to game (Banyai et al., 2019). Therefore, it is important for counselors to assess gaming motivations to discern between gaming enthusiasts and those who may have a gaming addiction (King & Delfabbro, 2018). Time spent gaming is not a sufficient determinant of addiction. Instead, clinicians can use the diagnostic criteria and psychometrically strong assessment instruments described in the following to help identify addiction.

HOW DO I IDENTIFY IT?

As evidence of the growing acceptance of internet gaming addiction, the research appendix of the fifth edition of the *Diagnostic and Statistical Manual of Mental Disorders* (5th ed.; *DSM-5*; American Psychiatric Association [APA], 2013) contains proposed criteria for IGD. The proposed diagnosis would be appropriate if five of the following criteria are met within a 12-month period: preoccupation with gaming, withdrawal symptoms when not gaming, tolerance (e.g., increased duration of gaming sessions, gaming more frequently), inability to control gaming, loss of interest in previously enjoyable hobbies or leisure activities, continued gaming despite negative consequences, lying about amount of time spent gaming, gaming to escape dysphoric moods, and risking significant relationships, jobs, or opportunities to game. Additionally, to meet diagnostic criteria, gaming must lead to significant distress or impairment of functioning (e.g., neglecting other responsibilities, personal hygiene, physical health, important relationships; APA, 2013). Note that these criteria reflect the four Cs of addiction (described in Chapter 1): compulsivity, loss of control, continued engagement despite negative consequences, and craving or mental preoccupation.

Although IGD is a condition for further study and not a formal diagnosis in the *DSM-5*, the World Health Organization (WHO; 2018) included gaming disorder in the 11th revision of the *International Classification of Diseases* (*ICD-11*). Listed in the section "Disorders due to Substance Use or Addictive Behaviors," gaming disorder is marked by loss of control over gaming, increased priority given to gaming to the neglect of other interests and activities, continuing to game despite negative consequences, and evidence of impaired functioning in the previous 12 months (WHO, 2018). The proposed (*DSM-5*) and adopted (*ICD-11*) criteria can help clinicians distinguish between social or casual gamers, gaming enthusiasts, professional gamers, and those with an internet gaming addiction.

NEGATIVE CONSEQUENCES OF GAMING ADDICTION

A primary way to identify addiction is to explore whether the behavior persists despite negative consequences; yet what are the potential negative consequences of internet gaming? Given that many online games persist even after the gamer has logged of, there is a constant pull to stay in or return to the virtual world. Addicted gamers often sacrifice sleeping, eating, showering, or other basic health-maintaining behaviors to continue their presence in the game. Thus, negative consequences may include sleep deprivation, poor nutrition, poor hygiene, excessive caffeine intake, isolation, and lack of appropriate physical activity and exercise (Griffiths & Meredith, 2009; King & Delfabbro, 2018; Young, 2009). Additionally, specific physical health concerns resulting from prolonged gaming include ailments of the skin, tendons, and joints in gamers' hands, elbows, wrists, and necks (Griffiths & Meredith, 2009).

Along with the aforementioned issues, researchers have found that those who met the proposed diagnostic criteria for IGD more frequently neglected social contacts (Wartberg et al., 2017). Indeed, Pontes et al. (2019) found a significant, positive correlation between disordered gaming and loneliness. Although many multiplayer games offer opportunities to socialize with other players, virtual contact alone may be insufficient for meeting the gamer's need for attachment and belonging. Additionally, among a sample of adolescents, those who engaged in problematic gaming reported poorer familial relationships and more family conflict (Bonnaire & Phan, 2017). Hence, a negative consequence of internet gaming addiction can be strained familial ties as time spent gaming or mental preoccupation with gaming becomes a point of contention between family members, particularly parents and adolescent gamers. Adults too, however, can sacrifice important family responsibilities (e.g., parenting or spousal roles) in lieu of gaming. In fact, the term "gamer widow" or "cyber widow" reflects a partner's sense of loss as the gamer invests more and more time gaming to the detriment of their relationship (Young, 1998).

Another important potential negative consequence of gaming addiction is financial problems. Through the monetization of gaming, gamers can spend real currency to purchase virtual items to enhance gameplay such as unlocking mystery loot boxes (which may contain items to enhance gaming performance) or buying skins to change the appearance of the gamer's avatar. Moreover, as gameplay becomes more challenging, gamers have the option to purchase in-game rewards that could make their character stronger or help them progress within a particular level. Indeed, the monetization of gaming presents the risk of excessive spending to advance in the game, which could result in financial problems for addicted gamers.

CLINICAL NOTE 3.3

According to a recent survey by Accredited Debt Relief (2020), 89.4% of a sample of MMO gamers spent real currency in online games, averaging $229 per person. Of note, 5.6% of the sample spent more than $1,000 on in-game purchases.

GAMING ADDICTION AND MENTAL HEALTH

Negative consequences related to gaming also include mental health symptomology. Andreassen et al. (2016) found that certain mental health symptoms (e.g., obsessive-compulsive disorder, depression, and attention deficit hyperactive disorder [ADHD]) significantly predicted internet gaming addiction. Additionally, researchers found those with internet gaming addiction had higher levels of depression, anxiety, and alexithymia (difficulty with emotional awareness) than gamers without addiction (Bonnaire & Baptista, 2019). Moreover, a negative consequence of gaming addiction is mood alteration (King & Delfabbro, 2018), which may include extreme anger (known as "gamer rage" or "raging") when a gamer performs poorly in a game.

Cross-sectional designs, however, cannot answer the question: Which came first, the mental health symptom or the problematic behavior? To answer this question, an important longitudinal study was conducted by Gentile et al. (2011) that followed students in Singapore for 2 years to assess mental health and gaming patterns over time. The researchers found that gaming significantly predicted mental health symptoms; specifically, those who became pathological gamers exhibited more depression, anxiety, and social phobia symptomology. Those students who stopped pathological gaming subsequently reported fewer mental health symptoms. Therefore, the researchers concluded that although some individuals may use gaming to cope with preexisting mental health concerns, others experience mental health symptoms as a result of their gaming behavior (Gentile et al., 2011). Continued gaming despite the development of mental health symptomology and other negative consequences can help counselors differentiate between clients with internet gaming addiction and nonaddicted gamers.

HOW DO I ASSESS IT?

Given the prevalence of internet gaming addiction and references in both the *DSM-5* and *ICD-11*, many assessment and screening instruments have been created to assess the disorder. The following are three examples of psychometrically sound measures that may be helpful in your clinical practice.

INTERNET GAMING DISORDER SCALE-SHORT FORM

The authors of the nine-item Internet Gaming Disorder Scale-Short Form (IGDS9-SF; Pontes & Griffiths, 2015) utilized the proposed IGD criteria in the *DSM-5* to assess internet gaming addiction. The IGDS9-SF was tested on a global sample (participants from 58 countries) recruited from 52 online gaming forums. Participants' ages ranged from 16 to 70 with an average age of 27. The majority of participants identified as male (85.1%) and 26.7% disclosed gaming for more than 30 hours per week. The scale demonstrated strong reliability (Cronbach's alpha = .87) and convergent validity. Items assess participants' experiences with gaming over the previous 12 months. Example items include: *Have you lost interest in previous hobbies and other entertainment activities as a result of your engagement with the* game and *Do you play in order to temporarily escape or relieve a negative mood (e.g., helplessness, guilt, anxiety)*. Each of the nine items corresponds with a five-point Likert-type scale ranging from *never* (1) to *very often* (5) with total scores spanning from 9 to 45. To obtain a total score on the IGDS9-SF, individual item scores are summed, with higher total scores reflecting stronger degrees of IGD (Pontes & Griffiths, 2015). Pontes and Griffiths (2015) suggested a potential cutoff score of 36 to reflect IGD, yet encouraged clinicians to use the yes/no format provided by the *DSM-5* (APA, 2013) for diagnostic purposes. The full IGDS9-SF is listed in Table 3 of the Pontes and Griffiths (2015) article and also on the lead author's website (www.halleypontes.com/igds9sf).

THE GAMING DISORDER TEST

The four-item Gaming Disorder Test (GDT; Pontes et al., 2019) was created to assess disordered gaming using the criteria developed by the WHO in the *ICD-11*. Using a British and Chinese sample of college students who gamed in the previous year, the authors found strong reliability (overall Cronbach's alpha: .84), convergent validity, and discriminant validity. Example items include: *I have had difficulties controlling my gaming activity* and *I have continued gaming despite the occurrence of negative consequences*. The four GDT items correspond with five-point Likert-type scales with answer choices ranging from *never* (1) to *very often* (5). Total scores are determined by summing the individual item scores (ranging from 4 to 20). Higher scores indicate more disordered gaming (Pontes et al., 2019). The full GDT scale can be found in the appendix of the Pontes et al. (2019) article and on the lead author's website (www.halleypontes.com/gdt).

MOTIVES FOR ONLINE GAMING QUESTIONNAIRE

Rather than assessing frequency and negative consequences of gaming, Demetrovics et al. (2011) developed the Motives for Online Gaming Questionnaire (MOGQ) to better understand individuals' reasons for gaming. The scale was normed on 3,818 gamers, of which 90.6% were male and had an average age of 20.9 years. The authors developed the 27-item scale assessing seven motivational factors: escape (to avoid offline issues or problems), coping (to improve mood when facing distress), fantasy (to become someone else and engage in new behaviors), skill development (to improve abilities such as coordination, cooperation, and concentration), recreation (for fun and relaxation), competition (to feel a sense of achievement by succeeding and defeating others), and social (forming new relationships and playing with others; Demetrovics et al., 2011). Example items include: *I play online games because it makes me forget real life* and *I play online games because I can get to know new people.* The 27 items correspond to five-point Likert-type scales ranging from *almost never/never* (1) to *almost always/always* (5). Each of the seven subscales has demonstrated adequate internal consistency with Cronbach's alpha scores ranging from .75 to .88 (Ballabio et al., 2017). The full MOGQ and scoring instructions can be found in the appendix of the Demetrovics et al. (2011) original article.

HOW DO I TREAT IT?

IGD can vary on a continuum ranging from mild to severe (APA, 2013); thus, treatment strategies will be contingent upon the client's level of severity. For those with severe internet gaming addiction who have neglected personal hygiene and physical health, and may be exhibiting extreme anger or suicidal ideation in response to gaming cessation or poor performance in the game, counselors must first focus on client health and safety. Clients may be under or over a healthy weight, experiencing depletion of essential vitamins and minerals, and may be struggling with day–night sleep reversal. Working with a primary care physician to perform appropriate physical exams can be a helpful supplemental resource to counseling. Counselors also should anticipate that the client will experience withdrawal symptoms when not gaming, such as cravings to game, irritability, and anxiety (APA, 2013), and therefore work with the client to develop appropriate coping mechanisms to navigate these adverse emotional states. Finally, a suicide assessment is recommended for clients with severe internet gaming addiction as researchers have found higher rates of suicidal ideation among those with internet addiction compared to healthy controls (Cheng et al., 2018).

Given the ubiquitous nature of the internet, counselors and clients will need to develop plans for how the client will interact with technology while abstaining from compulsive internet gaming. Examples of technological plans include clients removing internet capabilities from their phones, using computers only in public spaces, and limiting the amount of time clients are online before logging off and taking a break. Clients with internet gaming addiction typically spend hours gaming each day; thus counselors and clients will need to identify and implement effective replacement activities to help the client reconnect to the offline world. Clients may need help relearning how to engage with peers (i.e., social skills training) as well as how to recognize and respond to their own physical cues (e.g., hunger, tiredness, restlessness, boredom).

As with all addictions, it is important for counselors to recognize that the treatment of one addictive behavior may lead to the development of a new addictive behavior. Indeed, in the study of 144 collegiate gamers, Giordano et al. (2020) found that if gaming was unavailable, 50% of participants indicated being slightly to much more likely to engage in sexual activity, 33.1% indicated being slightly to much more likely to drink alcohol, 11.9% indicated being slightly to much more likely to use illicit substances, 8.3% indicated being slightly to much more likely to gamble/bet, and 5.6% indicated being slightly to much more likely to self-injure. Recall that clients with behavioral addictions often rely on the addictive behaviors to change the way that they feel (e.g., emotion regulation). Therefore, as counselors work with a particular manifestation of addiction, it is important to simultaneously monitor other potentially addictive behaviors that may emerge as a means of regulating emotions.

VOICES FROM THE FIELD: Clinical Work With Internet Gaming Addiction

Working with internet and video game addicts is pioneering work. Digital culture is new territory for many clinicians who did not grow up as digital natives. Getting to understand the life experiences of digital natives requires being open to their experiences and really taking the time to research what clients are doing online. Because so many of them started in early childhood, their developmental trajectories are different from so many other addicts. Coming to understand this well is essential for the work to be successful.

At reSTART, we try to understand the online culture and experiences of our clients and, by putting clients together who share similar experiences, they feel understood and accepted within the therapeutic milieu. Our approach is broad and holistic, meaning that we address not only the addiction and other mental health concerns, but we also are working to improve their physical health, help them with skills that they lack, work to help the whole family system, and support them as they transition into an independent life with balanced technology use.

Behaviors can be just as addictive as ingested chemicals. So many people find it hard to accept that common behaviors, like gaming or other online activities, have the very real potential to devastate a person's life when a person loses control, yet we see it again and again: a life in tatters because of a digital addiction. The young people who come to us have failed out of college, lost jobs, lost relationships, lost health, become violent, stolen, lost thousands of dollars paying for loot boxes, and the list goes on. It is every bit as devastating as a chemical addiction and can even end in death, as we have learned from those who died at their computers after 40+ hours of gaming without a break. Yet, because gaming and internet use are ubiquitous and normal in our culture, this addiction is hard to recognize. Until there is formal, wide recognition by governmental, educational, and medical bodies, this is not likely to change. Our educational system does not do a good job of preparing mental health professionals for work with addictions; so therapists must do their due diligence and learn about it through their own research and training opportunities.

Hilarie Cash, PhD, LMHC, CSAT, WSGC; Founding Member, Chief Clinical Officer, Education Director; reSTART Life, PLLC, restartlife.com

COGNITIVE BEHAVIORAL THERAPY-INTERNET ADDICTION

Young (2011) developed cognitive behavioral therapy-internet addiction (CBT-IA) as a specific way to implement cognitive behavioral techniques when working with clients addicted to the internet (which includes internet gaming addiction). The approach has three phases: behavior modification, cognitive therapy, and harm reduction therapy. Applied to internet gaming specifically, the behavior modification phase consists of helping clients develop new goals to reduce problematic gaming. Clients may track their internet gaming experiences over the course of a week by completing a gaming log and identifying precipitating events, duration of gameplay, and subsequent consequences. Given this information, counselors and clients can begin identifying patterns of problematic gaming, including triggers and negative consequences. In the cognitive therapy phase, counselors help clients identify distorted thoughts that perpetuate their gaming addiction. For example, counselors and clients may identify maladaptive beliefs such as: "I am only worthwhile in the virtual world," "My virtual friends won't betray me, but my offline friends will," "My virtual self is desirable and my offline self is not," and "The virtual world is safe and the offline world is dangerous." Using cognitive techniques, counselors and clients can examine the validity of these thoughts and replace them with more realistic and adaptive beliefs. Finally, in the harm reduction therapy phase, counselors and clients begin to address co-occurring mental health concerns or underlying psychological distress that contribute to internet gaming addiction. Specifically, as the client takes incremental steps toward reducing problematic gaming, the counselor and client can explore and address reasons for disordered gaming, coexisting issues, and work to increase coping and emotion regulation skills. In this phase, the counselor and client identify the purpose of gaming in the client's life and find alternative ways to meet those needs (Young, 2011).

Young (2013) tested the efficacy of CBT-IA on 128 clients meeting criteria for internet addiction (23% identified online gaming as their most problematic online activity). After 12 sessions of CBT-IA, participants showed marked decreases in internet addiction symptomology (including preoccupation, loss of control, using the internet to escape, and concealing internet use). Follow-up testing at 1 month, 3 months, and 6 months demonstrated that 70% of clients maintained their treatment gains over time (Young, 2013).

INTERNET AND VIDEO GAME ADDICTION TREATMENT

Greenfield (2018) described a seven-step treatment approach for addressing internet and video game addiction. Step one is to engage the client in the process by creating a collaborative therapeutic relationship. Counselors can work to understand the client's relationship with gaming from a curious and nonjudgmental posture. Step two entails disrupting the problematic behavior, which may include abstinence from all screens, the internet, and gaming, or substantially limiting the behavior. The cessation of the problematic behavior provides opportunities to establish new, adaptive patterns of behavior as well as new neurological connections. Step three is to identify triggers (e.g., emotional, situational, behavioral) that serve as antecedents to the gaming addiction cycle. During this stage, the counselor and client work to develop trigger management skills to navigate triggers as they emerge. Step four includes managing urges, cravings, and compulsions to use internet games. Psychoeducation about the neurobiology of gaming, cognitive behavioral work, and social reengagement may be effective strategies during this step. Medication, such as bupropion, also may be a helpful adjunct to counseling, particularly for clients with gaming addiction and co-occurring depression (Greenfield, 2018).

Next, step five entails blocking, monitoring, and filtering problematic internet content (Greenfield, 2018). Using information technology support, the counselor and client (and when appropriate, members of the client's family) can discover and employ a variety of technological services to block gaming content and remove gaming applications from the client's devices. It is important to note that when those with gaming addiction are unable to game, they may replace the behavior by watching others game on streaming sites like Twitch and YouTube. Counselors and clients can decide which sites are helpful to the client's recovery and which sites should be blocked. Step six is to implement real-time living strategies (i.e., coping strategies and ways to enhance enjoyment of nongaming, healthy life activities). Counselors and clients can develop a list of numerous alternative behaviors and coping strategies to employ when the client is faced with triggers or cravings to game. Real-time living strategies should be realistic, attainable behaviors to aid in "the redevelopment of naturalistic reward stimulation" (Greenfield, 2018, p. 339) such as engaging with peers, spiritual practices, physical activity, listening to music, artistic projects, contacting a member of one's support system, changing one's environment, or reading. Finally, step seven includes cultivating relapse prevention strategies to help clients plan how to navigate a relapse and resume their recovery plan (e.g., contact their counselor, utilize 12-step support, employ a predetermined coping strategy, engage in in-person activities to increase offline social connectivity). Greenfield (2018) developed these steps after years of clinical work with clients struggling with internet and video game addiction.

12-STEP SUPPORT

In addition to counseling, there are 12-step support programs for internet gaming addiction that may be helpful resources for clients. Computer Gaming Addicts Anonymous (CGAA) is a program modeled after Alcoholics Anonymous that offers community for those who share the desire to stop gaming. Complete with meetings (online and in-person), sponsorship, literature, working the 12 steps (Step one states, "we admitted that we were powerless over gaming addiction, and that our lives had become unmanageable" [CGAA, 2020, The Twelve Steps, para. 4]), and spiritual components, CGAA seeks to help those with internet gaming addiction reach complete abstinence from gaming. CGAA does not provide a formal definition of "gaming" but encourages members to avoid "interactive forms of electronic entertainment" (CGAA, 2020, The Basic Program of Recovery, para. 6) and cautions against watching others game, which can trigger cravings and urges to game. CGAA provides a list of 20 questions to help individuals determine if the program may be a helpful resource for them. Example items include: *Have you ever used sick days or vacation days or skipped work or class just for gaming* and *Do you set rules or limits with gaming and then break them, playing longer or more frequently than intended* (CGAA, 2020, Self Test to Assess Video Game Addiction, para. 2). Endorsing several of these 20 questions indicates a potential gaming addiction. For more information about CGAA, including pamphlets and flyers for mental health professionals, visit cgaa.info.

DIAGNOSTIC CONSIDERATIONS

Gaming disorder is now recognized in the *ICD-11*. Therefore, clinicians who utilize this classification system for diagnostic purposes can apply the appropriate code for clients with internet gaming addiction (WHO, 2018). Counselors who do not use the *ICD-11* often diagnose the co-occurring mental illnesses that may exist with gaming addiction (e.g., depression, generalized anxiety, ADHD, autism spectrum disorder; Andreassen et al., 2016; Gentile et al., 2011). Currently, IGD is a condition warranting further study in the appendix of the *DSM-5*, and, with the proliferation of gaming addiction research, may be included in the *DSM* proper in future editions.

HOW CAN I LEARN MORE?

If you are working with clients with internet gaming addiction or would like to learn more about the condition, consider the following resources.

BOOKS

- King, D., & Delfabbro, P. (2018). *Internet gaming disorder: Theory, assessment, treatment, and prevention.* Elsevier.
- Roberts, K. (2010). *Cyber junkie: Escape the gaming and internet trap.* Hazelden.
- Young, K. (1998). *Caught in the net.* John Wiley & Sons.

PEER-REVIEWED ARTICLES

- Gorman, T. E., Gentile, D. A., & Green, C. S. (2018). Problem gaming: A short primer. *American Journal of Play, 10,* 309–327.
- Greenfield, D. N. (2018). Treatment considerations in internet and video game addiction: A qualitative discussion. *Child and Adolescent Psychiatric Clinics of North America, 27,* 327–344. https://doi.org/10.1016/j.chc.2017.11.007
- Zhang, J., & Brand, M. (Eds.). (2018). Neural mechanisms underlying internet gaming disorder. Frontiers Media. doi:10.3389/978-2-88945-655-0

WEBSITES

- Computer Gaming Addicts Anonymous (CGAA): cgaa.info
- Game Quitters: gamequitters.com
- National Association of Collegiate Esports (NACE): nacesports.org

REFERENCES

Accredited Debt Relief. (2020). *MMO money, MMO problems: The spending habits of online gamers.* https://www.accrediteddebtrelief.com/blog/mmo-money-mmo-problems

American Psychiatric Association. (2013). *Diagnostic and statistical manual of mental disorders* (5th ed.). Author.

Andreassen, C. S., Griffiths, M. D., Kuss, D. J., Mazzoni, E., Billieux, J., Demetrovics, Z., & Pallesen, S. (2016). The relationship between addictive use of social media and video games and symptoms of psychiatric disorders: A large-scale cross-sectional study. *Psychology of Addictive Behaviors, 30,* 252–262. https://doi.org/10.1037/adb0000160

Ballabio, M., Griffiths, M. D., Urban, R., Quartiroli, A., Demetrovics, Z., & Kiraly, O. (2017). Do gaming motives mediate between psychiatric symptoms and problematic gaming? An empirical survey study. *Addiction Research and Theory, 25,* 397–408. https://doi.org/10.1080/16066359.2017.1305360

Banyai, F., Griffiths, M. D., Kiraly, O., & Demetrovics, Z. (2019). The psychology of esports: A systemic literature review. *Journal of Gambling Studies, 35,* 351–365. https://doi.org/10.1007/s10899-018-9763-1

Bonnaire, C., & Baptista, D. (2019). Internet gaming disorder in male and female young adults: The role of alexithymia, depression, anxiety and gaming type. *Psychiatry Research, 272,* 521–530. https://doi.org/10.1016/j.psychres.2018.12.158

Bonnaire, C., & Phan, O. (2017). Relationships between parental attitudes, family functioning, and internet gaming disorder in adolescents attending school. *Psychiatry Research, 255,* 104–110. https://doi.org/10.1016/j.psychres.2017.05.030

Burleigh, T. L., Stavropoulos, V., Liew, L. W. L., Adams, B. L. M., & Griffiths, M. D. (2017). Depression, internet gaming disorder, and the moderating effect of the gamer-avatar relationship: An exploratory longitudinal study. *International Journal of Mental Health and Addiction, 16,* 102–124. https://doi.org/10.1007/s11469-017-9806-3

Carlisle, K. L., Neukrug, E., Pribesh, S., & Krahwinkel, J. (2019). Personality, motivation, and internet gaming disorder: Conceptualizing the gamer. *Journal of Addiction and Offender Counseling, 40,* 107–122. https://doi.org/10.1002/jaoc.12069

Centers for Disease Control and Prevention. (2012). *Principles of epidemiology in public health practice* (3rd ed.). Author.

Chen, K. H., Oliffe, J. L., & Kelly, M. T. (2018). Internet gaming disorder: An emergent health issue for men. *American Journal of Men's Health, 12,* 1151–1159. https://doi.org/10.1177/1557988318766950

Cheng, Y. S., Tseng, P. T., Lin, P. Y., Chen, T. Y., Stubbs, B., Carvalho, A. F., Wu, C. K., Chen, Y. W., & Wu, M. K. (2018). Internet addiction and its relationship with suicidal behaviors: A meta-analysis of multinational observational studies. *Journal of Clinical Psychiatry, 79,* e1–e15. https://doi.org/10.4088/JCP.17r11761

Computer Gaming Addicts Anonymous. (2020). *The basic program of recovery.* https://cgaa.info

Demetrovics, Z., Urban, R., Nagygyorgy, K., Farkas, J., Zilahy, D., Mervo, B., Reindl, A., Ágoston, C., Kertész, A., & Harmath, E. (2011). Why do you play? The development of the motives for online gaming questionnaire (MOGQ). *Behavior Research Methods, 43,* 814–825. https://doi.org/10.3758/s13428-011-0091-y

Entertainment Software Association. (2019). *2019 Essential facts about the computer and video game industry.* https://www.theesa.com/wp-content/uploads/2019/05/2019-Essential-Facts-About-the-Computer-and-Video-Game-Industry.pdf

eSports Earnings. (2019). *Overall eSports stats for 2019.* https://www.esportsearnings.com/history/2019/top_players

Gentile, D. A., Choo, H., Liau, A., Sim, T., Li, D., Fung, D., & Khoo, A. (2011). Pathological video game use among youths: A two-year longitudinal study. *Pediatrics, 127,* e319–e329. https://doi.org/10.1542/peds.2010-1353

Giordano, A. L., Prosek, E. A., Bain, C., Malacara, A., Turner, J., Schunemann, K., & Schmit, M. K. (2020). Withdrawal symptoms among American collegiate internet gamers. *Journal of Mental Health Counseling, 42,* 63–77. https://doi.org/10.17744/mehc.42.1.05

Gorman, T. E., Gentile, D. A., & Green, C. S. (2018). Problem gaming: A short primer. *American Journal of Play, 10,* 309–327.

Greenfield, D. N. (2018). Treatment considerations in internet and video game addiction: A qualitative discussion. *Child and Adolescent Psychiatric Clinics of North America, 27,* 327–344. https://doi.org/10.1016/j.chc.2017.11.007

Griffiths, M. D., & Meredith, A. (2009). Video-game addiction and its treatment. *Journal of Contemporary Psychotherapy, 39,* 247–253. https://doi.org/10.1007/s10879-009-9118-4

King, D., & Delfabbro, P. (2018). *Internet gaming disorder: Theory, assessment, treatment, and prevention.* Elsevier.

Kiraly, O., Griffiths, M. D., King, D. L., Lee, H., Lee, S., Banyai, F., Zsila, A., Takacas, Z. K., & Demetronics, Z. (2018). Policy responses to problematic video game use: A systematic review of current measures and future possibilities. *Journal of Behavioral Addictions, 7,* 503–517. https://doi.org/10.1556/2006.6.2017.050

Kiraly, O., Griffiths, M. D., Urban, R., Farkas, J., Kokonyei, G., Elekes, Z., Tamás, D., & Demetrovics, Z. (2014). Problematic internet use and problematic online gaming are not the same: Findings from a large nationally representative adoeslcent sample. *Cyberpsychology, Behavior, and Social Networking, 17,* 749–754. https://doi.org/10.1089/cyber.2014.0475

Kiraly, O., Urban, R., Griffiths, M. D., Agoston, C., Nagygyorgy, K., Kokonyei, G., & Demetrovics, Z. (2015). The mediating effect of gaming motivation between psychiatric symptoms and problematic online gaming: An online survey. *Journal of Medical Internet Research, 17,* e88. https://doi.org/10.2196/jmir.3515

Kuss, D. J., Pontes, H. M., & Griffiths, M. D. (2018). Neurobiological correlates in Internet Gaming Disorder: A systematic literature review. *Frontiers in Psychiatry, 9,* 166. https://doi.org/10.3389/fpsyt.2018.00166

Macey, J., & Hamari, J. (2019). eSports, Skins, and loot boxes: Participants, practices, and problematic behavior associated with emergent forms of gambling. *New Media and Society, 21,* 20–41. https://doi.org/10.1177/1461444818786216

Martoncik, M., & Loksa, J. (2016). Do World of Warcraft (MMORPG) players experience less loneliness and social anxiety in online world (virtual environment) than in real world (offline)? *Computers in Human Behavior, 56,* 127–134. https://doi.org/10.1016/j.chb.2015.11.035

Menegas, W., Babayan, B. M., Uchida, N., & Watabe-Uchida, M. (2017). Opposite initialization to novel cues in dopamine signaling in ventral and posterior striatum in mice. *eLife, 6,* e21886. https://doi.org/10.7554/eLife.21886

Mihara, S., & Higuchi, S. (2017). Cross sectional and longitudinal epidemiological studies of internet gaming disorder: A systematic review of the literature. *Psychiatry and Clinical Neurosciences, 71,* 425–444. https://doi.org/10.1111/pcn.12532

National Association of Collegiate Esports. (2019). *What is NACE?* https://nacesports.org/about

Newzoo. (2019a). *Global games market report.* https://newzoo.com/solutions/standard/market-forecasts/global-games-market-report

Newzoo. (2019b). *Esports audience growth.* https://newzoo.com/key-numbers

Paik, S., Choi, M. R., Kwak, S. M., Bang, S. H., & Kim, D. (2018). Decreased serum glutamate levels in male adults with internet gaming disorder: A pilot study. *Clinical Psychopharmacology and Neuroscience, 16,* 276–281. https://doi.org/10.9758/cpn.2018.16.3.276

Paulus, F. W., Ohmann, S., Von Gontard, A., & Popow, C. (2018). Internet gaming disorder in children and adolescents: A systematic review. *Developmental Medicine and Child Neurology, 60,* 645–659. https://doi.org/10.111/dmcn.13754

Pontes, H. M., & Griffiths, M. D. (2015). Measuring DSM-5 internet gaming disorder: Development and validation of a short psychometric scale. *Computers in Human Behavior, 45*, 137–143. https://doi.org/10.1016/j.chb.2014.12.006

Pontes, H. M., Schivinski, B., Sindermann, C., Li, M., Becker, B., Zhou, M., & Montag, C. (2019). Measurement and conceptualization of gaming disorder according to the World Health Organization framework: The development of the gaming disorder test. *International Journal of Mental Health and Addiction*. http://dx.doi.org/10.1007/s11469-019-00088-z

Sanchez, J. (2009). A social history of virtual worlds. *Library Technology Reports, 45*, 9–12.

Saunders, J. B., Hao, W., Long, J., King, D. L., Mann, K., Fauth-Buhler, M., Rumpf, H. J., Bowden-Jones, H., Rahimi-Movaghar, A., Chung, T., Chan, E., Bahar, N., Achab, S., Lee, H. K., Potenza, M., Petry, N., Spritzer, D., Ambekar, A., Derevensky, J., . . . Poznyak, V. (2017). Gaming disorder: Its delineation as an important condition for diagnosis, management, and prevention. *Journal of Behavioral Addictions, 6*, 271–279. https://doi.org/10.1556/2006.6.2017.0039

Simpkins, C. A., & Simpkins, A. M. (2013). *Neuroscience for clinicians: Evidence, models, and practice*. Springer Publishing.

Skinner, B. F. (1969). *Contingencies of reinforcement: A theoretical analysis*. Meredith Corporation.

Skinner, B. F. (1976). *About behaviorism*. Vintage Books.

Sourmelis, T., Ioannou, A., & Zaphiris, P. (2017). Massively Multiplayer Online Role Playing Games (MMORPGs) and the 21st century skills: A comprehensive research review from 2010 to 2016. *Computers in Human Behavior, 67*, 41–48. https://doi.org/10.1016/j.chb.2016.10.020

Wartberg, L., Kriston, L., & Thomasius, R. (2017). The prevalence and psychosocial correlates of Internet Gaming Disorder: Analysis in a nationally representative sample of 12 to 25 year olds. *Deutsches Aerzreblatt International, 114*, 419–424. https://doi.org/10.3239/arztebl.2017.0419

Weinstein, A., Livny, A., & Weizman, A. (2017). New developments in brain research of internet and gaming disorder. *Neuroscience and biobehavioral review, 75*, 314–330. https://doi.org/10.1016/j.neurobiorev.2017.01.040

World Health Organization. (2018). *International statistical classification of diseases and related health problems* (11th Rev.). https://icd.who.int/browse11/l-m/en

Yao, Y., Liu, L., Ma, S., Shi, X., Zhou, N., Zhang, J., & Polenza, M. N. (2017). Functional and structural neural alterations in internet gaming disorder: A systematic review and meta analysis. *Neuroscience & Biobehavioral Reviews, 83*, 313–324. https://doi.org/10.1016/j.neubiorev.2017.10.029

Yee, N. (2006). Motivations for play in online games. *Cyber Psychology and Behavior, 9*, 772–775. https://doi.org/10.1089/cpb.2006.9.772

Young, K. (1998). *Caught in the net*. John Wiley & Sons.

Young, K. (2009). Understanding online gaming addiction and treatment issues for adolescence. *The American Journal of Family Therapy, 37*, 355–372. https://doi.org/10.1080/01926180902942191

Young, K. S. (2011). CBT-IA: The first treatment model for internet addiction. *Journal of Cognitive Psychotherapy, 25*, 304–312. https://doi.org/10.1891/0889-8391.25.4.304

Young, K. S. (2013). Treatment outcomes using CBT-IA with internet-addicted patients. *Journal of Behavioral Addictions, 2*, 209–215. https://doi.org/10.1556/JBA.2.2013.4.3

4

Social Media Addiction

HOW DO I CONCEPTUALIZE IT?

The internet has become an indispensable component of social functioning. Reconnecting with old friends, staying connected with current friends, and developing new relationships can all occur online, particularly via social media platforms. Social media is a broad term referring to applications that allow user generated content to be shared with others in a virtual space (Kuss & Griffiths, 2017). Therefore, social media includes video sharing (e.g., TikTok, YouTube), photo or image sharing (e.g., Snapchat, Instagram, Facebook), message sharing (e.g., WhatsApp, Twitter), bookmarking (e.g., Pinterest, Reddit), blogs (e.g., WordPress), dating apps (e.g., Hinge, Tinder), chatrooms (e.g., Chatous), discussion boards and forums (e.g., Quora, Reddit), and comments related to online content (e.g., news, stories). Social networking is a specific type of social media that allows for the creation of user profiles connected to a network of social contacts (Kuss & Griffiths, 2017). Some of the current popular social networking sites include LinkedIn (established in 2002), Facebook (established in 2004), Twitter (established in 2006), Instagram (established in 2010), Snapchat (established in 2011), and TikTok (established in 2017). Social networking sites allow for the dissemination of text, images, and videos to the virtual world, yet this is only part of the appeal. One of the most addictive features of social networking is the *feedback* component. Once content is posted, social media users await feedback from the online community in the form of likes, retweets, shares, and comments. The process of uploading content and receiving immediate social feedback through a variety of metrics can be extremely rewarding. Indeed, Alter (2017) wrote, "Instagram is addictive, for example, because some photos attract many likes, while others fall short. Users chase the next big hit of likes by posting one photo after another" (p. 9). Thus, the feedback features on social media platforms create a drive for achieving positive social reinforcement, which, for some users, can lead to addictive behavior.

Another potentially addictive feature of social media is the fact that, unlike reading a book or watching a movie, there is no natural stopping point. Users can spend hours scrolling content without reaching an end. Social media is marked by continuous novelty, as there is always another tweet to read, video to watch, or profile to explore. Moreover, social media is available anywhere with internet access; thus in technologically advanced (i.e., wired) countries, social media is easily accessible, free to use, and can provide unlimited distractions from one's present reality. Many individuals use social media without experiencing problems, yet for a small percentage of users, social media use becomes compulsive, they lose control over their use, they continue to use social media despite negative consequences, and they crave social media or are mentally preoccupied with it when they are not using it. Taken together, using social media can be a beneficial, rewarding behavior, yet it also has the potential to be addictive for vulnerable individuals.

CLINICAL NOTE 4.1

Consider your own experience with social media (or, if you do not use social media, the experiences you have heard from close friends or family members). In your opinion, what are the most appealing or rewarding features? What keeps you (or your close friends and family members) using social media?

SMARTPHONE ADDICTION VERSUS SOCIAL MEDIA ADDICTION

The introduction of the smartphone in the early 1990s dramatically changed the world's relationship with technology. Suddenly, people did not need to use computers to access the internet, but instead, could carry the internet with them in their pockets or purses. Unlimited, easy access to the internet via smartphones has made the devices all but indispensable in today's society. In fact, the public's reliance on smartphones has become so strong that a new condition, coined *nomophobia* (derived from "no mobile phone phobia"), was proposed for consideration in the fifth edition of the *Diagnostic and Statistical Manual of Mental Disorders* (5th ed.; *DSM-5*; American Psychiatric Association [APA], 2013; Bragazzi & Del Puente, 2014). Although not included in the *DSM-5*, nomophobia denotes the fear of being without one's smartphone. It was proposed that those with nomophobia experience extreme distress when they do not have access to their smartphones and are disconnected from the online world (King et al., 2010). Nomophobia can lead to anxiety, panic attacks, and impaired functioning when the smartphone is inaccessible and individuals may hear or feel phantom sounds or vibrations, even when their smartphones are not present (Bragazzi & Del Puente, 2014; King et al., 2010).

In contrast to focusing on the captivating nature of the smartphone itself, scholars began investigating specific smartphone activities and applications that can lead to pathological or addictive use. Given that smartphones have the basic capabilities of computers, it is a medium for many potentially addictive online behaviors such as shopping, gambling, gaming, cybersex, and social media use. In light of these diverse activities, researchers proposed that it is more helpful to explore the nature of the addictive content itself, rather than focus on the mobile device. Indeed, Kuss and Griffiths (2017) wrote, "It could be argued that mobile phone addicts are no more addicted to their phones than alcoholics are addicted to bottles" (p. 8). Thus, when a client presents with excessive smartphone use, counselors should explore the function of their use and identify those aspects that are compulsive, difficult to control, create negative consequences, and produce cravings. The remainder of this chapter focuses on the experience of individuals who display addictive behaviors related specifically to social media use, via smartphones or other electronic devices.

MOTIVES FOR SOCIAL MEDIA USE

Andreassen and Pallesen (2014) described social media addiction as being preoccupied or deeply concerned with social networking activity, experiencing strong urges to use social networking sites and applications, spending time and energy on social media to the detriment of offline activities and relationships, and trying unsuccessfully to control or cut back use. As we seek to understand this behavioral addiction, it is important to examine individuals' motives for using social media. Nadkarni and Hofmann (2012) reviewed 42 studies examining psychological factors influencing Facebook use. The scholars concluded that Facebook use was primarily motivated by two needs: (a) the need to belong (i.e., obtain acceptance and social connection) and (b) the need for self-presentation (i.e., impression management). Thus, Facebook users often seek belonging through virtual connections and attempt to project their ideal self-image via their user profile (Nadkarni & Hofmann, 2012). It is important to note that although social media users may be striving for belonging, the virtual realm may not be an effective means of meeting that need. Indeed, Savci and Aysan (2017) found that social media addiction was associated with decreased social connectedness among adolescents. Moreover, in their discussion of limbic resonance (i.e., the experience in which the neuronal patterns of two human beings become synchronized when they are attuned to one another), Lewis et al. (2001) reported that the internet is a poor substitute for in-person and face-to-face connections. Thus, evidence suggests that online, virtual connections may not be as fulfilling as offline relationships.

In addition to the aforementioned motives, those diagnosed with social media addiction are driven by the desire for mood modification. Social media use can produce euphoric feelings as users receive positive feedback from their peers and the online community. Escaping one's daily stressors by getting lost in newsfeeds, forums, anonymous chats, and Instagram stories can be a powerful form of regulating one's emotions. In fact, there is some evidence to suggest that those with poor emotion regulation skills may be at higher risk of developing an addiction to social media. Hormes et al. (2014) studied undergraduates with Facebook profiles and found that those who met criteria for Facebook addiction experienced significantly more difficulty regulating their emotions. Furthermore, among social media users, those with lower levels of emotional intelligence had higher problematic social media use (Sural et al., 2019). Therefore, social media use could be a means of coping with negative emotions among those with less developed emotion regulation skills or lower levels of emotional intelligence.

Finally, research indicates that social media addiction may be motivated by the desire to experience immediate gratification. Turel et al. (2018) examined 33 adult Facebook users and found that Facebook addiction was associated with greater delay discounting, or the preference for small immediate rewards over larger delayed awards. Like other addictions, those with Facebook addiction demonstrated greater impulsivity (Turel et al., 2018). Thus, the motive to experience immediate gratification on social media by receiving likes or positive comments may outweigh motives to pursue larger, future rewards such as cultivating strong, offline relationships. In sum, it is important for counselors to explore the reasons why their clients use social media and their clients' perceived benefits of social media use. Understanding the function of the compulsive behavior can help counselors identify clients' unmet needs and work to find alternative, more adaptive, strategies to meet those needs.

PREVALENCE OF SOCIAL MEDIA ADDICTION

According to the Pew Research Center, 69% of American adults use Facebook and 51% report checking Facebook several times per day (Perrin & Anderson, 2019). Among adolescents, 85% use YouTube, 72% use Instagram, 69% use Snapchat, 51% use Facebook, and 32% use Twitter (Anderson & Jiang, 2018). The median age of first social media use is 14 years old, with 28% of adolescents using social media before turning 13 (Rideout & Robb, 2019). Interestingly, 24% of adolescents reported that social media has a mostly negative effect on their lives, citing reasons such as bullying, spreading rumors, creating unrealistic perceptions of others' experiences, distractions, and mental health symptomology (Anderson & Jiang, 2018).

CLINICAL NOTE 4.2

In a recent study of 440 adolescents, researchers found that participants used social media for a median of 6 hours per day (Watson et al., 2020). The most preferred social media platform among participants was Snapchat (35.2% of the sample reported using it the most), followed by Instagram (24.9%), Facebook (17.5%), Twitter (8.4%), Pinterest (3.4%), Tumblr (3.2%), Musical.ly (1.6%), and WhatsApp (1.4%). Only 3.4% of the adolescent sample reported not using social media (Watson et al., 2020).

The frequency of social media addiction varies across the globe. Hou et al. (2019) found that 14.7% of a sample of college students in China met criteria for social media addiction. Among a national sample of Hungarian adolescents, researchers classified 4.5% as problematic social media users (Banyai et al., 2017). In the United States, researchers modified the criteria for alcohol dependence and found that 9.7% of undergraduates demonstrated social networking dependence (Hormes et al., 2014). Many researchers confirm that women experience higher rates of social media addiction than men (Andreassen et al., 2017; Banyai et al., 2017; He et al., 2017), yet counselors should be aware that men also experience social media addiction. Without an official diagnosis and universally accepted criteria, it is difficult to ascertain exact prevalence rates of social media addiction.

NEUROSCIENCE OF SOCIAL MEDIA ADDICTION

Researchers have found neurobiological similarities between individuals with social media addiction and other forms of addiction (Turel et al., 2018). For example, in the study of Facebook users, researchers found that higher social media addiction scores were associated with less gray matter volume in the amygdala (He et al., 2017). This reduction in amygdala gray matter is found among individuals with other forms of addiction and is indicative of neural pruning (i.e., the removal of unused neural connections to increase the brain's efficiency), creating strong associations between environmental cues (e.g., a social media notification) and the reward system (He et al., 2017). The amygdala is responsible for learning what environmental stimuli lead to both positive and negative responses by storing emotional memories (e.g., happiness associated with a friend request on social media; Simpkins & Simpkins, 2013), and individuals are motivated to seek cues and stimuli associated with rewards (Arias-Carrion et al., 2010). Learned associations between environmental stimuli and rewards occur through the process of *conditioning*.

Behaviorist B. F. Skinner (1976) introduced the idea of operant conditioning, which posits that reinforced behavior gets repeated. Reinforcements are rewards; actions, objects, or internal states to which an individual assigns positive value (Shultz et al., 1997). If a particular behavior is followed by a reward, it increases the probability that an individual will repeat the action. For example, if you praise a client for engaging in a desired behavior (e.g., driving from one destination to another without checking social media), your praise serves to reinforce the behavior, thereby increasing the probability that the client will repeat it (of course, a counselor's praise cannot be the only reinforcement for a client's desirable behavior and part of behavioral counseling is increasing positive reinforcements within the client's environment).

It is important to note that rewards can occur on different schedules. *Fixed ratio schedules* refer to rewards that accompany a behavior after a certain number of repetitions (Skinner, 1969). Consider giving a woman a voucher for food and hygiene products after three negative drug tests (thus, the reinforcement occurs after every third response). Fixed ratio schedules are predictable because the reward follows a set number of responses held constant over time. This reinforcement schedule leads to steady engagement in the behavior, yet over time, the excitement of receiving the reward may diminish due to predictability. *Variable ratio reinforcement schedules*, however, refer to instances in which a behavior is reinforced in an unpredictable manner (Skinner, 1969, 1976). Gambling is the best example of a variable ratio reinforcement schedule (see Chapter 8); gamblers know a reward is coming (the percentage of a slot machine's payouts are regulated), but they do not know how many times they must engage in the behavior (i.e., press the button on the electronic gambling machine) to get the reward. Without a set pattern or predictability, individuals continue to engage in the behavior in anticipation of the reward. Variable ratio reinforcement schedules are powerful, and the associated behaviors often are the most difficult to extinguish (Greenfield, 2011; Skinner, 1969).

So, what does all of this have to do with social media addiction? Social media applications operate on variable ratio reinforcement schedules. Social rewards (e.g., a new friend request, a like, a positive comment, a message from an exciting person; Sherman et al., 2018) can be reinforcing, just like primitive rewards (e.g., food, sex) and activate the same neural circuitry in the brain (Platt et al., 2010). The schedule of these rewards on social media is unpredictable (i.e., variable ratio), thus driving users to check the sites or applications again and again for possible notifications of rewards.

Researchers have found that when individuals receive a notification of a like on social media (or another form of positive social feedback), the reward circuitry of the brain is stimulated (Sherman et al., 2016). One of the primary neurotransmitters implicated in the brain's reward system is dopamine, which is theorized to be responsible for the "wanting" aspect of reward (Berridge & Robinson, 2016). Specifically, dopamine release affects motivation and goal-directedness as the brain learns what stimuli elicit dopaminergic responses. At first, dopamine is released upon the delivery of a reward (e.g., reading a positive comment on a Facebook status), but as learning (i.e., conditioning) transpires and the brain recognizes predictive cues (like a notification symbol), dopamine is released upon *seeing the cue*, rather than receiving the reward itself (Shultz et al., 1997). The size of the dopaminergic release in response to a cue is contingent upon the salience of the reward and the probability of receiving the reward (Platt et al., 2010). Therefore, every time an individual sees a symbol (or hears a sound) associated with a social media notification, the reward pathway is activated in anticipation of the potential reward, stimulating desire, "wanting," and motivation. The activation of reward circuitry in response to social media use can lead to compulsive, out-of-control behavior for susceptible individuals (see Chapter 2). Indeed, Greenfield (2011) wrote, "In essence, what we become addicted to is the intermittent and unpredictable flooding of dopamine that becomes classically associated with the substance or behavior being utilized" (p. 136).

An important component of treatment for social media addiction, therefore, is psychoeducation. It is imperative for counselors to provide information related to the role of reward circuitry in compulsive social media use and aspects of social media that trigger dopaminergic responses (e.g., notifications). With this knowledge, clients can feel empowered as they begin to understand the neurobiological processes of social media addiction and make intentional choices about their use (rather than being driven by internal cravings and the possibility of rewards).

FEAR OF MISSING OUT

Given that social media content is constantly updating, coupled with the emerging cultural expectation that individuals should always be available online (Kuss & Griffiths, 2017), social media users feel pressured to frequently check social media to avoid missing something important. Particularly among those who seek to meet their needs for belonging via social media, the risk of missing a gratifying experience creates a very real form of anxiety. Thus, some social media users experience a *fear of missing out* (FoMO), when they do not have access to the internet (Przybylski et al., 2013). FoMO is a feeling of anxiety predicated on the thought that others may be engaging in pleasurable activities in which an individual is not included (Przybylski et al., 2013).

The construct of FoMO has been linked to many undesirable consequences such as decreased life satisfaction and general mood, increased propensity to use Facebook during university lectures, and greater attention to one's mobile phone (e.g., email, texting, social media) while driving (Przybylski et al., 2013). Researchers also have found a direct link between social media addiction and FoMO. Specifically, among more than 500 social networking site users, researchers found that FoMO was the strongest predictor of social networking addiction among other variables (Pontes et al., 2018).

Moreover, FoMO significantly predicted increased Facebook engagement among adults in Great Britain (Przybylski et al., 2013). Finally, among 1,468 adolescents from Latin American countries, researchers found that FoMO, depression, and social network intensity had direct effects on negative consequences of social media use via mobile devices (Oberst et al., 2017). Therefore, it is clear that FoMO is linked to both social media addiction and negative consequences stemming from social media use.

Exploring clients' FoMO, or anxiety related to being left out of social experiences, can help counselors understand their clients' cognitions associated with compulsive social media use. For example, consider clinical work with an adolescent female who has experienced substantial negative consequences related to social media addiction (e.g., diminished academic performance, conflict with parents, decreased sleep quality, and a car accident caused by checking social media while driving). When assessing cognitions that precipitate social media use, the client discloses the thoughts: "I need to know what others are doing so I can be a part of it," "Everyone is having fun without me," and "I don't want to be abandoned." Further exploration reveals that these thoughts are underlain by the client's fear of not being included and thereby losing her social capital among her peers. Given the importance of peer relationships during adolescence, these cognitions are understandable. The counselor and client can begin exploring the validity of these thoughts and examine alternative, adaptive beliefs related to the client's inherent worth and the nature of healthy peer relationships. Replacing thoughts that lead to FoMO with thoughts that lead to self-acceptance can be a helpful therapeutic approach for clients with social media addiction.

CYBERBULLYING

An important consideration in the conceptualization of clients with social media addiction is *cyberbullying*. The term cyberbullying refers to harmful acts committed against others using technology (Bauman, 2011). Cyberbullying can include flaming (angry personal attacks), harassment (culturally influenced hostility), denigration (demeaning or defaming another), masquerading (pretending to be another person), outing and trickery (sharing confidential information), social exclusion (intentionally leaving someone out), and cyberstalking (threatening and terrorizing another; Bauman, 2011). Cyberbullying is prevalent, as researchers have found that 19% of adolescents experienced cyberbullying in the previous year (Sampasa-Kanyinga & Hamilton, 2015). Furthermore, among a sample of middle school students who had been cyberbullied, 46% experienced cyberbullying on social networking sites (Holfeld & Grabe, 2012). A meta-analysis of cyberbullying research studies concluded that engaging in bullying offline strongly predicted cyberbullying perpetration (Guo, 2016). Moreover, being victimized offline strongly predicted cyberbullying victimization (Guo, 2016). Therefore, in many ways, cyberbullying is an extension of offline bullying, but with several important distinctions. Cyberbullying perpetration requires access to and familiarity with technology, it can be anonymous (thus decreasing the risk of experiencing consequences), it does not allow the perpetrator to witness the immediate reaction of the victim (thus decreasing opportunities for empathic responses or remorse), it can occur anytime and anywhere, and the cyberbullying acts are observed by a wide and virtual audience (Li et al., 2012).

Researchers have found that increased frequencies of online activity correlate with both cyberbullying perpetration and victimization (Guo, 2016). Specifically, Sampasa-Kanyinga and Hamilton (2015) found those who used social media had greater odds of cyberbullying victimization. Additionally, Giordano et al. (2021) found that higher social media addiction scores significantly predicted increased cyberbullying perpetration. It is possible that individuals who compulsively use social media may adopt the social norms of online environments, which may be more aggressive than offline environments (Rost et al., 2016). Thus, when working with clients who report symptoms of social media addiction, it is important for counselors to explore clients' experience with both cyberbullying perpetration and victimization.

HOW DO I IDENTIFY IT?

Social media addiction is not currently represented in the *DSM-5* (APA, 2013) or the *International Classification of Diseases*, 11th Revision (*ICD-11;* World Health Organization [WHO], 2018). Therefore, no accepted, uniform diagnostic criteria exist. Young (1998a), however, proposed diagnostic criteria for internet addiction (which includes social media addiction) that could be helpful when working with clients who have lost control over their social media use. Young (1998a) adapted the diagnostic criteria for pathological gambling by applying them to internet use. The eight criteria are: (a) demonstrating preoccupation with the internet; (b) using the internet for longer amounts of time to achieve satisfaction; (c) unsuccessful attempts to control or cut back internet use; (d) experiencing withdrawal symptoms when the internet cannot be accessed (e.g., restlessness, depression, irritability); (e) using the internet longer than intended; (f) jeopardized relationships, educational pursuits, or career opportunities due to internet use; (g) deceiving others about amount of time spent online; and (h) using the internet to escape dysphoric moods or problems in life. According to Young (1998a), endorsing five or more criteria is indicative of internet addiction, of which social media addiction is a subcategory.

Rather than internet addiction that can occur on any device, Lin et al. (2016) developed criteria specifically for smartphone addiction. Using the criteria for both internet addiction and internet gaming addiction, the scholars proposed three diagnostic categories for smartphone addiction. Criterion A consists of six symptoms, of which an individual must endorse at least three within the same 3-month period: (a) repeated failure to resist the urge to use a smartphone, (b) withdrawal symptoms when not using a smartphone (e.g., irritability, dysphoria, anxiety), (c) use of a smartphone for longer than intended, (d) unsuccessful attempts to cut down smartphone use, (e) excessive time spent using or attempting to quit using a smartphone, and (f) continued smartphone use despite problems. Criterion B describes functional impairment with four symptoms, of which an individual must endorse at least two: (a) persistent or recurrent problems from smartphone use (physical or psychological); (b) using a smartphone in hazardous situations (e.g., crossing the street, while driving); (c) experiencing impairments in relationships, academic pursuits, or job performance due to smartphone use; and (d) experiencing subjective distress from smartphone use or use is time-consuming. Criterion C excludes a diagnosis for smartphone addiction if the symptoms are better accounted for by obsessive-compulsive disorder or bipolar 1 disorder (Lin et al., 2016). Although these two sets of criteria (internet addiction and smartphone addiction) have not been officially endorsed by the APA or WHO, they may provide a helpful starting place for counselors as they explore social media addiction among clients.

NEGATIVE CONSEQUENCES OF SOCIAL MEDIA ADDICTION

Another way to identify addictive behavior is to assess associated negative consequences. There are many ways in which compulsive social media use can lead to negative outcomes. Social media sites have no end, meaning scrolling through stories, images, and comments could go on indefinitely. The time spent on social media, or thinking about social media, is time not invested in other activities such as work (in fact, "cyberloafing" refers to using social media during work hours for nonwork-related purposes), academic pursuits, face-to-face interactions with family members or peers, and other offline responsibilities. Thus, social media addiction can lead to decreased academic and work performance as well as family conflict and deteriorating offline relationships (Andreassen & Pallesen, 2014).

Additionally, it has been proposed that social media addiction can negatively impact an individual's sleep cycle by affecting melatonin levels via blue light emission from smartphone screens and exposure to electromagnetic fields (Alter, 2017; Heo et al., 2017; Jiaxin et al., 2019), yet results from empirical studies on this topic are mixed (Singh & Pati, 2016). To assess the relationship between smartphone use and sleep, researchers conducted a meta-analysis of 14 articles with participants from six different countries. The results of the meta-analysis indicated that problematic smartphone use was significantly associated with poor sleep quality, as well as depression and anxiety. The majority of studies in the meta-analysis were cross-sectional, however, so implications regarding the cause of sleep disturbances cannot be determined (Jiaxin et al., 2019). Interestingly, many smartphones now offer a night shift function, which changes the light spectrum of the screen from blue light (which denotes daytime) to warmer colors (reflective of nighttime). Thus, in light of the potential association with sleep disturbance (from blue light emission, exposure to low-frequency electromagnetic field, or scrolling social media content instead of sleeping), clients with an addiction to social media may experience the detrimental effects of insufficient or disrupted sleep.

Finally, social media addiction has negative psychological impacts. Researchers found that adolescents with social media addiction disclosed lower self-esteem and higher depressive symptoms compared to those without addiction (Banyai et al., 2017). Additionally, in a longitudinal study of adolescents conducted over a 2-year period, researchers found that increases in social media use significantly predicted increases in depression (Raudsepp, 2019). Moreover, Andreassen et al. (2017) found that social media addiction was related to higher levels of narcissism and lower levels of self-esteem. In light of these findings, counselors should consider the potential impact of social media use on clients' views of themselves. Social media users work hard to present the best aspects of themselves and portray only the happiest moments of their lives online. The use of filters and photoshop applications can remove undesirable physical features and enhance desirable traits in images shared on social media. Typing one's thoughts and comments (rather than speaking) allows time to choose the perfect words and create the wittiest or most intelligent messages. Therefore, clients who use social media are constantly bombarded with other users' enhanced and edited realities, which they then compare to their own imperfect lives. This frequent comparison can lead to feelings of inadequacy, diminished self-esteem, envy, and self-doubt.

CLINICAL NOTE 4.3

Among a sample of collegiate female social media users, researchers found that staking one's self-worth in social media was linked to more depressive symptoms and stress and less resilience and self-kindness (Sabik et al., 2020). How might gender norms and stereotypes affect female clients' experience with social media?

HOW DO I ASSESS IT?

There are many helpful assessment tools for exploring social media addiction and related conditions such as FoMO. In what follows, you will find descriptions of three scales that may be useful in your work with clients with social media addiction.

BERGEN SOCIAL MEDIA ADDICTION SCALE

Andreassen et al. (2012) developed a six-item scale to screen for Facebook addiction (Bergen Facebook Addiction Scale [BFAS]) based on the components model of addiction proposed by Brown (1993) and Griffiths (1996, 2005). Specifically, the components model indicates that addiction involves: (a) salience, (b) mood modification, (c) tolerance, (d) withdrawal, (e) conflict, and (f) relapse. Items on the BFAS reflect each of the six components of addiction and correspond to Likert-type scales ranging from *very rarely* (1) to *very often* (5). Total scores range from 6 to 30, with higher scores indicative of more Facebook addiction symptomology. Later, Andreassen et al. (2016) adapted the BFAS to be inclusive of all social networking sites and thus changed the name to the Bergen Social Media Addiction Scale (BSMAS). Scale items remained the same with the exception of replacing the word "Facebook" with "social media." Example items of the BSMAS include: *How often during the last year have you used social media to forget about personal problems* and *How often during the last year have you tried to cut down on the use of social media without success* (Andreassen et al., 2016). The BSMAS demonstrated acceptable internal consistency among a large Norwegian sample (Cronbach's alpha = .88). The items of the BSMAS are listed in the appendix of the Andreassen et al. (2016) article.

SOCIAL MEDIA ADDICTION SCALE

The Social Media Addiction Scale (SMAS; Al-Menayes, 2015) is an adapted version of the Internet Addiction Test created by Kimberly Young (1998b), which assessed all online activity. Originally written in Arabic, the items of the SMAS reflect social media use specifically. Example items include: *I find life boring without SM* (social media) and *School grades deteriorated because of SM*. Each item is assessed using a five-point Likert-type scale ranging from *strongly disagree* (1) to *strongly agree* (5). Using a sample of undergraduate students, Al-Menayes (2015) determined that the scale had three factors: social consequences (five items), time displacement (three items), and compulsive feelings (four items). The subscale scores demonstrated Cronbach's alpha levels ranging from .61 to .75. Higher scores on each subscale are indicative of more social media addiction symptomology. The scale also demonstrated concurrent validity (Al-Menayes, 2015). All items of the SMAS are found in the original Al-Menayes (2015) article.

PROBLEMATIC SOCIAL NETWORKING SERVICES USE SCALE

The Problematic Social Networking Services Use Scale (PSUS; Lou et al., 2017) was designed to assess social networking use among college students.

The 25-item scale corresponds with four-point Likert-type scales ranging from *totally true of me* (1) to *totally not true of me* (4). The PSUS provides a total score or scores on five subscales: impaired social functioning (six items), withdrawal (six items), deviant behavior (five items), attention state (five items), and tolerance (three items). Example items include: *I am able to control my SNS use* and *When the internet is not available, I will become anxious about whether someone has contacted me online or if there are any updates on my online chat sites.* The scale was normed on a large sample of young adult students in Beijing, China. The authors found a Cronbach's alpha level of .92 for total PSUS scores and subscale scores ranging from .79 to .89. Lower scores indicate more problematic social networking service use (Lou et al., 2017). The items of the PSUS can be found in the original Lou et al. (2017) article.

HOW DO I TREAT IT?

Social media addiction is a complex issue given the potential benefits of social media use and the growing popularity of utilizing social media to manage and develop relationships. Treatment often involves helping clients reconfigure their relationship with technology (rather than abstaining completely), and determining which internet activities should be reduced or discontinued. Counselors can help clients be mindful and intentional about their internet use by creating a detailed technology plan (described later in this section) to guide future behavior.

As with any addiction, the cessation of a compulsive behavior must be accompanied by the development of alternate, replacement behaviors. Therefore, as clients abstain from social media, they must be prepared to engage in more adaptive ways to meet their needs of belonging, connection, self-presentation, and self-worth. Counselors and clients can work to enhance clients' social skills, foster meaningful offline social connections, and cultivate an intrinsic sense of self-worth (rather than relying on external validation via positive social feedback). Clients also may benefit from the development of effective coping strategies to navigate feelings of boredom, loneliness, or dysphoric mood states.

Of note, it is important for counselors to consider that social media also can be a medium for other potentially addictive or harmful behaviors. Indeed, many social networking sites have had to create policies against posts that encourage or glorify self-injury (see Chapter 9) and/or suicide. Additionally, social media sites offer opportunities for online gaming (see Chapter 3), online shopping (see Chapter 13), and can be used for cybersex (see Chapter 6). Therefore, treatment for social media addiction may also include the simultaneous treatment of additional behavioral addictions.

VOICES FROM THE FIELD: Clinical Work With Social Media Addiction

Working with clients who present with social media addiction is very similar to working with clients with drug, alcohol, or sex addiction. In some cases, the client may present with the same type of guilt and shame and they may be wrestling with the same social stigma that corresponds with the more common types of addiction. Also, the seriousness of the social media addiction can be downplayed by the client, often because they do not recognize the critical nature of their addiction. When someone is addicted to drugs, for instance, they may lose weight, lose money, lose friends and family, and therefore their addiction issues come front and center. This is not always the case with someone addicted to social media; therefore, it may be harder for them to recognize, or come to terms with, their addiction. As a clinician, I approach therapy with these clients in the same manner as I would someone with other addiction issues.

For many clients, quitting their social media platform of choice and/or setting up boundaries to reduce, taper off, and then to completely eliminate their social media use (for a time or forever) works best. However, there is a give-and-take to this process that is specific to the personality of the client. Some clients have to exit the social media platform or deactivate their accounts altogether because there is no safe or minimal consumption for them. Others can taper down their social media use with the right type of accountability. In either case, there has to be some time of abstinence from social media, followed by an assessment of whether the social media platform is necessary or beneficial, and then a final determination of whether or not to continue with limited exposure to social media or end their use completely. In my experience, helping clients come to a place where they value connecting with people, nature, or things outside of the cyber universe has been of great help.

Many people do not see social media addiction as a problem and may try to rationalize their use (even when it is clearly problematic). Counselors are not immune; therefore, they must assess their own value system as it relates to addiction—and social media addiction in particular. Counselors must try to step into the worlds of their clients as much as possible to gain perspective on how their addiction is affecting them and the costs of social media use.

Jon Anderson Parker, MAMFT, LPC, NCC; www.jonparker.me

POSITIVE PSYCHOLOGY FOR INTERNET ADDICTION

Khazaei et al. (2017) tested the efficacy of using group-based positive psychology interventions to treat internet addiction (including social media addiction). Positive psychology interventions are designed to enhance positive emotions, strengthen social relationships, and identify individuals' capabilities, while reducing negative emotions. Using a sample of Iranian undergraduate students with internet addiction, the researchers created two groups: the experimental group, composed of participants who received the positive psychology intervention, and the control group, composed of participants who were on a waitlist for the intervention. The positive psychology intervention consisted of 10 group counseling sessions aimed to help participants do the following: nurture positive emotions, identify capabilities and strengths, express emotions, cultivate forgiveness and thankfulness, write letters of gratitude, apply capabilities and strengths, and distinguish between satisfaction and perfectionism. The researchers found that undergraduates in the experimental group demonstrated improvement in social adjustment, quality of relationships, and a decrease in the severity of internet use. Indeed, after the positive psychology intervention, 71% of participants no longer met criteria for internet addiction (Khazaei et al., 2017). Therefore, the use of positive psychology interventions, including strengthening the quality of offline social relationships, identifying strengths, and cultivating gratitude, may be effective treatment strategies for those with social media addiction.

DEVELOP A TECHNOLOGY PLAN

Another component of treatment for social media addiction is to construct a realistic plan for internet and technology use. Clients may benefit from developing concrete goals and boundaries to guide their engagement with technology. The technology plan should be co-constructed between the counselor and client, and the client must have the knowledge and skills necessary to complete the plan (e.g., client should effectively learn and develop alternative coping strategies prior to implementing the plan). A technology plan may include the following guidelines: (a) identify times of day when the client will not use technology (e.g., first thing in the morning, during meals, within 2 hours of bed), (b) keep client's smartphone out of reach while driving (e.g., in the glove compartment, backseat) to prevent use, (c) refrain from checking social media during employment- or education-related activities, (d) prioritize face-to-face interactions over online interaction (e.g., refrain from *phubbing*, or snubbing those in one's immediate environment to engage with others on a smartphone; Chotpitayasunondh & Douglas, 2016), (e) only use technology for preset durations of time (e.g., 10- or 15-minute intervals), (f) only use technology when the resulting emotion is positive (e.g., engage in periodic emotional check-ins and end technology use when feelings of depression, envy, anger, or loneliness emerge), and (g) utilize nontechnological coping mechanisms to navigate negative mood states (e.g., spiritual practices, mindfulness exercises, physical activity, face-to-face conversations, gratitude lists, positive self-statements, playing or listening to music, journaling, drawing, calling a supportive person).

Another component of a technology plan may include making modifications to a client's devices. Indeed, among a sample of undergraduate students in the United States, researchers explored methods of controlling social media use (Brevers & Turel, 2019). The most commonly utilized control strategy among participants was to modify the device (such as putting one's phone on airplane mode so that the internet is inaccessible) followed by preventing access to social media (going to a location without Wi-Fi or putting one's phone in another room). Interestingly, only 3% of the sample reported not utilizing some form of control strategies for social media use, indicating that the overwhelming majority of participants felt the need to control their use (Brevers & Turel, 2019). Clients also may choose to remove social media applications from their smartphones and devices or forego using certain social media platforms altogether. Clients may benefit from turning off all social media notifications, which serve as reward cues. Additionally, changing the smartphone color scheme to gray scale can dampen the effects of rewarding color notifications. Finally, clients may choose to download apps on their devices designed to help limit smartphone usage (e.g., Offtime).

GROUP COUNSELING

Group counseling may be a particularly effective treatment strategy for clients with social media addiction (Pluhar et al., 2019). The group format creates opportunities to increase social interactions, enhance communication skills, and develop an off-line support network (Pluhar et al., 2019). Group counseling is a popular modality to treat internet addiction, particularly in Asian countries. Liu et al. (2017) conducted a meta-analysis of 30 studies examining the effectiveness of group counseling for internet addiction. The researchers found significant effects of group counseling including reduction in internet addiction symptoms, obsessive-compulsive symptoms, depressive symptoms, anxious symptoms, and aggression among participants. In light of the motives influencing social media addiction (need for belonging and self-presentation; Nadkarni & Hofmann, 2012), the group modality may provide a corrective social experience for clients to find belonging and learn to present themselves authentically without the use of social media features.

12-STEP SUPPORT

A 12-step support program may be a helpful resource for clients with social media addiction. Internet and Technology Addicts Anonymous (ITAA, 2020) was founded in 2017 to help those with the desire to stop compulsive internet use. Following the format of Alcoholics Anonymous, members of ITAA work the 12 steps (Step one states, "we admitted that we were powerless over our addiction, and that our lives had become unmanageable" [ITAA, 2020, The Twelve Steps and Twelve Traditions of ITAA, para. 2]), attend meetings via conference calls (connecting members in over 30 different countries), and rely on program literature from other 12-step fellowships (such as the literature used by Overeaters Anonymous). Like other 12-step programs for behavioral addictions, members are intentional about defining what abstinence entails for them (given that some internet and technology use is necessary in today's society). To do this, many members utilize the bottom lines, middle lines, and top lines model (ITAA, 2020, Tools of Recovery, para. 12). Bottom lines signify those behaviors over which an individual has lost control (e.g., social networking site use, Netflix binging, using Reddit or Pinterest, watching YouTube videos, commenting on online content), middle lines signify triggering behaviors (e.g., boredom, interpersonal conflict, insomnia, loneliness, long car rides), and top lines signify aspirational uses of one's time (mediation, prayer, exercise, interacting with friends, listening to music, rewarding hobbies). By identifying bottom, middle, and top lines, ITAA members have a concrete plan for recovery (abstain from bottom lines, avoid or employ coping strategies for middle lines, and increase engagement in top lines). For more information about ITAA, visit their website (internetaddictsanonymous.org).

DIAGNOSTIC CONSIDERATIONS

Although the *DSM-5* includes internet gaming disorder as a condition for further study (listed in the appendix) and the *ICD-11* includes gaming disorder (WHO, 2018), no diagnostic codes presently exist for social media addiction or internet addiction, more broadly. When working with clients with social media addiction, therefore, counselors may choose to diagnose a co-occurring mental health concern, if applicable. Researchers have identified common comorbid mental disorders among those with internet addiction including depression, attention deficit hyperactivity disorder, autism spectrum disorder, and social anxiety (Pluhar et al., 2019). Additionally, clients' behavior may meet *DSM-5* criteria for unspecified disruptive, impulse-control, and conduct disorder if social media use is causing functional impairment and distress, is out of control, and is harming others or is in conflict with societal norms (APA, 2013).

HOW CAN I LEARN MORE?

If you are working with clients with social media addiction or would like to learn more about the condition, consider the following resources.

BOOKS

- Alter, A. (2017). *Irresistible: The rise of addictive technology and the business of keeping us hooked*. Penguin Books.
- Bauman, S. (2011). *Cyberbullying: What counselors need to know*. American Counseling Association.
- Young, K. S., & de Abreu C. N. (Eds.). *Internet addiction: A handbook and guide to evaluation and treatment*. Wiley & Sons.

PEER-REVIEWED ARTICLES

- Andreassen, C. S., & Pallesen, S. (2014). Social network site addiction: An overview. *Current Pharmaceutical Design, 20*, 4053–4061. https://doi.org/10.2174/13816128113199990616
- Kuss, D. J., & Griffiths, M. D. (2017). Social networking sites and addiction: Ten lessons learned. *International Journal of Environmental Research and Public Health, 14*, 1–17. https://doi.org/10.3390/ijerph14030311
- Pluhar, E., Kavanaugh, J. R., Levinson, J. A., & Rich, M. (2019). Problematic interactive media use in teens: Comorbidities, assessment, and treatment. *Psychology Research and Behavior Management, 12*, 447–455. https://doi.org/10.2147/PRBM.S208968

WEBSITES

- Center for Humane Technology: humanetech.com
- Center for Internet and Technology Addiction: virtual-addiction.com
- Internet and Technology Addicts Anonymous: internetaddictsanonymous.org

REFERENCES

Al-Menayes, J. (2015). Psychometric properties and validation of the Arabic social media addiction scale. *Journal of Addiction, 2015*, 1–6. https://doi.org/10.1155/2015/291743

Alter, A. (2017). *Irresistible: The rise of addictive technology and the business of keeping us hooked*. Penguin Books.

American Psychiatric Association. (2013). *Diagnostic and statistical manual of mental disorders* (5th ed.). Author.

Anderson, M., & Jiang, J. (2018). *Teens, social media & technology 2018.* https://www.pewresearch.org/internet/2018/05/31/teens-social-media-technology-2018

Andreassen, C. S., Billieux, J., Griffiths, M. D., Kuss, D. J., Demetrovics, Z., Mazzoni, E., & Pallesen, S. (2016). The relationship between addictive use of social media and video games and symptoms of psychiatric disorders: A large scale cross sectional study. *Psychology of Addictive Behaviors, 30,* 252–262. https://doi.org/10.1037/adb0000160

Andreassen, C. S., & Pallesen, S. (2014). Social network site addiction: An overview. *Current Pharmaceutical Design, 20,* 4053–4061. https://doi.org/10.2174/13816128113199990616

Andreassen, C. S., Pallesen, S., & Griffiths, M. D. (2017). The relationship between addictive use of social media, narcissim, and self-esteem: Findings from a large national survey. *Addictive Behaviors, 64,* 287–293. https://doi.org/10.1016/j.addbeh.2016.03.006

Andreassen, C. S., Torsheim, T., Brunborg, G. S., & Pallesen, S. (2012). Development of a facebook addiction scale. *Psychological Reports, 110,* 501–517. https://doi.org/10.2466/02.09.18.PR0.110.2.501-517

Arias-Carrion, O., Stamelou, M., Murillo-Rodriguez, E., Menendez-Gonzalez, M., & Poppel, E. (2010). Dopaminergic reward system: A short integrative review. *International Archives of Medicine, 3,* 24. https://doi.org/10.1186/1755-7682-3-24

Banyai, F., Zsila, A., Kiraly, O., Maraz, A., Elekes, Z., Griffiths, M. D., Andreassen, C. S., & Demetrovics, Z. (2017). Problematic social media use: Results from a large-scale nationally representative adolescent sample. *PLoS One, 12,* 1–13. https://doi.org/10.1371/journal.pone.0169839

Bauman, S. (2011). *Cyberbullying: What counselors need to know.* American Counseling Association.

Berridge, K. C., & Robinson, T. E. (2016). Liking, wanting and the incentive-sensitization theory of addiction. *The American Psychologist, 71,* 670–679. https://doi.org/10.1037/amp0000059

Bragazzi, N. L., & Del Puente, G. (2014). A proposal for including nomophobia in the new DSM-V. *Psychology Research & Behavior Management, 7,* 155–160. https://doi.org/10.2147/PRBM.S41386

Brevers, D., & Turel, O. (2019). Strategies for self-controlling social media use: Classification and role in preventing social media addiction symptoms. *Journal of Behavioral Addictions, 8,* 554–563. https://doi.org/10.1556/2006.8.2019.49

Brown, R. I. F. (1993). Some contributions of the study of gambling to the study of other addictions. In W. R. Eadington & J. A. Cornelius (Eds.), *Gambling behaviour and problem gambling* (pp. 341–272). University of Nevada Press.

Chotpitayasunondh, V., & Douglas, K. M. (2016). How 'phubbing' becomes the norm: The antecedents and consequences of snubbing via smartphone. *Computers in Human Behavior, 63,* 9–8. https://doi.org/10.1016/j.chb.2016.05.018

Giordano, A. L., Prosek, E. A., & Watson, J. (2021). Understanding adolescent cyberbullies: Exploring social media addiction and psychological factors. *Journal of Child and Adolescent Counseling, 7,* 42-55. https://doi.org/10.1080/23727810.2020.1835420

Greenfield, D. (2011). The addictive properties of internet usage. In K. S. Young & C. N. de Abreu (Eds.), *Internet addiction: A handbook and guide to evaluation and treatment* (pp. 135–153). Wiley & Sons.

Griffiths, M. D. (1996). Behavioural addiction: An issue for everybody? *Journal of Workplace Learning, 8,* 19–25. https://doi.org/10.1108/13665629610116872

Griffiths, M. (2005). A "components" model of addiction within a biopsychosocial framework. *Journal of Substance Use, 10,* 191–197. https://doi.org/10.1080/14659890500114359

Guo, S. (2016). A meta-analysis of the predictors of cyberbullying perpetration and victimization. *Psychology in the Schools, 53,* 432–453. https://doi.org/10.1002/pits.21914

He, O., Turel, O., & Bechara, A. (2017). Brain anatomy alterations associated with social networking site (SNS) addiction. *Scientific Reports, 7,* 45064. https://doi.org/10.1038/srep45064

Heo, J. Y., Kim, K., Fava, M., Mischoulon, D., Papakostas, G. I., Kim, M. J., Chang, K. J., Oh, Y., Yu, B. H., & Jeon, H. J. (2017). Effects of smartphone use with and without blue light at night in healthy adults: A randomized double-blind, cross-over, placebo-controlled comparison. *Journal of Psychiatric Research, 87,* 61–70. https://doi.org/10.1016/j.jpsychires.2016.12.010

Holfeld, B., & Grabe, M. (2012). An examination of the history, prevalence, characteristics, and reporting of cyberbullying in the United States. In Q. Li, D. Cross, & P. K. Smith (Eds.), *Cyberbullying in the global playground: Research from international perspectives* (pp.117–142). Blackwell Publishing Ltd.

Hormes, J. M., Kearns, B., & Timko, C. A. (2014). Craving Facebook? Behavioral addiction to online social networking and its association with emotion regulation deficits. *Addiction, 109,* 2079–2088. https://doi.org/10.1111/add.12713

Hou, Y., Xiong, D., Jiang, T., Song, L., & Wang, Q. (2019). Social media addiction: Its impact, mediation, and intervention. *CyberPsychology, 13,* 4. https://doi.org/10.5817/cp2019-1-4

Internet and Technology Addicts Anonymous. (2020). *Tools of recovery.* https://internetaddictsanonymous.org

Jiaxin, Y., Xi, F., Xiaoli, L., & Yamin, L. (2019). Association of problematic smartphone use with poor sleep quality, depression, and anxiety: A systematic review and meta analysis. *Psychiatry Research, 284,* 112686. https://doi.org/10.106/j.psychres.2019.112686

Khazaei, F., Khazaei, O., & Ghanbari, H. B. (2017). Positive psychology interventions for internet addiction treatment. *Computers in Human Behavior, 72,* 304–311. https://doi.org/10.1016/j.chb.2017.02.065

King, A. L. S., Valenca, A. M., & Nardi, A. E. (2010). Nomophobia: The mobile phone in panic disorder with agoraphobia: Reducing phobias or worsening of dependence? *Cognitive and Behavioral Neurology, 23,* 52–54. https://doi.org/10.1097/WNN.ob013e3187b7eabc

Kuss, D. J., & Griffiths, M. D. (2017). Social networking sites and addiction: Ten lessons learned. *International Journal of Environmental Research and Public Health, 14,* 1–17. https://doi.org/10.3390/ijerph14030311

Lewis, T., Amini, F., & Lannon, R. (2001). *A general theory of love.* Vintage Books.

Li, Q., Smith, P. K., & Cross, D. (2012). Research into cyberbullying. In Q. Li, D. Cross, & P. K. Smith (Eds.), *Cyberbullying in the global playground: Research from international perspectives* (pp. 3–12). Blackwell Publishing Ltd.

Lin, Y. H., Chaing, C. L., Lin, P. H., Change, L. R., Ko, C. H., Lee, Y. H., & Lin, S. H. (2016). Proposed diagnostic criteria for smartphone addiction. *PLoS One, 11,* 1–11. https://doi.org/10.1371/journal.pone.0163010

Liu, J., Nie, J., & Wang, Y. (2017). Effects of group counseling programs, cognitive behavioral therapy, and sports intervention on internet addiction in East Asia: A systematic review and meta analysis. *International Journal of Environmental Research and Public Health, 14,* 1470. https://doi.org/10.3390/ijerph.14121470

Lou, J., Liu, H., & Liu, X. (2017). Development of the problematic social networking services uses scale with college students. *Social Behavior and Personality, 45,* 1889–1904. https://doi.org/10.2224/sbp.6179

Nadkarni, A., & Hofmann, S. G. (2012). Why do people use facebook? *Personality and Individual Differences, 52,* 243–249. https://doi.org/10.1016/j.paid.2011.11.007

Oberst, U., Wegmann, E., Stodt, B., Brand, M., & Chamarro, A. (2017). Negative consequences from heavy social networking in adolescents: The mediating role of fear of missing out. *Journal of Adolescence, 55,* 51–60. https://doi.org/10.1016/j.adolescence.2016.12.008

Perrin, A., & Anderson, M. (2019). *Share of U.S. adults using social media, including Facebook, is mostly unchanged sing 2018.* https://www.pewresearch.org/fact-tank/2019/04/10/share-of-u-s-adults-using-social-media-including-facebook-is-mostly-unchanged-since-2018

Platt, M. L., Watson, K. K., Hayden, B. Y., Shepherd, S. V., & Klein, J. T. (2010). Neuroeconomics: Implications for understanding the neurobiology of addiction. In C. M. Kuhn & G. F. Koob (Eds.), *Advances in the neurobiology of addiction* (pp. 193–227). Taylor & Francis Group.

Pluhar, E., Kavanaugh, J. R., Levinson, J. A., & Rich, M. (2019). Problematic interactive media use in teens: Comorbidities, assessment, and treatment. *Psychology Research and Behavior Management, 12,* 447–455. https://doi.org/10.2147/PRBM.S208968

Pontes, H. M., Taylor, M., & Stavropoulos, V. (2018). Beyond "Facebook addiction": The role of cognitive-related factors and psychiatric distress in social networking site addiction. *Cyberpsychology, Behavior, and Social Networking, 21,* 240–247. https://doi.org/10.1089/cyber.2017.0609

Przybylski, A. K., Murayama, K., Deltaan, C. R., & Gladwell, V. (2013). Motivational, emotional, and behavioral correlates of fear of missing out. *Computers in Human Behavior, 29,* 1841–1848. https://doi.org/10.1016/j.chb.2013.02.014

Raudsepp, L. (2019). Brief report: Problematic social media use and sleep disturbances are longitudinally associated with depressive symptoms in adolescents. *Journal of Adolescence, 76,* 197–201. https://doi.org/10.1016/j.adolescence.2019.09.005

Rideout, V., & Robb, M. B. (2019). *The common sense consensus: Media use by tweens and teens, 2019.* Common Sense Media.

Rost, K., Stahel, L., & Frey, B. S. (2016). Digital social norm enforcement: Online firestorms in social media. *PLoS One, 11,* 1–26. https://doi.org/10.1371/journal.pone.0155923

Sabik, N. J., Falat, J., & Magagnos, J. (2020). When self-worth depends on social media feedback: Associations with psychological well-being. *Sex roles, 82,* 411–421. https://doi.org/10.1007/s11199-019-01062-8

Sampasa-Kanyinga, H., & Hamilton, H. A. (2015). Use of social networking sites and risk of cyberbullying victimization: A population-level study of adolescents. *CyberPsychology, Behavior, and Social Networking, 18,* 704–710. https://doi.org/10.1089/cyber.2015.0145

Savci, M., & Aysan, F. (2017). Technological addictions and social connectedness: Predictor effect of Internet addiction, social media addiction, digital game addiction and smartphone addiction on social connectedness. *The Journal of Psychiatry and Neurological Sciences, 30,* 202–216. https://doi.org/10.5358/DAJPN2017300304

Sherman, L. E., Hernandez, L. M., Greenfield, P. M., & Dapretto, M. (2018). What the brain 'likes': Neural correlates of providing feedback on social media. *Social Cognitive and Affective Neuroscience, 13*, 699–707. https://doi.org/10.1093/scan/nsy051

Sherman, L. E., Payton, A. A., Hernandez, L. M., Greenfield, P. M., & Dapretto, M. (2016). The power of the like in adolescence: Effects of peer influence on neural and behavioral responses to social media. *Psychological Science, 27*, 1027–1035. https://doi.org/10.1177/0956797616645673

Shultz, W., Dayan, P., & Montague, P. R. (1997). A neural substrate of prediction and reward. *Science, 275*, 1593–1599. https://doi.org/10.1126/science.275.5306.1593

Simpkins, C. A., & Simpkins, A. M. (2013). *Neuroscience for clinicians: Evidence, models, and practice*. Springer Publishing.

Singh, M. M., & Pati, A. K. (2016). Effects of radiation emanating from base transceiver station and mobile phone on sleep, circadian rhythm and cognition in humans: A review. *Biological Rhythm Research, 47*, 353–388. https://doi.org/10.1080/09291016.2015.1116741

Skinner, B. F. (1969). *Contingencies of reinforcement: A theoretical analysis*. Meredith Corporation.

Skinner, B. F. (1976). *About behaviorism*. Vintage Books.

Sural, I., Griffiths, M. D., Kircaburun, K., & Emirtekin, E. (2019). Trait emotional intelligence and problematic social media use motives. *International Journal of Mental Health and Addiction, 17*, 336–345. https://doi.org/10.1007/s11469-018-0022-6

Turel, O., He, Q., Brevers, D., & Bechara, A. (2018). Delay discounting mediates the association between posterior insular cortex volume and social media addiction symptoms. *Cognitive, Affective, and Behavioral Neuroscience, 18*, 644–704. https://doi.org/10.3758/s13415-018-0597-1

Watson, J. C., Prosek, E. A., & Giordano, A. L. (2020). Investigating psychometric properties of social media addiction measures among adolescents. *Journal of Counseling and Development, 98*, 458-466. https://doi.org/10.1002/jcad.12347

World Health Organization. (2018). *International statistical classification of diseases and related health problems* (11th Rev.). https://icd.who.int/browse11/l-m/en

Young, K. S. (1998a). Internet addiction: The emergence of a new clinical disorder. *CyberPsychology and Behavior, 1*, 237–244. https://doi.org/10.1089/cpb.1998.1.237

Young, K. (1998b). *Caught in the net*. John Wiley & Sons.

5

Sex Addiction

HOW DO I CONCEPTUALIZE IT?

Sex is a naturally rewarding behavior (i.e., activates reward circuitry in the brain) and is necessary for the propagation of our species. Individuals' sexual activity can be conceptualized on a continuum with healthy sexual behavior in the middle (Carnes, 1997). The two ends of the continuum represent extreme sexual activity: On one end is sexual anorexia (i.e., extreme aversion to sex) and on the other end is sexual addiction (i.e., sexual behavior that has become out of control and continues despite negative consequences; Carnes, 1997). Although those with both sexual anorexia and sex addiction are struggling with sexual behavior, the focus of this chapter is on sexual addiction (yet interested readers are encouraged to review Carnes's [1997] book *Sexual anorexia: Overcoming sexual self-hatred* to learn more about compulsive sexual avoidance).

In his pioneering research, Patrick Carnes (1989, 1991) popularized the idea that sex can be an addictive behavior for some individuals. Rather than identifying specific addictive sexual acts, Carnes (1991) noted that it is one's *relationship* with sexual activity that signifies addiction. Specifically, when an individual compulsively engages in sexual acts, experiences a loss of control over sex, continues to engage despite negative consequences, and craves or is mentally preoccupied with sex, they may have a sex addiction. Like other behavioral addictions, those with sex addiction use sex to regulate emotions: to experience pleasure, to escape pain, to experience emotional numbness, or to simply feel *something* (Weiss, 2015). The authors of the Sex Addicts Anonymous (SAA) text noted that compulsive sexual behavior "altered our feelings and consciousness, and we found this altered state very desirable. The obsession and rituals that led up to the sex act itself were part of the 'high.' We sought this addictive high repeatedly" (International Service Organization of SAA, Inc., 2005, p. 3). Indeed, Goodman (1993) described sex addiction as serving the function of producing pleasure and reducing discomfort; thus the behavior is both positively and negatively reinforcing.

In support of the mood modification role of sex addiction, researchers examined emotion regulation difficulties among college students with and without sex addiction (Cashwell et al., 2017). Those students with sex addiction (16.9% of the sample) had significantly higher difficulties in emotion regulation, specifically in the nonacceptance of their emotions, limited affect regulation strategies, and difficulty carrying out goal-directed activities when experiencing negative affect (Cashwell et al., 2017). Therefore, those with sex addiction likely are engaging in sexual acts as a means of regulating their emotional experiences via naturally rewarding sexual behavior. Insight into the emotion regulation function of sexual activity can be helpful for clients and a starting place for treatment and recovery.

SEX ADDICTION CYCLE

Carnes (2001) described a four-part cycle of sex addiction, which serves as a useful tool for conceptualizing the experience of clients. The cycle begins with *preoccupation*, in which individuals are mentally consumed with thoughts and fantasies related to sexual behavior. This mental preoccupation interferes with other life tasks as sexual thoughts override all other cognitions. The trance-like state of preoccupation leads to the engagement in *ritualistic behavior*, as individuals prepare for sexual acts. Those with sex addiction engage in familiar routines in anticipation of sexual behavior. These rituals could include using illicit drugs, going to particular locations, turning on a computer or electronic device, or engaging in behaviors such as cruising for potential sexual partners. The ritualistic behavior then leads to *acting out*, or engaging in the compulsive sexual act. This is the sexual behavior over which individuals have lost control (Carnes, 2001). It is important to remember that any act of sexual stimulation (partnered or solo) can become addictive; a sex addiction diagnosis is not contingent upon the *type* of sexual behavior, but upon the *role* of the behavior in the client's life (Goodman, 1993). Consequently, acting out behaviors can entail compulsive masturbation, pornography use, frequenting strip clubs, hiring prostitutes, engaging in anonymous sex with consenting adults, indecent liberties, voyeurism, exhibitionism, rape, or sexual assault (Carnes, 2001). Indeed, researchers examining 87 men in treatment for hypersexual disorder reported that 86% engaged in compulsive masturbation, 81% identified as dependent on pornography, 22% engaged in extramarital affairs, 16% hired sex workers, and 15% engaged in excessive, unprotected sexual behavior with anonymous adults (Reid et al., 2010).

The fourth and final component of the sex addiction cycle is *despair*. Like other addictive behaviors, sex addiction is characterized by a loss of control (powerlessness), which can lead to feelings of hopelessness and shame. The individual with sex addiction wants to stop the secrecy, isolation, violation of personal values, deception, and acting out, but is unable to do so. Unsuccessful attempts to control or stop the behavior lead to despair and shame. Importantly, shame is categorically different than guilt. Shame refers to negative perceptions of the self (i.e., "I am a bad person"), while guilt refers to negative perceptions of a behavior (i.e., "What I did was bad"; Lewis, 1971; Tangney & Dearing, 2002). Shame is a salient component of the sex addiction cycle for many clients. In the study of hypersexuality and self-directed emotions among undergraduates, researchers found that among male participants, higher levels of shame proneness and externalization (i.e., the propensity to blame others for behavior) and lower levels of guilt proneness and detachment (i.e., a state of minimal emotional investment) predicted hypersexual behavior among males (Giordano et al., 2015). The only self-directed emotion that predicted hypersexual behavior among female participants was detachment (which has implications for attachment work, described later in this chapter). Thus, along with highlighting potential gender differences in sex addiction, the scholars identified shame as a predictor of male hypersexuality (Giordano et al., 2015). Furthermore, Gilliland et al. (2011) studied those in treatment for compulsive pornography use (96% men) and found shame to be a significant predictor of hypersexuality.

It is important to note that shame can be both a precursor and consequence of the sex addiction cycle (Hall, 2011). In fact, unresolved shame can be the catalyst for mental preoccupation about sex (i.e., shame can trigger thoughts of sex as a coping response), and shame often follows sexual acting out (along with self-loathing, despair, and hopelessness). Therefore, it is important for counselors to create spaces devoid of evaluation or judgment and to be "virtually unshockable" when working with clients with sex addiction (Hagedorn & Juhnke, 2005, p. 82). This type of nonevaluative, supportive relationship can be a transformative, corrective experience for those encumbered by shame.

CLINICAL NOTE 5.1

Consider the cycle of sex addiction (preoccupation, ritualistic behavior, acting out, and despair). What clinical interventions might effectively interrupt the cycle at each stage? For example, what strategies might a client employ to interrupt the cycle during preoccupation? Create a list of potential interventions for each component of the cycle.

SEXUAL ADDICTION VERSUS SEXUAL OFFENDING

There are important distinctions between sex addiction and sexual offending of which counselors should be aware. Sexual offending is a legal construct and sex addiction is a psychological construct, so although there are some overlapping features, there are important differences (Schneider, 1999). An individual with sex addiction may become a sexual offender if the sexual acting out behavior violates the law. Additionally, a sex offender may have a sex addiction, especially if they demonstrate compulsivity, a loss of control, continued engagement despite negative consequences, and craves or is mentally preoccupied with sex. Therefore, some sexual offenders may have a sex addiction, but not all, and some individuals with sexual addiction may be offenders, but not all. In the study of 114 incarcerated male sex offenders, researchers found that less than half (43.9%) met criteria for sex addiction (Marshall et al., 2008).

To help differentiate between sex addiction and sexual offending, Delmonico and Griffin (1997) proposed a four-quadrant model to classify individuals with sexual behavior issues. The authors defined the first quadrant, *the sexually addicted sex offender*, as encompassing individuals who progress in their sexual acting out behaviors from legal forms of sexual stimulation (e.g., compulsive masturbation, sex with consenting adults) to illegal forms of sexual behavior (e.g., sexual victimization, voyeurism). These sexually addicted sex offenders often experience shame and remorse as a result of their sexual acts. The second quadrant describes *the sexual offender* (without sex addiction), characterized by violence, hatred, anger, low remorse, low victim empathy, and narcissism (Delmonico & Griffin, 1997). Indeed, sexual offenses often are driven by the desire to control and exert power, rather than sexual desire (Blum et al., 2012). The third quadrant, *the sexual addict* (non-offending), represents those who have lost control over their sexual behavior, yet have not engaged in illegal sexual activity (Delmonico & Griffin, 1997). Their behavior causes distress and impairment, yet has not crossed the line of legality. Finally, the fourth quadrant, the *sexually concerned*, describes those who do not yet meet criteria for sex addiction and have not committed a sexual offense, yet have sex-related presenting concerns (e.g., sexual dysfunction, disapproval of sexual behaviors, guilt over legal sexual acts, or disturbing sexual fantasies). Although individuals in this quadrant may benefit from counseling, they would not be conceptualized as sexual offenders or as having a sex addiction (Delmonico & Griffin, 1997). Therefore, it is imperative for counselors to do a thorough assessment of clients' sexual histories and behaviors to offer the best treatment options. Of note, most states require clinicians to earn a sex offender treatment provider credential in order to offer services to sex offenders, so counselors should investigate the specific regulations of their state.

PREVALENCE OF SEX ADDICTION

Without a uniform definition of sex addiction, it is not surprising to find a variety of proposed prevalence rates. Karila et al. (2014) reviewed the literature and found reported prevalence rates ranging from 3% to 16.8%. Moreover, Carnes (2005) suggested that up to 6% of the population in the United States has a sex addiction. Prevalence rates also vary according to subgroup. For example, among clients in treatment for substance use disorders, 21% met criteria for sex addiction (Deneke et al., 2015). Additionally, among clients with gambling addiction, researchers found that 19.6% also demonstrated compulsive sexual behavior (Grant & Steinberg, 2005). Researchers also have found substantial rates of sex addiction among collegiate populations. In the study of 235 college students (men and women), Giordano and Cecil (2014) found that 11.1% of all participants (16.2% of males) exceeded the clinical cutoff score for hypersexual behavior. Furthermore, using a short screening instrument (PATHOS; Carnes et al., 2012), researchers found that 21.2% of college men and 6.7% of college women endorsed three or more items, indicating a need for further assessment of sex addiction (Cashwell et al., 2015). Finally, among a sample of college counselors, scholars found that 84.4% worked with at least one client presenting with sex addiction in the previous year (Giordano & Cashwell, 2018).

It is clear that compulsive sexual behavior is a concern for a notable portion of the population. Although men tend to have higher prevalence rates than women (Kaplan & Krueger, 2010; Karila et al., 2014), counselors can advocate for clients by refuting the idea that sex addiction is a "man's problem," as many women also are impacted by the disorder (Ferree, 2001). Women with sex addiction may experience multiple layers of stigma: one layer for having an addiction and another for having a *sexual* addiction, specifically. By regularly assessing for sex addiction among both male and female clients, counselors can help reduce gender-related stigma.

NEUROSCIENCE OF SEX ADDICTION

For counselors to provide effective services, it is helpful to understand the neurobiological and physiological components of sex addiction. Sex is a naturally rewarding behavior that activates reward circuitry in the brain, specifically stimulating the release of dopamine into the nucleus accumbens (Blum et al., 2012). Reward system activation through sexual activity (and other behaviors such as eating, drinking, exercise, gambling, drugs of abuse, etc.) impacts motivation and learning as individuals actively seek stimuli that induce reward (Blum et al., 2012; Hall, 2011). It is theorized that reward system dysfunction contributes to individuals' susceptibility to behavioral addictions, including sex addiction (Blum et al., 2014; Comings & Blum, 2000; Gold et al., 2014; Goodman, 1993). Indeed, Blum et al. (2012) noted, "malfunctioning of the brain's reward center is increasingly understood to underline all addictive behaviors" (p. 41). Thus, it has been proposed that individuals with addiction (including sex addiction) may have a genetic predisposition caused by hypodopaminergic functioning in the brain's reward circuitry (Blum et al., 1996).

Along with genetic susceptibility, scholars have theorized that sex addiction is influenced, at least in part, by attachment ruptures and trauma in early childhood (Karila et al., 2014; Katehakis, 2009). Specifically, individuals who never developed self-regulatory skills due to chronic stress, disengaged caregivers, and/or traumatic experiences may be more prone to addictive behaviors as a means of emotion regulation. Self-regulation is a skill learned in early childhood as the child's needs are met by attuned caregivers, yet this is not the experience of every child. Some children never experience a secure relationship with a caregiver who responds consistently to their emotional and physical needs. In those instances, the child does not have the opportunity to learn self-regulation skills or experience co-regulation with their parent/guardian. Katehakis (2009) wrote, "Infants whose distress has not been interactively regulated by an attuned caregiver have not begun to learn how to manage their feelings, or even that feelings can be managed" (p. 8).

Additionally, when children face trauma in the absence of attuned, responsive caregivers, their stress response systems can remain chronically activated, releasing stress hormones such as cortisol and adrenaline (Burke Harris, 2018; Katehakis, 2009; van der Kolk, 2014). This chronic activation of the stress response system is known as *toxic stress*, a nonnormative state that "occurs when a child's stress response systems are activated in the absence of supportive, calming relationships, and stay activated for prolonged periods of time" (Nakazawa, 2015, pp. 66–67). A child experiencing toxic stress is in a constant state of hypervigilance with a perpetually activated hypothalamic–pituitary–adrenal (HPA) axis (known as the stress axis), creating states of hypervigilance, distractibility, anxiety, and fear (Nakazawa, 2015).

In light of these physiological changes, children who experience toxic stress are more susceptible to a variety of negative psychological and physical outcomes (Burke Harris, 2018; Felitti et al., 1998; Nakazawa, 2015), one of which may be self-regulation through sexual behaviors (Hall, 2011; Katehakis, 2009). Researchers examined the functioning of the HPA axis among men with sex addiction and healthy controls and found evidence of HPA axis dysregulation among those in the sex addiction group (Chatzittofis et al., 2016). Moreover, Carnes's (1991) landmark study of adults with sex addiction discovered that 97% of participants reported histories of emotional abuse, 81% reported histories of sexual abuse, and 72% reported histories of physical abuse. Additionally, the study of adult internet users who reported having an addiction (to either drugs of abuse, gambling, or sex) revealed that childhood emotional trauma significantly predicted adult sex addiction (yet childhood sexual or physical abuse did not; McPherson et al., 2013). Finally, in the groundbreaking adverse childhood experiences (ACEs) study, Felitti et al. (1998) found that as individuals' ACE scores increased, so too did the prevalence of having 50 or more sexual intercourse partners and risk of sexually transmitted diseases (STDs).

Thus, it is clear that early childhood trauma, lack of self-regulation skills, and histories of toxic stress can play a role in the development of sex addiction among some individuals. Specifically, some adults with attachment ruptures and trauma histories may be seeking to self-regulate their emotional experiences through sexual activity (Katehakis, 2009). Treatment for sex addiction, therefore, often involves trauma-informed care, enhancing and supporting the development of self-regulation skills, and processing ACEs.

SEX ADDICTION AND ATTACHMENT

Given the connection between childhood trauma and sex addiction, it is not surprising that *insecure attachment styles* also are linked to addictive sexual behavior. Attachment behaviors refer to a person "attaining or retaining proximity to some other differentiated and preferred individual, who is usually conceived as stronger and or wiser" (Bowlby, 1978, p. 5). According to Bowlby (1988), attachment involves the development of an emotional bond between a child and the primary caregiver who is perceived to provide support and protection. During the attachment process, infants develop mental representations (known as *working models*) of themselves and their attachment figures. Bowlby (1988) suggested that these working models of the self and attachment figures are key features of personality development and functioning.

Although originating in infancy, attachment behaviors are activated across the life span, particularly in times of distress (Bowlby, 1978, 1988). Ainsworth et al. (Ainsworth & Bell, 1970; Ainsworth et al., 1978) studied 1-year-old infants during the groundbreaking Strange Situation study and classified their attachment styles as secure, ambivalent, or avoidant; the latter two representing insecure attachment styles. Bowlby (1988) built on this work and described the three types of attachment as secure, anxious-resistant, and anxious-avoidant. Secure attachment is characterized by a child's confidence that the parent/guardian will be responsive and available when needed by the child. Anxious-resistant attachment is characterized by the child's uncertainty related to the parent/guardian's responsiveness and availability, leading to separation anxiety and hesitancy to explore new situations. Anxious-avoidant attachment is characterized by the expectation that help from a parent/guardian is not likely, leading to emotional detachment (Bowlby, 1988).

Researchers have identified a relationship between insecure attachment styles and compulsive sexual behavior (Crocker, 2015; Faisandier et al., 2012; Hall, 2011; Zapf et al., 2008). Indeed, in the study of 104 adults, researchers found a significant, positive correlation between sex addiction and ACEs, and determined that the relationship between ACEs and sex addiction was mediated by anxious adult attachment (Kotera & Rhodes, 2019). Faisandier et al. (2012) studied sex addiction and attachment styles among 621 adults in New Zealand and found that individuals with sex addiction had significantly higher insecure attachment styles and lower secure attachment styles than individuals without sex addiction. Moreover, in a study comparing male clients with and without sex addiction, researchers found that men with sex addiction had higher avoidant attachment scores than those without sex addiction (Crocker, 2015). Finally, Giordano et al. (2017) examined attachment styles and religious coping between male and female college students in and outside the clinical range for sex addiction. Anxious attachment styles and negative religious coping (i.e., struggle and tension in one's relationship with God; Pargament & Abu-Raiya, 2007) were significantly higher among participants in the clinical range for sex addiction (Giordano et al., 2017). Therefore, identifying clients' attachment style and engaging in attachment work may be particularly important among clients with sex addiction. In fact, Benfield (2018) noted, "if the individual can learn to form secure attachments and to regulate their own emotions, they may no longer need sexual acting-out for that purpose" (p. 13).

HOW DO I IDENTIFY IT?

There are multiple sets of criteria by which counselors can identify sex addiction. Kafka (2010) proposed criteria for hypersexual disorder for consideration in the *Diagnostic and Statistical Manual of Mental Disorders* (5th ed.; *DSM-5*; American Psychiatric Association [APA], 2013). Although not accepted in the *DSM-5*, the criteria are useful in the identification of sex addiction. Kafka (2010) proposed that the diagnosis for hypersexual disorder is appropriate when individuals experience at least three of the following symptoms for 6 months or more: (a) time allotted for individual responsibilities and activities is spent engaging in sexual fantasies, urges, and behaviors, (b) initiating sexual activity as a result of dysphoric mood, (c) initiating sexual activity as a result of stressful or difficult events, (d) inability to limit or control sexual behavior, and (e) continuing to engage in sexual behavior despite posing a risk to oneself or others. To meet criteria for the diagnosis, individuals must be experiencing significant impairment or emotional distress and the behavior cannot be the result of psychoactive drug use or medications. Finally, Kafka (2010) suggested specifying if the hypersexual disorder primarily manifested in masturbation, cybersex, pornography use, sexual engagement with consenting adults, strip clubs, telephone sex, or other forms of sexual activity. According to Kafka (2014), hypersexual disorder was not included in the *DSM-5* due to concerns related to the sufficiency of research, misclassifying developmentally appropriate sexual exploration in youth, and potential misuse in cases pertaining to sexual offenders in the criminal justice system. In response to these critiques, the diagnosis now requires endorsement of four of the five symptoms and is contraindicated for individuals younger than 18 years of age (Kafka, 2014).

Although not included in the *DSM-5*, the *International Classification of Diseases*, 11th Revision (*ICD-11*; World Health Organization [WHO], 2018) included compulsive sexual behavior disorder within the section for impulse-control disorders. Compulsive sexual behavior disorder is classified by the centrality of sexual behavior in an individual's life (to the detriment of other responsibilities), inability to reduce, limit, or stop sexual behavior, continued engagement despite negative consequences, and emotional distress and functional impairment lasting at least 6 months due to the sexual behavior (WHO,

2018). Importantly, compulsive sexual behavior disorder and hypersexual disorder are distinct from paraphilic disorders (Kafka, 2010, 2014; WHO, 2018).

NEGATIVE CONSEQUENCES OF SEX ADDICTION

In his seminal study of those with sex addiction, Carnes (1991) identified several negative consequences of compulsive sexual behavior including contracting STDs, unwanted pregnancies, physical injuries, financial difficulties, job loss, shame, despair, and loss of meaningful relationships. Additionally, 17% of those with sex addiction reported engaging in a suicide attempt (Carnes, 1991). Subsequent researchers confirmed the prevalence of negative consequences among those with sex addiction. Reid et al. (2012) studied the extent to which detrimental outcomes of hypersexual behavior were endorsed by those with sex addiction. Participants disclosed that their hypersexual behavior contributed to: negative mental health outcomes (endorsed by 93.7% of the sample), causing a loved one emotional pain (89.1%), hindering the ability to engage in healthy sexual activity (77.9%), financial loss (52.7%), ending a romantic relationship (39.3%), contraction of an STD (27.5%), job loss (17.3%), and legal issues (17.3%; Reid et al., 2012).

Moreover, in the study of hypersexual men and women in Sweden, researchers found that hypersexual men were more likely to engage in drug use, heavy alcohol consumption, and gambling, had less satisfaction with their sexual activities, more problems in romantic relationships, were more likely to have an STD, and had less physical and psychological health and life satisfaction compared to their nonhypersexual male counterparts (Langstrom & Hanson, 2006). In addition, hypersexual women were more likely to engage in drug use, heavy alcohol consumption, have comorbid psychiatric disorders, have an STD, and demonstrate low psychological health and life satisfaction compared to their nonhypersexual female counterparts (Langstrom & Hanson, 2006). Therefore, one way to identify sex addiction is to assess clients' continuation of sexual behaviors despite negative consequences.

CLINICAL NOTE 5.2

In a study comparing men with hypersexual disorder and healthy male controls, researchers found that participants with hypersexual disorder had more depressive symptoms, impulsivity, symptoms of attention deficit hyperactivity disorder, alexithymia (i.e., difficulty identifying emotions), maladaptive emotion regulation strategies, and anxious and avoidant attachment styles (Engel et al., 2019). If a client came to you with any of the preceding presenting concerns, how might you broach and assess sexual activity to rule out sex addiction?

HOW DO I ASSESS IT?

There are many helpful tools for assessing sex addiction. In what follows are descriptions of three assessment instruments, yet readers are encouraged to review Karila et al. (2014) for a complete list of existing sex addiction measures.

SEXUAL ADDICTION SCREENING TEST-REVISED

The Sexual Addiction Screening Test-Revised (SAST-R; Carnes et al., 2010) served to update the original SAST (Carnes, 1989) by adding culturally relevant questions and subscales specific to gender and sexual orientation differences. Specifically, the SAST-R is composed of a 20-item core scale assessing elements of sex addiction common across genders and sexual orientations. Example core scale items include: *Have you ever sought help for sexual behavior you did not like* and *Do you feel controlled by your sexual desire*. Each item has a dichotomous, yes or no answer choice. Endorsing six or more items on the core scale is indicative of sex addiction. The core scale of the SAST-R has demonstrated strong internal reliability with Cronbach's alpha scores ranging from .78 to .92 across samples. Additional subscales of the SAST-R include a six-item internet scale (cutoff 3), a six-item heterosexual men's scale (cutoff 2), a six-item heterosexual women's scale (cutoff 2), and a six-item homosexual men's scale (cutoff 3; Carnes et al., 2010). An online version of the SAST-R is available at recoveryzone.com and the full scale is printed in the appendix of the Carnes et al. (2010) article.

SEXUAL COMPULSIVITY SCALE

The Sexual Compulsivity Scale (SCS; Kalichman et al., 1994) is a 10-item measure with items derived from sex addiction literature. The authors of the scale defined sexual compulsivity as "an insistent, repetitive, intrusive, and unwanted urge to perform specific acts often in ritualized or routinized fashions" (Kalichman & Rompa, 1995, p. 587). The SCS includes items such as: *I feel that my sexual thoughts and feelings are stronger than I am* and *My desires to have sex have disrupted my daily life*. Respondents select the extent to which they agree with each statement on a four-point Likert-type scale ranging from *not at all like me* (1) to *very much like me* (4). Final SCS scores are derived by summing the scores of all 10 items (Kalichman et al., 1994; Kalichman & Rompa, 2001). Among a sample of gay men, SCS scores positively correlated with sexual sensation-seeking and loneliness, and negatively correlated with self-esteem and sexual control (Kalichman et al., 1994). The scale has demonstrated acceptable reliability among samples of gay men (Cronbach's alpha = .86) and inner-city men and women (Cronbach's alpha = .87;

Kalichman & Rompa, 1995). The full 10-item SCS can be found in Kalicham and Rompa's original (2001) article.

HYPERSEXUAL BEHAVIOR INVENTORY

The Hypersexual Behavior Inventory (HBI; Reid et al., 2011) was designed to measure partnered and solo compulsive sexual behavior. The 19-item HBI offers a total scale score as well as scores on three subscales: coping (using sex as a means of managing emotions; seven items), control (diminished control over sexual urges, fantasies, and actions; eight items), and consequences (continued engagement in sexual behavior in spite of detrimental outcomes; four items). Example items include: *My attempts to change my sexual behavior fail* and *Doing something sexual helps me cope with stress*. Participants respond to each item on a five-point Likert-type scale ranging from *never* (1) to *very often* (5). Scores are determined by summing the total scale or subscale items. The scale's scores demonstrated adequate reliability with a sample of men in treatment for sex addiction (Cronbach's alpha = .95 for total scale, .94 for control subscale, .90 for coping subscale, and .87 for consequences subscale; Reid et al., 2011). Additionally, among male and female college students, Giordano and Cecil (2014) found good reliability for HBI total scale scores (Cronbach's alpha = .93). The full 19-item HBI is listed in the appendix of the Reid et al. (2011) article.

> ### CLINICAL NOTE 5.3
>
> An easy way to begin conversations about sex addiction with clients is to include an item on your clinical intake form related to compulsive or addictive sexual activity. Consult your current intake form; to what degree do you have items representing behavioral addictions (including, but not limited to, sex addiction)?

HOW DO I TREAT IT?

The treatment of sex addiction, like other forms of addiction, is multifaceted. Counselors and clients will need to determine if residential, intensive outpatient, or outpatient treatment is most advisable, and whether family counseling or couples counseling should be included in the process. Rather than a quick fix, Carnes (1991) noted that the recovery process for sex addiction can span 3 to 5 years. Along with abstaining from compulsive sexual behaviors, clients need to address attachment ruptures, childhood trauma, shame, emotion dysregulation, and develop new, adaptive ways of coping with life's adversities. Treatment usually begins with a period of abstinence from all sexual stimulation so that the dysregulated reward system in the brain can begin to heal and return to baseline. Weiss (2015) wrote, "In much the same way that drug detox is a first step toward recovery from a substance addiction, this short period of complete sexual abstinence—a 'detox' from addictive sex—is a first step toward recovery" (p. 130).

Without sexual behavior as a means of regulating affect, clients will need to cultivate alternative coping strategies for negative mood states. It is at this point that the client may be in heightened risk of developing a new addictive behavior such as gambling, eating, substance use, internet gaming, or non-suicidal self-injury to manage emotions (Weiss, 2015). Indeed, multiple addictions are the norm rather than the exception among those with sex addiction. In the study of clients with sexual disorders (both sexual anorexia and sex addiction), Carnes et al. (2005) found that 69% of heterosexual men, 80% of homosexual men, and 79% of heterosexual women met criteria for another addiction (e.g., substance use, compulsive spending, compulsive eating, compulsive working, compulsive gambling). These researchers posited that "addictions do more than coexist. They in fact interact, reinforce, and become part of one another" (Carnes et al., 2005, p. 87). Rather than addressing each addiction separately, counselors are encouraged to address the addictions simultaneously as a unit of interacting behaviors (Carnes et al., 2005).

Along with multiple addictions, clients with sex addiction often also have co-occurring mental health disorders such as depression, phobias, anxiety, and personality disorders (Kaplan & Krueger, 2010). In the study of German therapists specializing in sex addiction, researchers found that female clients with sex addiction often had anxiety or eating disorders and male clients with sex addiction often had substance use disorders and sexual dysfunctions (Briken et al., 2007). Moreover, Raymond et al. (2003) interviewed 24 individuals with sex addiction and discovered that 88% met criteria for a current axis I disorder (i.e., 42% anxiety disorder, 33% mood disorder, 25% impulse-control disorder, 4% eating disorder) and 46% met criteria for a current axis II disorder. Therefore, counselors must be prepared to address both co-occurring disorders and multiple addictions in their treatment of sex addiction.

VOICES FROM THE FIELD: Clinical Work With Sex Addiction

Working with clients with sex addiction is full of paradox for me; it is simultaneously endlessly rewarding and frustrating. Clients with sex addiction desperately want to be known and are also desperately afraid of being seen. They lie to others, yet they often do not realize that the person they lie to, and hide from, the most is actually themselves. Helping clients break through the crippling denial and shame can be painfully slow and maddening for counselors, but once the breakthrough happens—the rewards are beyond anything else I have ever experienced in all my years of counseling.

There are several things that can help counselors be successful in their work with clients with sex addiction. First and foremost, counselors need a solid poker face. They will hear things they have never heard of before and they must respond with empathy. I have stopped saying, "I've heard everything, you can't shock me," because clients still do—but I have developed an amazing poker face! Second, counselors need patience—lots and lots of patience—when working with sex addiction. The recovery process takes time. Third, counselors need an overwhelming amount of compassion and curiosity for their clients. Fourth, they need to have the ability to confront clients and highlight discrepancies caused by their addiction. Fifth, counselors need a deep understanding of trauma and possess the skills necessary to help those with sex addiction process the overwhelming amounts of trauma they have experienced.

Treatment for sex addiction also involves addressing clients' toxic shame. Toxic shame is the most crippling and isolating emotion in the known universe. When counselors can shake shame loose from their clients with sex addiction, their clients begin to find freedom and the ability to form healthy emotional attachments—which is what they have wanted from the beginning.

My hope for counselors working with sex addiction is that they understand this is a very specific disease. It is in clients' best interest to work with someone with specific training in the treatment of sex addiction. If there is no one in the counselor's area who has this training, I strongly recommend pursuing certification as a Certified Sex Addiction Therapist (CSAT).

Tal Prince, LPC, CSAT, NCC; Director, Insights Counseling Center, Birmingham, AL

CARNES'S 30-TASK MODEL

A popular component of sex addiction treatment is the task model developed by Patrick Carnes. Based on his research, Carnes (2005) developed a list of 30 recovery tasks to guide sex addiction treatment and long-term recovery. These tasks include understanding sexual addiction, involvement in a 12-step program, grieving losses, financial planning, addressing family issues, restoring healthy sexual behaviors, and cultivating a spiritual life, among others (Carnes, 2005). Carnes has written several workbooks (e.g., *Facing the Shadow* and *Recovery Zone,* Volume 1) that counselors and clients can use to work through the recovery tasks of the model. Each task corresponds with performables (i.e., concrete actions) for clients to carry out. For example, the fifth task, *establish sobriety,* is accompanied by performables including writing sobriety statements (e.g., defining abstinence), completing relapse prevention plans and contracts, and establishing a sobriety date (Carnes, 2005). The 30-task model can provide a helpful structure for counselors and clients to utilize in the treatment of sex addiction.

ATTACHMENT AND EMOTION REGULATION WORK

Attachment ruptures and childhood trauma exist in the histories of many clients with sex addiction, which lead to difficulties in emotion regulation (Katehakis, 2009; Riemersma & Sytsma, 2013). Therefore, both attachment work and emotion regulation enhancement strategies are necessary components of sex addiction treatment (Katehakis, 2009). When addressing attachment issues, Bowlby (1988) suggested that counselors work to provide a secure base from which the client can explore potentially painful past and present experiences. The concept of a secure base entails being emotionally responsive, aware of clients' experiences, available, and sensitive to clients' needs. As a secure base, counselors can encourage clients to explore the nature of their relationships, including their expectations and belief about themselves and how others will treat them (thus uncovering clients' working models of self and attachment figures). Next, counselors can help clients become aware of how their working models influence their current relationships. As clients gain insight into the origin of their working models, they can recognize the effects of those models on their current relationships and attachments with others. In light of this awareness, clients can assess the accuracy of the models and replace them with new, adaptive perceptions of themselves and others (Bowlby, 1988). This type of attachment work can be conducted in both individual and group counseling with clients with sex addiction. A benefit of group counseling is that it allows the counselor to witness how clients interact with others and the opportunity to provide immediate feedback. Additionally, sex addiction is marked by isolation and secrecy; therefore, group counseling allows clients to be known by others who have shared similar experiences and can challenge the clients' hidden, distorted beliefs.

With regard to emotion regulation work, Katehakis (2009) suggested that neuroaffective treatment could be helpful for those with sex addiction. Specifically, neuroaffective treatment includes: (a) an initial assessment in which the counselor identifies the client's attachment style and extent of parental attunement in early childhood, (b) early interventions including the formation of a strong therapeutic alliance marked by the counselor's attunement to the client's experience, (c) intermediate interventions including interactive regulation of the client's emotions, and (d) tailoring clinical interventions to match the client's attachment style and engagement in affect regulation strategies (e.g., awareness of bodily reactions and sensations, tracking affect, identifying and expressing emotions, applying self-soothing strategies, and increasing self-regulation; Katehakis, 2009). With regard to affect regulation, Adams and Robinson (2002) noted that an individual with sex addiction "does not succeed in developing the ability to identify, differentiate, and express emotion" (p. 76). Therefore, counselors working with sex addicted clients must help them "bridge the gap" between their emotions and behaviors (Adams & Robinson, 2002, p. 76). Specifically, counselors can aid clients in the recognition of their emotions by increasing awareness of their internal states and cultivating appropriate responses to those internal states (Adams & Robinson, 2002). Thus, both attachment and emotion regulation work are integral to sex addiction treatment.

12-STEP SUPPORT

Several 12-step fellowships exist for those with sex addiction. Among them is SAA, founded in 1977. SAA offers in-person, online, and phone meetings to help those with sex addiction find recovery in community. The only requirement for membership is a desire to end compulsive sexual acting out. SAA follows the 12 steps of Alcoholics Anonymous with the first step stating, "We admitted we were powerless over addictive sexual behavior—that our lives had become unmanageable" (International Service Organization of SAA, Inc., 2005, p. 20). SAA is open to all genders and sexual orientations with approximately 1,900 meetings in 33 countries (International Service Organization of SAA, Inc., 2019). A recent survey of SAA members revealed that 30.26% of members were introduced to SAA by a mental health professional, which was the most frequently reported referral source (International Service Organization of SAA, Inc., 2019). SAA developed a 12-item questionnaire to help individuals determine if they have a sex addiction. Items on the questionnaire include: *Have your sexual practices caused you legal problems* and *Does your preoccupation with sexual fantasies cause problems in any area of your life—even when you do not act out your fantasies* (International Service Organization of SAA, Inc., 2015). Endorsing two or more of the items may be indicative of sexual addiction. The questionnaire has some empirical support as researchers have found that it could correctly distinguish between those with sex addiction, sexual offenders, and participants from the general community (Mercer, 1998).

Oftentimes, those with behavioral addictions have questions about the definition of abstinence or sobriety. For example, are they expected to abstain from all sexual activity for the rest of their lives? SAA clarifies the concept of abstinence by positing that each individual member is responsible for determining their own definition of sexual sobriety. To do this, members and sponsors often use the Three Circles technique (International Service Organization of SAA, Inc., 2000). This technique includes drawing three concentric circles and listing all compulsive, sexual behaviors in the innermost circle. These are the sexual acts over which the member has lost control and desires to abstain, such as compulsive masturbation, pornography use, hiring prostitutes, anonymous sex, or using hook-up apps. Abstaining from inner circle behaviors constitutes sexual sobriety. The middle circle contains any behavior that could lead to inner circle behaviors. These behaviors are neither ideal nor addictive, but should be closely monitored. Middle circle behaviors can include acting seductively, contacting old sexual partners, cruising for sexual partners, specific forms of sexual fantasy, isolating from others, substance use, or viewing movies with graphic sexual scenes. Engaging in a middle circle behavior is not a relapse, but, instead, is considered a warning sign that a member is nearing inner circle behaviors. When they engage in a middle circle behavior, the member should take steps to seek support by talking to a sponsor, attending an SAA meeting, engaging in spiritual practices, or enacting another component of their recovery plan. Finally, the outer circle contains healthy behaviors that support the member's recovery goals. Outer circle behaviors can include nonsexual friendships and relationships, SAA involvement and working the 12 steps, consensual sex within the bounds of a meaningful, committed relationship, respectful dating practices, developing nonsexual hobbies and activities, and supporting other SAA members. The Three Circles technique is foundational to defining sexual sobriety and fostering relapse prevention strategies (International Service Organization of SAA, Inc., 2000).

Leaders and members of SAA are dedicated to working with counselors and mental health professionals to best serve those with sex addiction. SAA offers a variety of resources for counselors including client referral packets, literature about the program, information related to events, retreats, workshops, and conventions, and telephone support. You can learn more about SAA by visiting their website (saa-recovery.org).

DIAGNOSTIC CONSIDERATIONS

Given that hypersexual disorder was not included in the *DSM-5*, clinicians must utilize other diagnostic criteria if a diagnosis is necessary. Some practitioners may use the compulsive sexual behavior code of the *ICD-11*. Alternatively, given the frequency of co-occurring disorders and comorbid addictions (Briken et al., 2007; Carnes, 1991), clinicians often choose to diagnose the co-occurring mental health concern (e.g., major depressive disorder, alcohol use disorder, bulimia nervosa, adjustment disorder with depressed mood), if applicable. Kafka (2014) also suggested the use of the diagnostic code for other specified disruptive, impulse-control, and conduct disorders with the specifier of hypersexual disorder.

HOW CAN I LEARN MORE?

Counselors who would like more training in sex addiction are encouraged to consider pursuing the Certified Sex Addiction Therapist (CSAT) credential. Information related to CSAT certification can be found on the website for the International Institute for Trauma and Addiction Professionals (iitap.com/page/csat). Additionally, the following are helpful books, articles, and websites to increase your knowledge related to sex addiction.

BOOKS

- Carnes, P. (2001). *Out of the shadows: Understanding sexual addiction* (3rd ed.). Hazelden.
- Carnes, P. (2005). *Facing the shadow: Starting sexual and relationship recovery* (2nd ed). Gentle Path Press.
- Weiss, R. (2015). *Sex addiction 101: A basic guide to healing from sex, porn, and love addiction.* Health Communications.

PEER-REVIEWED ARTICLES

- Carnes, P. J., Murray, R. E., & Charpentier, L. (2005). Bargains with chaos: Sex addicts and addiction interaction disorder. *Sexual Addiction and Compulsivity, 12,* 79–120. https://doi.org/10.1080/10720160500201371
- Hall, P. (2011). A biopsychosocial view of sex addiction. *Sexual and Relationship Therapy, 26,* 217–228. https://doi.org/10.1080/14681994.2011.628310
- Katehakis, A. (2009). Affective neuroscience and the treatment of sexual addiction. *Sexual Addiction and Compulsivity, 16,* 1–31. https://doi.org/10.1080/10720160802708966
- Rosenberg, K. P., Carnes, P., & O'Connor, S. (2014). Evaluation and treatment of sex addiction. *Journal of Sex and Marital Therapy, 40,* 77–91. https://doi.org/10.1080/0092623X.2012.701268

WEBSITES

- International Institute for Trauma and Addiction Professionals (IITAP): iitap.com
- Recovery Zone: recoveryzone.com
- Sex Addicts Anonymous (SAA): saa-recovery.org

REFERENCES

Adams, K. M., & Robinson, D. W. (2002). Shame reduction, affect regulation, and sexual boundary development: Essential building blocks of sexual addiction treatment. In P. J. Carnes & K. M. Adams (Eds.), *Clinical management of sex addiction* (pp. 67–88). Brunner-Routledge.

Ainsworth, M. D. S., & Bell, S. M. (1970). Attachment, exploration, and separation: Illustrated by the behavior of one-year-olds in a strange situation. *Child Development, 41,* 49–67. https://doi.org/10.2307/1127388

Ainsworth, M. D. S., Blehar, M. C., Waters, E., & Wall, S. N. (1978). *Patterns of attachment: A psychological study of the strange situation.* Erlbaum.

American Psychiatric Association. (2013). *Diagnostic and statistical manual of mental disorders* (5th ed.). Author.

Benfield, J. (2018). Secure attachment: An antidote to sex addiction? A thematic analysis of therapists' experiences of utilizing attachment-informed treatment strategies to address sexual compulsivity. *Sexual Addiction and Compulsivity, 25,* 12–27. https://doi.org/10.1080/10720162.2018.1462746

Blum, K., Cull, J. G., Braverman, E. R., & Comings, D. E. (1996). Reward deficiency syndrome. *American Scientist, 84,* 132–146.

Blum, K., Oscar-Berman, M., Demetrovics, Z., Barh, D., & Gold, M. S. (2014). Genetic addiction risk score (GARS): Molecular neurogenetic evidence for predisposition to reward deficiency syndrome (RDS). *Molecular Neurobiology, 50,* 765–796. https://doi.org/10.1007/s12035-014-8726-5

Blum, K., Werner, T., Carnes, S., Carnes, P., Bowirrat, A. Giordano, J., Oscar-Berman, M., & Gold, M. (2012). Sex, drugs, and rock 'n' roll: Hypothesizing common mesolimbic activation as a function of reward gene polymorphisms. *Journal of Psychoactive Drugs, 44,* 38–55. https://doi.org/10.1080/02791072.2012.662112

Bowlby, J. (1978). Attachment theory and its therapeutic implication. *Adolescent Psychiatry, 6,* 5–33.

Bowlby, J. (1988). *A secure base.* Routledge.

Briken, P., Habermann, N., Berner, W., & Hill, A. (2007). Diagnosis and treatment of sexual addiction: A survey among German sex therapists. *Sexual Addiction and Compulsivity, 14,* 131–143. https://doi.org/10.1080/10720160701310450

Burke Harris, N. (2018). *The deepest well: Healing the long-term effects of childhood adversity.* Bluebird.

Carnes, P. (1989). *Contrary to love: Helping the sexual addict.* CompCare Publishers.

Carnes, P. (1991). *Don't call it love: Recovery from sexual addiction.* Bantam Books.

Carnes, P. (1997). *Sexual anorexia: Overcoming sexual self-hatred.* Hazeldon.

Carnes, P. (2001). *Out of the shadows: Understanding sexual addiction* (3rd ed.). Hazeldon.

Carnes, P. (2005). *Facing the shadow: Starting sexual and relationship recovery* (2nd ed.). Gentle Path.

Carnes, P., Green, B., & Carnes, S. (2010). The same yet different: Refocusing the sexual addiction Screening Test (SAST) to reflect orientation and gender. *Sexual Addiction and Compulsivity, 17,* 7–30. https://doi.org/10.1080/10720161003604084

Carnes, P. J., Green, B. A., Merlo, L. J., Polles, A., Carnes, S., & Gold, M. S. (2012). PATHOS: A brief screening application for assessing sexual addiction. *Journal of Addiction Medicine, 6,* 29–34. https://doi.org/10.1097/ADM.ob013e313182251a28

Carnes, P. J., Murray, R. E., & Charpentier, L. (2005). Bargains with chaos: Sex addicts and addiction interaction disorder. *Sexual Addiction and Compulsivity, 12,* 79–120. https://doi.org/10.1080/10720160500201371

Cashwell, C. S., Giordano, A. L., King, K., Lankford, C., & Henson, R. K. (2017). Emotion regulation and sex addiction among college students. *International Journal of Mental Health and Addiction, 15,* 16–27. https://doi.org/10.1007/s11469-016-9646-6

Cashwell, C. S., Giordano, A. L., Lewis, T. F., Wachtel, K. A., & Bartley, J. L. (2015). Using the PATHOS questionnaire for screening sexual addiction among college students: A preliminary exploration. *Sexual Addiction and Compulsivity, 22,* 154–166. https://doi.org/10.1080/10720162.2015.1037481

Chatzittofis, A., Arver, S., Oberg, K., Hallberg, J., Nordstrom, P., & Jokinen, J. (2016). HPA axis dysregulation in men with hypersexual disorder. *Psychoneuroendocrinology, 63,* 247–253. https://doi.org/10.1016/j.psyneuen.2015.10.002

Comings, D. E., & Blum, K. (2000). Reward deficiency syndrome: Genetic aspects of behavioral disorders. *Progress in Brain Research, 126,* 325–341. https://doi.org/10.1016/S0079-6123(00)26022-6

Crocker, M. M. (2015). Out-of-control sexual behavior as a symptom of insecure attachment in men. *Journal of Social Work Practice in the Addictions, 15,* 373–393. https://doi.org/10.1080/1533256X.2015.1091000

Delmonico, D. L., & Griffin, E. (1997). Classifying problematic sexual behavior: A working model. *Sexual Addiction and Compulsivity, 4,* 91–104. https://doi.org/10.1080/10720169708400133

Deneke, E., Knepper, C., Green, B. A., & Carnes, P. J. (2015). Comparative study of three levels of care in a substance use disorder inpatient facility on risk for sexual addiction. *Sexual Addiction and Compulsivity, 22,* 109–125. https://doi.org/10.1080/10720162.2014.979382

Engel, J., Veit, M, Sinke, C., Heitland, I, Kneer, J., Hillemacher, T., Hartmann, U., & Kruger, T. H. C. (2019). Same same but different: A clinical characterization of men with hypersexual disorder in the sex@brain study. *Journal of Clinical Medicine, 8,* 157. https://doi.org/10.3390/jcm8020157

Faisandier, K. M., Taylor, J. E., & Salisbury, R. M. (2012). What does attachment have to do with out-of-control sexual behavior? *New Zealand Journal of Psychology, 41,* 19–29.

Felitti, V. J., Anda, R. F., Nordenberg, D., Williamson, D. F., Spitz, A. M., Edwards, V., Koss, M. P., & Marks, J. S. (1998). Relationship of childhood abuse and household dysfunction to many of the leading causes of death in adults: The Adverse Childhood Experiences (ACE) study. *American Journal of Preventive Medicine, 14,* 245–258. https://doi.org/10.1016/S0749-3797(98)00017-8

Ferree, M. C. (2001). Females and sex addiction: Myths and diagnostic implications. *Sexual Addiction and Compulsivity, 8,* 287–300. https://doi.org/10.1080/107201601753459973

Gilliland, R., South, M., Carpenter, B. N., & Hardy, S. A. (2011). The roles of shame and guilt in hypersexual behavior. *Sexual Addiction and Compulsivity, 18,* 12–29. https://doi.org/10.1080/10720162.2011.551182

Giordano, A. L., & Cashwell, C. S. (2018). An examination of college counselors' work with student sex addiction: Training, screening, and referrals. *Journal of College Counseling, 21,* 43–57. https://doi.org/10.1002/jocc.12086

Giordano, A. L., Cashwell, C. S., Lankford, C., King, K., & Henson, R. (2017). Collegiate sexual addiction: Exploring religious coping and attachment. *Journal of Counseling and Development, 95*, 135–144. https://doi.org/10.1002/jcad.12126

Giordano, A. L., & Cecil, A. L. (2014). Religious coping, spirituality, and hypersexual behavior among college students. *Sexual Addiction and Compulsivity, 21*, 225–239. https://doi.org/10.1080/10720162.2014.936542

Giordano, A. L., Prosek, E. A., Cecil, A. L., & Brown, J. (2015). Predictors of hypersexual behavior among college men and women: Exploring self-conscious emotions. *Journal of Addictions and Offender Counseling, 36*, 113–125. https://doi.org/10.1002/jaoc.12007

Gold, M. S., Blum, K., Febo, M., McLaughlin, T., Cronje, F. J., & Han, D. (2014). Hatching the behavioral addiction egg: Reward deficiency solution system (RDSS) as a function of dopaminergic neurogenetics and brain functional connectivity linking all addictions under a common rubric. *Journal of Behavioral Addictions, 3*, 149–156. https://doi.org/10.556/JBA.3.2014.019

Goodman, A. (1993). Diagnosis and treatment of sexual addiction. *Journal of Sex and Marital Therapy, 19*, 225–251. https://doi.org/10.1080/00926239308404908

Grant, J. E., & Steinberg, M. A. (2005). Compulsive sexual behavior and pathological gambling. *Sexual Addiction & Compulsivity, 12*, 235–244. https://doi.org/10.1080/10720160500203856

Hagedorn, B. W., & Juhnke, G. A. (2005). Treating the sexually addicted client: Establishing a need for increased counselor awareness. *Journal of Addiction and Offender Counseling, 25*, 66–86. https://doi.org/10.1002/j.2161-1874.2005.tb00194.x

Hall, P. (2011). A biopsychosocial view of sex addiction. *Sexual and Relationship Therapy, 26*, 217–228. https://doi.org/10.1080/14681994.2011.628310

International Service Organization of SAA, Inc. (2000). *Three circles: Defining sexual sobriety in S.A.A.* https://saa-recovery.org/literature/three-circles-defining-sexual-sobriety-in-saa

International Service Organization of SAA, Inc. (2005). *Sex addicts anonymous.* https://saa-recovery.org/literature/sex-addicts-anonymous-green-book-saas-basic-text

International Service Organization of SAA, Inc. (2015). *Getting started in sex addicts anonymous: A beginner's packet for recovering sex addicts.* https://saa-recovery.org/literature/getting-started-in-sex-addicts-anonymous-a-beginners-packet-for-recovering-sex-addicts

International Service Organization of SAA, Inc. (2019). *Sex addicts anonymous: 2019 membership survey.* https://saa-iso.org/docs/survey/SAA-2019-SurveyResults.pdf

Kafka, M. P. (2010). Hypersexual disorder: A proposed diagnosis for DSM-V. *Archives of Sexual Behavior, 39*, 377–400. https://doi.org/10.1007/s10508-009-9574-7

Kafka, M. P. (2014). What happened to hypersexual disorder? *Archives of Sexual Behavior, 43*, 1259–1261. https://doi.org/10.1007/s10508-014-0326-y

Kalichman, S. C., Johnson, J. R., Adair, V., Rompa, D., Multhauf, K., & Kelly, J. A. (1994). Sexual sensation seeking: Scale development and predicting AIDS-risk behavior among homosexually active men. *Journal of Personality Assessment, 62*, 385–397. https://doi.org/10.1207/s15327752jpa6203_1

Kalichman, S. C., & Rompa, D. (1995). Sexual sensation seeking and sexual compulsivity scales: Validity, and predicting HIV risk behavior. *Journal of Personality Assessment, 65*, 586–601. https://doi.org/10.1207/s15327752jpa6503_16

Kalichman, S. C., & Rompa, D. (2001). The sexual compulsivity scale: Further development and use with HIV-positive persons. *Journal of Personality Assessment, 76*, 379–395. https://doi.org/10.1207/S15327752JPA7603_02

Kaplan, M. S., & Krueger, R. B. (2010). Diagnosis, assessment, and treatment of hypersexuality. *Journal of Sex Research, 47*, 181–198. https://doi.org/10.1080/00224491003592863

Karila, L., Wery, A., Weinstein, A., Cottencin, O., Petit, A., Reynaud, M., & Billieux, J. (2014). Sexual addiction or hypersexual disorder: Different terms for the same problem? A review of the literature. *Current Pharmaceutical Design, 20*, 4012–4020. https://doi.org/10.2174/13816128113199990619

Katehakis, A. (2009). Affective neuroscience and the treatment of sexual addiction. *Sexual Addiction and Compulsivity, 16*, 1–31. https://doi.org/10.1080/10720160802708966

Kotera, Y., & Rhondes, C. (2019). Pathways to sex addiction: Relationships with adverse childhood experience, attachment, narcissism, self-compassion, and motivation in a gender-balanced sample. *Sexual Addiction and Compulsivity, 26*, 54–76. https://doi.org/10.1080/10720162.2019.1615585

Langstrom, N., & Hanson, R. K. (2006). High rates of sexual behavior in the general population: Correlates and predictors. *Archives of Sexual Behavior, 35*, 37–52. https://doi.org/10.1007/s10508-006-8993-y

Lewis, H. B. (1971). *Shame and guilt in neurosis*. International Universities Press.

Marshall, L. E., Marshall, W. L., Moulden, H. M., & Serran, G. A. (2008). The prevalence of sexual addiction in incarcerated sexual offenders and matched community nonoffenders. *Sexual Addiction and Compulsivity, 15*, 271–283. https://doi.org/10.1080/10720160802516328

McPherson, S., Clayton, S., Wood, H., Hiskey, S., & Andrews, L. (2013). The role of childhood experiences in the development of sexual compulsivity. *Sexual Addiction and Compulsivity, 20*, 259–278. https://doi.org/10.1080/10720162.2013.803213

Mercer, J. T. (1998). Assessment of the sex Addicts anonymous questionnaire: Differentiating between the general population, sex addicts, and sex offenders. *Sexual Addiction and Compulsivity, 5*, 107–117. https://doi.org/10.1080/10720169808400153

Nakazawa, D. J. (2015). *Childhood disrupted: How your biography becomes your biology, and how you can heal*. Atria.

Pargament, K. I., & Abu-Raiya, H. (2007). A decade of research on the psychology of religion and coping: Things we assumed and lessons we learned. *Psyche and Logos, 28*, 742–766.

Raymond, N. C., Coleman, E., & Miner, M. H. (2003). Psychiatric comorbidity and compulsive/impulsive traits in compulsive sexual behavior. *Comprehensive Psychiatry, 44*, 370–380. https://doi.org/10.1016/S0010-440X(03)00110-X

Reid, R. C., Carpenter, B. N., Hook, J. N., Garos, S., Manning, J. C., Gilliland, R., & Fong, T. (2012). Report of findings in a DSM-5 field trial for hypersexual disorder. *Journal of Sexual Medicine, 9*, 2868–2877. https://doi.org/10.1111/j.1743-6109.2012.02936.x

Reid, R. C., Garos, S., & Carpenter, B. N. (2011). Reliability, validity, and psychometric development of the Hypersexual Behavior Inventory in an outpatient sample of men. *Sexual Addiction and Compulsivity, 18*, 30–51. https://doi.org/10.1080/10720162.2011.555709

Reid, R. C., Karim, R., McCrory, E., & Carpenter, B. N. (2010). Self-reported differences on measures of executive function and hypersexual behavior in a patient and community sample of men. *International Journal of Neuroscience, 120*, 120–127. https://doi.org/10.3109/00207450903165577

Riemersma, J., & Sytsma, M. (2013). A new generation of sexual addiction. *Sexual Addiction and Compulsivity, 20*, 306–322. https://doi.org/10.1080/10720162.2013.843067

Schneider, J. P. (1999). New paradigms for treating sex offenders. *Sexual Addiction and Compulsivity, 6*, 267–269. https://doi.org/10.1080/10720169908400196

Tangney, J. P., & Dearing, R. L. (2002). *Shame and guilt*. Guilford Press.

van der Kolk, B. A. (2014). *The body keeps the score: Brain, mind, and body in the healing of trauma*. Penguin Books.

Weiss, R. (2015). *Sex addiction 101: A basic guide to healing from sex, porn, and love addiction*. Health Communications Inc.

World Health Organization. (2018). *International statistical classification of diseases and related health problems* (11th Rev.). https://icd.who.int/browse11/l-m/en

Zapf, J. L., Greiner, J., & Carroll, J. (2008). Attachment styles and male sex addiction. *Sexual Addiction and Compulsivity, 15*, 158–175. https://doi.org/10.1080/10720160802035832

6

Pornography and Cybersex Addiction

HOW DO I CONCEPTUALIZE IT?

Sexual material on the internet can take a variety of forms ranging from educational information about sexual practices to real-time, virtual sex shows. Doring (2009) identified six realms of *online sexual behavior*: (a) pornography (sexually stimulating material), (b) sex shops (purchasing sexual toys and materials), (c) sex work (live online broadcasting of sexual activity or marketing offline sex work), (d) sex education (information related to sex), (e) sex contacts (finding partners for cybersex activities or offline sexual activities in chat rooms, games, dating apps, and other online communities), and (f) sexual subcultures (connecting with others with similar sexual preferences). Some forms of online sexual behavior can be utilized in healthy ways, while others have the potential to become addictive for a portion of users, constituting cybersex addiction. Specifically, *cybersex* refers to all sexual activity conducted via the internet or with the use of a computer or mobile device (Carnes, 2007; Jones & Tuttle, 2012). Although pornography is one type of cybersex, several other forms exist. Carnes (2007) identified additional cybersex categories as: (a) real-time partnered sexual acts, (b) other cybersex venues (sexual activity facilitated by social networking sites, dating apps, internet games), and (c) multimedia software (watching erotic content on a computer offline via shared files).

Pornography use is arguably the most common form of cybersex and is a massive global industry. Although difficult to define, many scholars agree that at the most basic level, pornography is any sexually arousing material used as a sexual outlet (Carroll et al., 2017; Grubbs et al., 2019; Maltz & Maltz, 2008). Pornographic material can include sexually explicit photographs in magazines, movies, internet images or online audio, webcam footage, computer generated pornography, and sexually explicit pictures texted via mobile devices. Furthermore, with the emergence of virtual reality (VR) came the arrival of VR porn, which creates unique experiences from two-dimensional pornography (Elsey et al., 2019). Pornography can be classified as softcore (simulations of sexual acts, nude images), hardcore (real sexual behaviors), and illegal/deviant (e.g., sexual acts with children or animals, fetishist, rape, and violence; Doring, 2009).

With the advent of the internet, new pornographic material can be continuously accessed, with an unending supply of novel subjects and behaviors. Indeed, decades ago, Cooper (1998) referred to the internet as the *Triple A Engine* for fueling pornography and cybersex given that it is anonymous, easily accessible, and affordable. According to data reported by the free pornography website, Pornhub, 92 million internet users visit the site each day (Pornhub Insights, 2018). In 2018, the site had 33.5 billion visits with over 207,000 pornographic videos watched each minute (Pornhub Insights, 2018). Moreover, statistics released by another free site, YouPorn, reported 4 billion visits to the site in 2018 with 14 billion pornographic videos viewed (YouPorn, 2020). The growing use of pornography has been recognized by many state legislatures. As of the date of this publication, 17 of the 50 U.S. states have passed resolutions declaring pornography a public health crisis (Nelson & Rothman, 2020). Furthermore, it appears that pornography users themselves have become concerned by their use as evidenced by the development of recovery websites such as RebootNation.org and NoFap.com complete with videos, discussion forums, and advice related to the cessation of pornography use.

Pornography and cybersex addiction are components of the broader term, *sex addiction* (Chapter 5), yet have some distinctions (Griffiths, 2012). Riemersma and Sytsma (2013) differentiated *classic sex addiction* (often corresponding with early trauma and insecure attachment) from *contemporary sex addiction* (often corresponding with early exposure to internet pornography). The authors noted that early pornography exposure among those with contemporary sex addiction affects both the reward circuitry in the brain and the individual's arousal template, which may lead to recurrent pornography-seeking behaviors (even in the absence of early trauma or attachment ruptures). Thus, classic and contemporary sex addiction can evolve from different preceding events and entail distinct motivations, and, consequently, treatment strategies for the two types of sex addiction may differ. While the treatment for classic sex addiction often entails trauma and attachment work, treatment for contemporary sex addiction often entails enhancing clients' interpersonal skills and altering clients' relationship with cybersex and pornography to restore neurochemical balance (Riemersma & Sytsma, 2013).

ADOLESCENT PORNOGRAPHY USE AND SEXTING

Given the affordability, accessibility, and anonymity provided by the internet (Cooper, 1998), it is not surprising that children and teens are being exposed (either intentionally or unintentionally) to pornography. Indeed, researchers found the average age of first pornography exposure was approximately 12 years (Kraus & Rosenberg, 2014). Moreover, among a nationally representative sample of 2,227 men and women, participants reported age of first pornography exposure to be 13.8 for men and 17.8 for women (Herbenick et al., 2020). In addition, among a nationally representative sample of over 600 American adolescents (ages 14–18), researchers found that 68.4% had viewed pornography (Wright et al., 2020). There appear to be specific strategies utilized by some pornography companies to attract young users to their sites. Specifically, the act of *cybersquatting*, or using domain names that can easily be mistaken for those of other trademark owners, has been used to funnel young internet users to pornographic websites. For example, in the past, pornography companies have taken on names associated with children's toys (e.g., Barbiesplaypen.com), which may cause accidental exposure among youth (DiSabatino, 2000). In the case of Barbiesplaypen.com, Mattel (a toy manufacturing company) won a case on trademark infringement against the pornography site forcing it to shut down (DiSabatino, 2000).

Another consideration related to youth and pornography is the act of *sexting*, or sending sexually explicit images (nude or seminude) to another person via one's smartphone or electronic device (Delmonico et al., 2017; Hasinoff, 2015). A review of 18 empirical studies of sexting practices among youth (10–18 years of age) revealed prevalence rates of active sexting (creating, posting, sending, or showing sexual texts) ranging from 0.9% to 27.6% across samples (Barrense-Dias et al., 2017). Moreover, a meta-analysis of 39 studies (totaling 110,380 participants) examining sexting among youth (younger than 18 years of age) found that 14% of the sample sent a sexual image, 27.4% received a sexual image, and 12% forwarded a sexual image without the sender's consent (Madigan et al., 2018).

Although some consider sexting a developmentally appropriate act among teenagers in a digital age, or a natural consequence of socialization in a highly sexualized society, others contend that sharing sexual images is distribution (and/or possession) of child pornography (if the subject of the image is a minor and the image is explicit) and thus, a criminal behavior (Barrense-Dias et al., 2017; Hasinoff, 2015; Lee & Darcy, 2020; Lorang et al., 2016). Indeed, minors engaged in sexting have been prosecuted and have faced civil and criminal charges, including registering as sex offenders (Lorang et al., 2016). It also has been argued that child pornography laws were not written for cases of consensual sexting among adolescents, and thus their application to sexting cases may be unreasonable (Lee & Darcy, 2020; Zhang, 2010). Several states have developed, or are in the process of developing, legislation specific to sexting, yet "the content of the current statutes demonstrates that there is no legal consensus" (Lorang et al., 2016, p. 75). While policies and regulations related to sexting evolve to catch up with technology, controversy still exists regarding the best response to reports of sexting, particularly among student populations. Rather than assuming sexting is a homogeneous act, some scholars argue that the nature, intent, and motives of sexting should be considered when determining the appropriate response (e.g., Was sexting consensual, coerced, or malicious?; Delmonico et al., 2017; Hasinoff, 2015; Lee & Darcy, 2020). Indeed, sexting behaviors can range from sharing sexual images with another consenting person (i.e., consensual sexting), sending sexual images to nonconsenting persons (i.e., nonconsensual sexting), or distributing sexual images without permission (e.g., creating sexual images of someone who is unaware, receiving a sexual image, then forwarding it to others unbeknownst to the sender, cyberbullying acts to deliberately humiliate or harm another person by disseminating sexual images; Hasinoff, 2015). Therefore, assessing the motives and intent of the behavior can be a helpful starting place for counselors working with clients who report sexting. Additionally, it is important to assess whether an adult was involved in cases of adolescent sexting (e.g., requesting images, taking pictures), as this has legal implications and should be reported.

School counselors, or counselors working with child or adolescent populations, should be familiar with the laws, statutes, and regulations of both their state and clinical or school setting to determine how to respond to students or clients who engage in sexting. One example of legislation is the *Jessica Logan Act* related to antibullying policies in public schools, which was signed into law in 2012 in Ohio. The legislation was developed in response to a high school student who committed suicide shortly after sexually explicit pictures of herself circulated around school, which led to subsequent bullying (Aldridge et al., 2013; Lorang et al., 2016). Thus, school counselors should be prepared to work with students who have sent sexual images, received sexual images, or forwarded sexual images without the owner's consent.

School counselors also may be involved in prevention planning or crisis teams to construct protocol for how to respond to sexting in their schools (Aldridge et al., 2013). In this role, it may be helpful for counselors to consult with law enforcement officials, lawyers, and state counseling associations to determine best practices for addressing sexting among minors. Additionally, educating students and families about the school's response to sexting cases may be an important role of school counselors. Overall, responding to adolescent clients who send sexually explicit images is a controversial and complicated issue. Delmonico et al. (2017) noted, "Clinicians should neither overreact nor underreact to youth sexting cases. Creating a trusting environment where youth can honestly discuss their thoughts, feelings, and behaviors related to sexting is the essential foundation for prevention at all levels" (pp. 80–81).

CLINICAL NOTE 6.1

Consider a situation in which your high school female client discloses sending nude images of herself to a male peer in her class. She then reports that the male peer sent the image to many other students and it has since been posted on social media and viewed hundreds of times. How might you respond to your client? What might this student need from you? What actions might you take in response to this situation?

PREVALENCE OF PORNOGRAPHY AND CYBERSEX ADDICTION

Data reveal that pornography and cybersex use is common in today's society. Among a sample of over 2,000 adult internet users in the United States, 70.4% reported viewing pornography at least one time (Grubbs et al., 2019). Additionally, data from a 2014 survey revealed that 40% of American men (aged 18–23) and 19% of women (aged 18–23) used pornography in the previous week (Regnerus et al., 2016). Furthermore, in the study of 2,690 college students from four countries, 30.8% reported being engaged in real-time partnered cybersex at some point in their lives (Doring et al., 2017).

Like other rewarding behaviors, simply engaging in pornography use or cybersex does not constitute addiction. Instead, Jones and Tuttle (2012) described three types of cybersex users: (a) recreational users (prefer offline sexual activity but occasionally use cybersex), (b) at-risk users (use cybersex as a primary coping strategy), and (c) sexually addicted users (loss of control, experience of negative consequences, failed attempts to cut back or stop). In light of the spectrum of cybersex use, coupled with the lack of a uniform definition of pornography and cybersex addiction, it is difficult to acquire consistent prevalence rates. For example, in the study of 339 college students, Giordano and Cashwell (2017) found that 10.3% met criteria for cybersex addiction. Additionally, Kraus et al. (2016) found that among 1,298 adult male pornography users, 27.7% met criteria for hypersexual disorder (Kafka, 2010). Finally, researchers asked adult internet users about their pornography use and 6.7% somewhat to strongly believed that they were addicted (Grubbs et al., 2019).

With regard to gender, researchers typically find that men use pornography and cybersex more than women (Doring et al., 2017; Herbenick et al., 2020; Hesse & Floyd, 2019; Wery & Billieux, 2017), yet important distinctions have been noted. Women more frequently engage in partnered cybersex (such as sexual text and video chats), while men engage in more solo cybersex (such as pornography use; Wery & Billieux, 2017). Additionally, in the study of cybersex partners, researchers found that men had significantly more cybersex experiences with strangers (rather than known partners) compared to women (Shaughnessy & Byers, 2014). Thus, both men and women can struggle with cybersex addiction and clinicians should inquire about a wide array of online sexual activities with their clients, rather than asking about pornography use only.

CLINICAL NOTE 6.2

In a recent study of 1,075 men and 1,152 women in the United States, researchers found that 94% of men and 87% of women viewed pornography at some point in their lifetimes (either intentionally or accidentally; Herbenick et al., 2020). Participants identified the most common means of accessing pornography was free pornography websites on their smartphones (Herbenick et al., 2020).

NEUROSCIENCE OF PORNOGRAPHY ADDICTION

Sex is a naturally rewarding activity, activating the release of several neurotransmitters such as dopamine during sexual arousal and endogenous opioids during sexual consummation (Doidge, 2007). This natural relationship between sexual activity and reward circuitry activation makes sense, given that partnered sexual activity is necessary for passing down genetic code and the continued survival of our species. The reward experienced during sexual activity encourages the continuation of the behavior (Christensen, 2017). Pornography use, however, does not contribute to survival, yet the activation of reward circuitry during use signals that it is important and should be repeated (Doidge, 2007; Wilson, 2014). Scholars have described pornography as a *supernormal stimulus*, or an artificial exaggeration of an evolutionarily developed instinct (Barrett, 2010; Hilton, 2013; Park et al., 2016). The term supernormal stimulus was first coined by Niko Tinberger, a researcher who found that male stickleback fish would ignore natural female stickleback fish to pursue artificial, exaggerated females (with rounder bellies; Barrett, 2010). Similarly, he discovered that birds would choose to care for fake, brightly colored eggs to the neglect of their own modestly colored eggs. Tinberger also found that male butterflies preferred exaggerated, cardboard butterflies over real female butterflies. Barrett (2010) noted, "The most interesting of Tinbergen's discoveries was that dummies could surpass the power of any natural stimuli" (p. 12).

These discoveries revealed much about the world around us. Any exaggerated, artificial creation that mimics a natural instinct, but is more concentrated or salient in its potency, can become a supernormal stimulus. Consider the way in which a piece of candy made with processed sugar can overpower the natural sweetness of a blueberry. Fast food and processed sugar products are supernormal stimuli that capitalize on our natural instincts for eating sweet and high-calorie food (Barrett, 2010). In the same way, pornography is an exaggerated, artificial creation that taps into our natural instinct for sexual activity. Pornographic videos and images can feature photoshopped or surgically enhanced individuals who are always available for sex and completely willing to perform a myriad of sexual behaviors—an artificial exaggeration of a natural sexual partner. Like the artificial brightly colored eggs, cardboard butterflies, or overly round stickleback fish of Tinberger's experiments, pornography can "surpass the power" of natural sexual stimuli, leading users to choose pornographic material over partnered sexual activity (Barrett, 2010, p. 12).

Indeed, as a supernormal stimulus, pornography elicits more reward pathway activation (specifically in the mesolimbic dopamine system) than a natural stimulus (Hilton, 2013; Love et al., 2015; Wilson, 2014). The fact that pornography can cause a surge of dopamine release is important, given that dopamine is implicated in the "wanting" or desire component of reward and influences goal-oriented, approach behaviors (Berridge & Kringelbach, 2015;

Berridge & Robinson, 2016). Moreover, the release of dopamine consolidates the neural pathways of behaviors, thus strengthening these neural connections (Doidge, 2007). Repeated pornography use accompanied by repeated dopamine release strengthens the neural networks that pair viewing pornography with reward (Doidge, 2007). In this way, the behavior can become compulsive and out of control. Additionally, it is important to note that dopamine is triggered by novelty (which evolutionarily may have contributed to reproductive fitness by creating sexual preference for nonfamilial partners; Hilton, 2013; Menegas et al., 2017; Park et al., 2016; Wilson, 2014). Indeed, novel sexual material can cause an increase in dopamine release, which fuels the drive for users to continually find new types of pornography. The novelty available on internet pornography sites is unmatched by offline sexual partners, another feature of the supernormal stimulus nature of pornography (Hilton, 2013).

Researchers purport that continued pornography use can lead to neuroplastic change (Doidge, 2007; Hilton 2013), particularly in the *arousal template* (Carnes, 2001; Carnes et al., 2007). In the 1980s, John Money introduced the idea of a lovemap, which "carries the program of a person's erotic fantasies and their corresponding practices" (Money, 1984, p. 165). According to Money (1984), the lovemap contains unique specifiers of what an individual finds attractive and is fairly stable after it is developed. Patrick Carnes (2001; Carnes et al., 2007) built upon the idea of a lovemap by introducing the arousal template, which he posited is flexible and malleable across time. Specifically, the arousal template is an individual's sexual beliefs about what they find sexually attractive. The template is influenced by genetics, experience (general and sexual), cultural norms, and family history (Carnes, 2001; Carnes et al., 2007). Carnes (2001) proposed that the arousal template can be altered by cybersex and pornography use, even to the point of eroticizing aspects of a mobile device or computer (mouse, keyboard, sound of clicking icons, interface properties) that are repeatedly paired with sexual stimuli. The endless novelty of sexual acts, scenes, scripts, and objects in pornography can influence individuals' arousal templates by exposing them to new sexually stimulating material, which they then incorporate into their sexual preferences (Carnes et al., 2007).

Psychiatrist Norman Doidge (2007) confirmed the notion that pornography can lead to changes in the brain in his groundbreaking work on *neuroplasticity*, or the brain's ability to change over time as a result of learning and experience. Doidge noted that pornography exposes an individual to new sexual acts that can become more salient to the user than their offline sexual partners. Over time, however, the pornography user develops tolerance to the sexual material (much like individuals with chemical addiction) and begins to seek out new forms of pornography to reach the same level of arousal. This novelty-seeking behavior may lead individuals to view types of pornography they never thought they would find stimulating, such as images deemed personally reprehensible. However, due to changes in their arousal templates, or what Doidge called *sexual maps*, these pornography users seek novelty to feel excitement and sexual stimulation. Doidge said, "When pornographers boast that they are pushing the envelope by introducing new, harder themes, what they don't say is that they must, because their customers are building up a tolerance to the content" (p. 105). Alterations to the brain's sexual map or arousal template can make it challenging for those who use pornography to find offline partners as desirable or arousing as they did prior to initiating pornography use (Doidge, 2007).

It can be very helpful for clients to learn about the neuroscience of pornography addiction including concepts such as supernormal stimuli, neuroplasticity, and arousal templates. This information moves pornography addiction from a moral model conceptualization to a biopsychosocial conceptualization, which can reduce clients' shame and provide insight into treatment planning and goal setting.

ETHICAL CONSIDERATIONS FOR PORNOGRAPHY ADDICTION TREATMENT

Given that a portion of pornography is illegal (e.g., child pornography), it is important for counselors to consider how they might respond to a client's disclosure of viewing illegal pornography (importantly, this refers to *viewing only*, rather than making or distributing, which requires a different response). Counselors should consult with a lawyer in their state to gain information related to the specifics of mandated reporting and privileged communication laws. Some states (e.g., California) require counselors to report clients who disclose viewing child pornography. Other states do not mandate reporting of this nature due to concern of creating a *chilling effect*, in which potential clients do not seek treatment out of fear of being reported. Counselors also must consider ethical codes related to the duty to warn if a client discloses viewing child pornography and sexual attraction to children while living with or working with minors. Other instances of viewing child pornography may fall under child abuse, which is always a mandated, ethical reason to break confidentiality. Any decision about breaking confidentiality must include consideration of both legal statutes in the counselor's state and relevant ethical codes (e.g., American Counseling Association [ACA] *Code of Ethics* [2014]). Consulting with legal professionals and the ACA ethical services (see www.counseling.org/knowledge-center/ethics) can help clinicians make informed and ethical choices. Additionally, specific information related to illegal pornography and confidentiality should be described in the counselor's informed consent document so that both clients and counselors are aware of relevant laws and ethical codes prior to the start of counseling.

HOW DO I IDENTIFY IT?

Pornography and cybersex addiction are components of sex addiction. Therefore, the proposed criteria for hypersexual disorder (Kafka, 2010, 2014) can be applied to pornography and cybersex addiction despite the decision not to include the diagnosis in the *Diagnostic and Statistical Manual of Mental Disorders* (5th ed.; *DSM-5*; American Psychiatric Association [APA], 2013). Additionally, the *International Classification of Diseases*, 11th Revision (*ICD-11*; World Health Organization [WHO], 2018) included criteria for compulsive sexual behavior, which counselors may find useful for identifying those with pornography or cybersex addiction (see Chapter 5 for details regarding both hypersexual disorder and the *ICD-11* code for compulsive sexual behavior). Furthermore, Goodman (2001) provided criteria for addictive disorder derived from the criteria for substance dependence utilized in the *Diagnostic and Statistical Manual of Mental Disorders* (4th ed.; *DSM-IV*; APA, 1994). Specifically, Goodman (2001) replaced the word "substance" with the word "behavior" and suggested that these criteria could be used to identify a range of addictive behaviors, including sex addiction (and therefore pornography and cybersex addiction). The criteria for addictive disorder include: (a) tolerance (need to increase intensity or frequency of behavior to reach desired effect); (b) withdrawal (physiological or psychological changes when not engaging in behavior); (c) engaging in behavior for longer, at higher degrees of intensity, or in greater amounts than intended; (d) unsuccessful attempts to control or cut down behavior; (e) large amounts of time dedicated to preparing for, engaging in, and recovering from the behavior; (f) engagement in the behavior negatively affects important relational, occupational, or leisure activities; and (g) continuing to engage in the behavior despite negative consequences (physical or psychological). According to Goodman (2001), individuals who meet three or more of these criteria in a 12-month period would be classified as having an addictive disorder.

With regard to pornography and cybersex addiction specifically, Carnes et al. (2007) proposed 10 criteria for problematic online sexual behavior. These criteria include: (a) mental preoccupation or obsession with online sexual content, (b) engaging in online sexual activities for longer than intended or more frequently than intended, (c) failed attempts to control or stop using cybersex or pornography, (d) withdrawal symptoms when not using online sexual activities (e.g., restlessness, irritability), (e) online sexual activity becomes a primary means of escaping problems or negative mood states (e.g., depression, guilt, anxiety), (f) searching for more intense online sexual content or seeking out higher risk experiences, (g) lying about online activities to hide pornography or cybersex use, (h) engaging in illegal sexual activity online, (i) losing or risking meaningful opportunities or relationships because of pornography or cybersex use, and (j) accruing significant debt or experiencing financial problems due to online sexual activity. Carnes et al. (2007) suggested that endorsing three or more of these criteria is indicative of problematic online sexual behavior. These signs, along with proposed diagnostic criteria for sex addiction, hypersexual disorder, and compulsive sexual behavior, can help counselors identify pornography and cybersex addiction in their clinical work.

NEGATIVE CONSEQUENCES OF PORNOGRAPHY OR CYBERSEX ADDICTION

A primary means of identifying addiction is to assess the persistence of the behavior in spite of problems or negative consequences. Research on pornography addiction documents several potential negative consequences associated with pornography use. In the study of 64 German adult males, researchers found a positive, significant relationship between hours of pornography use per week and depression and alcohol use (Kuhn & Gallinat, 2014). It is important to note, however, that the correlation found in this study does not indicate causality (i.e., the researchers cannot know if pornography use contributed to alcohol use and depression, or if depression and alcohol use contributed to pornography use). Nevertheless, it appears that pornography use and alcohol use could be means of emotion regulation associated with depression. Another potential problem associated with pornography addiction is relational discord with romantic partners. In the study of married couples, 13.7% of males and 18.0% of females agreed that pornography was a source of marital conflict and 21% of males and 32.9% of females believed pornography use constituted infidelity (Carroll et al., 2017). Additionally, Hesse and Floyd (2019) found a significant association between more pornography consumption and less relationship satisfaction and relationship closeness. Moreover, more pornography consumption correlated with increased loneliness and depression (Hesse & Floyd, 2019). Other possible negative consequences include the loss of time designated for engaging in other responsibilities (e.g., work, home, school) or offline relationships due to cybersex, the development of unrealistic expectations for sexual experiences and sexual partners, and engaging in illegal online sexual activities (Doring, 2009). Furthermore, in light of the supernormal stimulus of pornography, individuals with pornography addiction may prefer cybersex and pornography use over partnered sexual experiences (Park et al., 2016). Those with cybersex or pornography addiction also may experience sexual difficulties or issues with arousal when engaging in sexual acts without pornography (Maltz & Maltz, 2008).

HOW DO I ASSESS IT?

Many formal measures exist to assess various aspects of pornography and cybersex addiction. The following are descriptions of three instruments you may find useful in your work. Of note, the assessments described in the previous chapter on sex addiction (Chapter 5) also are appropriate for clients using pornography or cybersex. For a more comprehensive review of 20 instruments used to assess problematic pornography use, see Fernandez and Griffiths (2019).

PROBLEMATIC PORNOGRAPHY USE SCALE

The 12-item Problematic Pornography Use Scale (PPUS; Kor et al., 2014) assesses four factors associated with compulsive pornography use, including distress and functional problems (three items), excessive use (three items), control difficulties (three items), and using to escape (three items). The PPUS was developed using samples of male and female Israeli adults who spoke Hebrew. Researchers created items for the PPUS by consulting existing measures, literature on pornography, and their operational definition of problematic pornography. Items correspond with six-point Likert-type scales ranging from *never true* (0) to *almost always true* (5). Example items include: *I feel I cannot stop watching pornography* and *I use pornographic materials to escape my grief or to free myself from negative feelings*. Possible total scores range from 0 to 60 with higher scores indicating more problematic use. PPUS scores demonstrated strong reliability with Cronbach's alpha level of .93 for the total score (12 items) and Cronbach's alpha levels ranging from .79 to .92 for the four subscales. Items of the PPUS are found in the original Kor et al. (2014) article.

PORNOGRAPHY CONSUMPTION EFFECTS SCALE-SHORT FORM

The Pornography Consumption Effects Scale-Short Form (PCES-SF; Miller et al., 2019) is a shortened, 14-item version of the original 47-item PCES. The scale was normed on 312 heterosexual adult men with a history of pornography use composed of both students and community members. The PCES-SF utilizes seven-point Likert-type scales ranging from *not at all* (1) to *an extremely large extent* (7). Items on the PCES-SF comprise two subscales: Positive Effects Dimension (PED; eight items) and Negative Effects Dimension (NED; six items). An example item on the PED scale is *pornography has positively influenced your opinions of sex*. An example item on the NED scale is *pornography has made your life more problematic*. The PCES-SF scores demonstrated good reliability with the Cronbach's alpha scores for both the PED and NED scales at .91 using the sample of heterosexual adult males. The short form version of the PCES strongly correlated with the long version, demonstrating concurrent validity. The shortened version of the scale may demonstrate more utility in clinical settings than the longer version (Miller et al., 2019). All items of the PCES-SF can be found in the original Miller et al. (2019) article.

PORNOGRAPHY CRAVING QUESTIONNAIRE

Rather than focusing on the frequency of pornography use and related negative consequences, the Pornography Craving Questionnaire (PCQ; Kraus & Rosenberg, 2014) assesses urges or cravings for using pornography. The authors of the scale described pornography craving as a "transient but intense urge or desire that waxes and wanes over time and as a relatively stable preoccupation or inclination to use pornography" (Kraus & Rosenberg, 2014, p. 452). The 12-item PCQ assesses five dimensions of pornography craving including: perceived control, desire, psychophysiological reactivity, intention to use, and mood changes. Items on the PCQ were adapted from substance craving questionnaires. Each item corresponds with a seven-point Likert-type scale ranging from *disagree completely* (1) to *agree completely* (7). Example items include: *If I were watching porn this minute, I would feel happier* and *If the situation allowed, I would watch porn right now*. The PCQ was normed on American male undergraduate students, and scores demonstrated strong reliability with a Cronbach's alpha level of .91 (Kraus & Rosenberg, 2014). Scores on the PCQ are obtained by summing the 12 items and finding the average. Higher scores indicate more cravings for pornography. The items of the PCQ are listed in the original Kraus and Rosenberg (2014) article.

HOW DO I TREAT IT?

Given the nature of pornography as a supernormal stimulus and subsequent sexual conditioning, it is important to help clients engage in a period of abstinence from sexual stimulation to allow the brain to return to original setpoints for sexual arousal. Counselors and clients can discuss a range of technological blocking and filtering systems to help prevent pornography use in the home and at work, as well as develop a computer use plan (Carnes, 2001). Clients may take actions such as moving their computer or laptop to a public space in the home (e.g., kitchen, living room), enabling content restrictions on smartphone settings, using a filtering system on the household's Wi-Fi network, and disabling the ability to download applications on smartphones without a password. These precautions may be helpful in early recovery, yet they are only supplementary to counseling, group therapy, and 12-step support.

CLINICAL NOTE 6.3

Given the prominence of sex and sexuality in American culture, what obstacles might a client face who is trying to achieve a period of abstinence from sexual stimulation? What triggers might the client encounter? How should the client prepare for pursuing a period of abstinence?

With regard to counseling modalities, individual, couple, family, and group counseling may be helpful for clients with cybersex and pornography addiction. One common thread across various forms of counseling for clients with pornography or cybersex addiction is the cultivation of emotion regulation skills. Along with other forms of addictive behaviors, it appears that many individuals with cybersex addiction engage in online sexual activities as a means of coping with difficult emotions or situations (Brahim et al., 2019; Wery & Billieaux, 2017). For example, among a sample of 306 adults using sexually related internet sites, researchers found a strong relationship between using cybersex as a means of coping and compulsive cybersex use (Brahim et al., 2019). In light of this finding, the authors noted, "these results suggest the importance of interventions that focus on emotion regulation to help people with compulsive cybersex" (Brahim et al., 2019, p. 447). Therefore, enhancing emotion regulation strategies, such as identifying, labeling, expressing, and coping with various emotions, may be an important component to pornography and cybersex addiction treatment.

VOICES FROM THE FIELD: Clinical Work With Porn Addiction

The majority of clients who present with pornography addiction walk into my office with immense shame and little hope. They have not lived up to their values, they may have been caught by a significant other, and they view themselves as irreversibly dirty or broken. As a clinician, I love having the opportunity to provide hope to clients who are not able to see it yet.

In my experience, the most important factor in pornography addiction treatment is helping the client establish real, genuine friendships in theirr life. Shame is a primary driver of pornography addiction; the only way to sustainably combat shame is through genuine relationships. Another important component of treatment is the assessment of sexual fantasies. The kinds of pornography clients watch tell a story about their deepest fears and deepest desires. I encourage counselors to pay attention to the details: Who shows up in the pornography? What sexual acts are being performed? If there is more than one person in the pornography, which person does the client resonate with? How do they want to feel? All of these details point to underlying issues driving the pornography use.

Finally, it is important for counselors to recognize that any time you work with clients regarding their sexuality, it is inevitable that your own feelings and beliefs about sexuality will be activated. That is okay! You are human. Do not avoid the things that are evoked in you; instead, invite them to the table (after your client leaves), and learn from them.

Uncovering sexual wounds and false sexual narratives in your own mind and body can illuminate the path toward your own sexual healing. If you do not believe you are in need of your own sexual healing, you may not be ready to go into this field yet. To be trusted with another's sexual story is a great privilege, and each story must be treated with dignity. As clinicians, we have the honor of bringing new life to the most hopeless parts of our client's lives.

Thorn Winkler, MA, APC, AMFT; Stonegate Counseling Associates

ACCEPTANCE AND COMMITMENT THERAPY

Acceptance and commitment therapy (ACT; Hayes et al., 2012) is an approach to counseling aimed at increasing clients' psychological flexibility. Developed in the 1980s, ACT is a third-generation cognitive behavioral therapy (CBT) intervention based on the tenets of relational frame theory (Hayes & Smith, 2005). At its core, ACT works to replace six processes of psychological inflexibility with six processes of psychological flexibility (Luoma et al., 2017). The processes of inflexibility include: (a) cognitive fusion (becoming attached to one's thoughts; awareness and cognitive narratives become fused together), (b) experiential avoidance (attempts to evade unwanted private events or experiences), (c) inflexible attention (rumination on the past or anxiety about the future without awareness of the present), (d) conceptualized self (attachment to stories about oneself that subsequently dictate behavior), (e) lack of contact with values (difficulty identifying or connecting with what makes life meaningful), and (f) inaction, impulsivity, and avoidant persistence (engaging in defensive or short-term actions to relieve psychological pain rather than long-term value-driven actions; Luoma et al., 2017). From an ACT perspective, counselors work with clients to choose alternatives to these psychological inflexible processes. These alternatives include: (a) acceptance (embracing private events), (b) cognitive defusion (observing thoughts dispassionately and with curiosity), (c) present-moment awareness (attending to the here and now and noticing private events), (d) self-as-context (accepting oneself as distinct from events and experiences), (e) defining valued directions (identifying those things that give life meaning), and (f) committed action (making behavior change toward value-based goals; Luoma et al., 2017). Thus, in ACT, acceptance of one's thoughts, feelings, and private events is a necessary step toward value clarification and value-consistent action (Hayes et al., 2012).

ACT has demonstrated effectiveness with clients with pornography addiction (Crosby & Twohig, 2016; Twohig & Crosby, 2010). Researchers examined the effects of a 12-session ACT intervention with adult males with problematic pornography use (Crosby & Twohig, 2016). Compared to clients on a waitlist, those in the ACT intervention group demonstrated significant reductions in pornography viewing and sexual compulsivity scores at the end of 12 weeks. All participants eventually completed the ACT intervention (the waitlist group completed the intervention after 12 weeks of serving as the control group), and the total sample ($N = 28$) demonstrated a 93% decrease in hours of pornography viewed at posttest and an 86% decrease at a 3-month follow-up (Crosby & Twohig, 2016).

The ACT intervention consisted of helping clients distinguish between urges to view pornography and the act of viewing pornography, insight into the ineffectiveness of trying to control urges, introducing the acceptance of urges to view pornography (willingness to experience them) as a replacement for trying to control urges, engaging in cognitive defusion (understanding the role of language in cognitive fusion; understanding one's relationship with thoughts), awareness of when the client is engaging in experiential avoidance, connection with the present moment, identifying personal values, choosing values, determining value-consistent goals, and applying ACT to relapse management strategies (Crosby & Twohig, 2009). Therefore, applying ACT to pornography addiction entails helping clients become aware of and alter the way they interact with their thoughts. Rather than trying to control urges to view pornography, clients can accept or be willing to experience the urge to use pornography. The acceptance of private experiences (such as feelings of loss stemming from ending their use of pornography) gives clients more freedom to pursue value-directed goals (Hayes & Smith, 2005). Thus, when clients accept, rather than try to control, private events and experiences, they are free to choose to live in value-consistent ways. The ACT manual for the pornography addiction intervention is available upon request from the authors of Crosby and Twohig (2016). To learn more about ACT, readers are encouraged to review Hayes et al. (2012) and visit contextualscience.org/act.

INTERNAL FAMILY SYSTEMS THERAPY

Internal family systems (IFS) therapy was developed by Richard Schwartz as a means of applying systems thinking to the intrapsychic domain (Schwartz, 2013; Schwartz & Sweezy, 2020). Just as family systems are made up of multiple people with roles, emotions, abilities, and perspectives, IFS counselors conceptualize an individual's psyche as being composed of parts (i.e., distinct mental systems), "each with their own idiosyncratic range of emotion, style of expression, abilities, desires, and views of the world" (Schwartz & Sweezy, 2020, pp. 30–31). Parts can take on multiple roles that fall into two categories: those who have been injured in the past and are vulnerable, sensitive, and carry emotional pain (exiles), and those who work to control the injured parts to keep them from becoming activated or to suppress their emotions when triggered (protectors). Thus, the roles of parts in an individual's intrapsychic system are purposeful and conducted with positive intentions. Amid the parts (i.e., exiles, protectors) is a core sense of consciousness called the Self, which is fully equipped to lead the intrapsychic system if the parts will trust its leadership. Thus, goals of IFS therapy include: speaking about the client's experience in terms of parts, assessing which parts are dominating the client's experience, freeing parts from extreme roles and encouraging new roles, reestablishing the leadership of the Self, and creating harmony among the parts to foster more integration (Schwartz, 2013; Schwartz & Sweezy, 2020).

Oftentimes, IFS counselors discover polarities among protectors who are trying to control or deactivate the emotions of an exile. Protectors tend to fall into two groups: managers, whose role is to control and preemptively strategize to keep exiles disconnected and deactivated, and firefighters, whose role is to respond immediately once exiles are activated (in any means necessary) to distract from or suppress the accompanying emotions. Firefighters and managers may be at odds in their roles, such as a firefighter who employs addictive behaviors to distract or numb from a triggered exile's emotional pain and a manager who responds with criticism and shaming tactics. The goal of IFS is not to eliminate parts, but to reestablish the Self as the leader so that the protectors' roles become less polarized and extreme. Once the Self has established leadership, it can attend to the needs of the exile, which often includes listening to the exile's experience of how it was injured in the past.

In the case of a client with pornography addiction, the counselor using IFS would conceptualize this behavior as a firefighter's attempt to numb, soothe, or distract from the emotional pain of an activated exile (Schwartz & Sweezy, 2020; Wonder, 2013). Typically, in situations of addiction, a firefighter is dominating the system (Schwartz & Sweezy, 2020). Managers may respond to the firefighter's efforts with extreme shame and criticism, leading to feelings of self-deprecation. Rather than adding to the client's felt shame and criticism, IFS counselors would try to understand and accept the firefighter (whose goal is to extinguish emotional pain). Indeed, Wonder (2013) noted, "The beginning of an addiction therapy always revolves around this polarity between firefighters and shaming managers. It is crucial not to side with the managers" (p. 165). Instead, counselors help clients separate from their protector and exile parts, accept and understand the parts, establish the leadership of the Self, heal or unburden the exile, and allow the protector parts to take on new roles. For more information about IFS and applying the approach to pornography addiction, review Wonder (2013) and Schwartz and Sweezy (2020), and visit IFS-institute.com.

12-STEP SUPPORT

With regard to 12-step support groups for pornography and cybersex addiction, several options exist including Sex Addicts Anonymous (12-step support group for sex addiction; saa-recovery.org; described in Chapter 5), Sexaholics Anonymous (12-step support group for sex, pornography, and lust addiction; www.sa.org), Sexual Compulsives Anonymous (12-step support group for sexual compulsion; sca-recovery.org/WP), and Celebrate Recovery (a Christian 12-step program for any form of addiction, including sex and pornography; www.celebraterecovery.com). Counselors are encouraged to attend open meetings, speak with support group volunteers, and read program literature to learn more about each fellowship as some distinctions exist. For example, Sexaholics Anonymous defines sobriety as engaging in sexual behavior only with one's spouse in the context of marriage, as well as working to progressively reduce lust (Sexaholics Anonymous Inc, 2020). Sexual Compulsives Anonymous, however, utilizes personalized Sexual Recovery Plans in which members construct plans for expressing their sexuality in a manner consistent with their values, thus defining sobriety for themselves (often in collaboration with a sponsor; International Service Organization of Sexual Compulsives Anonymous, n.d.). Although there are distinctions, many of the 12-step fellowships for sex, pornography, and cybersex addiction share similarities such as being spiritual programs, utilizing meetings, sponsors, and program literature, emphasizing the importance of community in recovery, and identifying specific acting out sexual behaviors from which to abstain (e.g., constructing bottom lines, middle lines, and top lines, utilizing the Three Circles technique; see Chapter 5). Before making referrals, counselors should become familiar with the fellowships in their area and provide their clients with information about various programs.

DIAGNOSTIC CONSIDERATIONS

Pornography and cybersex addiction fall under the umbrella of sex addiction or hypersexual disorder (Wery & Billieux, 2017), which currently is not represented in the *DSM-5*. An *ICD-11* code, however, exists for compulsive sexual behavior disorder (WHO, 2018). Without a *DSM* diagnosis, counselors working with clients with pornography and cybersex addiction often diagnose co-occurring mental health disorders (e.g., depression, anxiety, substance use disorders, gambling disorder). If no comorbid disorders exist, counselors may consider using the code for other specified disruptive, impulse-control, and conduct disorders and specify pornography, cybersex, or hypersexual disorder.

HOW CAN I LEARN MORE?

If you are working with clients with pornography and cybersex addiction and desire to learn more about the condition, consider the following resources.

BOOKS

- Carnes, P., Delmonico, D. L., & Griffin, E. (2007). *In the shadows of the net: Breaking free of compulsive online sexual behavior* (2nd ed.). Hazelden.
- Maltz, W., & Maltz, L. (2008). *The porn trap: The essential guide to overcoming problems caused by pornography*. Harper Collins Publishers.
- Wilson, G. (2014). *Your brain on porn: Internet pornography and the emerging science of addiction*. Commonwealth.

PEER-REVIEWED ARTICLES

- Doring, N. M. (2009). The internet's impact on sexuality: A critical review of 15 years of research. *Computers in Human Behavior, 25*, 1089–1101. https://doi.org/10.1016/j.chb.2009.04.003
- Hilton, D. L. (2013). Pornography addiction – A supranormal stimulus considered in the context of neuroplasticity. *Socioaffective Neuroscience and Psychology, 3*, 20767. https://doi.org/10.3402/snp.v3i0.20767
- Riemersma, J., & Sytsma, M. (2013). A new generation of sexual addiction. *Sexual Addiction and Compulsivity, 20*, 306–322. https://doi.org/10.1080/10720162.2013.843067

WEBSITES

- Sexaholics Anonymous: www.sa.org
- Sexual Compulsives Anonymous: sca-recovery.org/WP
- Your Brain on Porn: www.yourbrainonporn.com

REFERENCES

Aldridge, M. J., Arndt, K. J., & Davies, S. C. (2013). Sexting: You found the sext, what to do next? How school psychologists can assist with policy, prevention, and intervention. *Counselor Education and Human Services Faculty Publications, 13*, 6–10.

American Counseling Association. (2014). *ACA code of ethics*. http://www.counseling.org/knowledge-center/ethics

American Psychiatric Association. (2013). *Diagnostic and statistical manual of mental disorders* (5th ed.). Author.

Barrense-Dias, Y., Berchtold, A., Suris, J. C., & Akre, C. (2017). Sexting and the definition issue. *Journal of Adolescent Health, 61*, 544–554. https://doi.org/10.1016/j.jadohealth.2017.05.009

Barrett, D. (2010). *Supernormal stimuli: How primal urges overran their evolutionary purpose*. W. W. Norton & Company.

Berridge, K. C., & Kringelbach, M. L. (2015). Pleasure systems in the brain. *Neuron, 86,* 646–664. https://doi.org/10.1016/j.neuron.2015.02.018

Berridge, K. C., & Robinson, T. E. (2016). Liking, wanting and the incentive-sensitization theory of addiction. *The American Psychologist, 71,* 670–679. https://doi.org/10.1037/amp0000059

Brahim, F. B., Rothen, S., Bianchi-Demicheli, F., Courtois, R., & Khazaal, Y. (2019). Contribution of sexual desire and motives to the compulsive use of cybersex. *Journal of Behavioral Addictions, 8,* 442–450. https://doi.org/10.1556/2006.8.2019.47

Carnes, P. J. (2001). Cybersex, courtship, and escalating arousal: Factors in addictive sexual desire. *Sexual Addiction and Compulsivity, 8,* 25–78. https://doi.org/10.1080/10720/60127560

Carnes, P., Delmonico, D. L., & Griffin, E. (2007). *In the shadows of the net: Breaking free of compulsive online sexual behavior* (2nd ed.). Hazelden.

Carroll, J. S., Busby, D. M., Willoughby, B. J., & Brown, C. C. (2017). The porn gap: Differences in men's and women's pornography patterns in couple relationships. *Journal of Couple and Relationship Therapy, 16,* 146–163. https://doi.org/10.1080/15332691.2016.1238796

Christensen, J. F. (2017). Pleasure junkies all around! Why it matters and why 'the arts' might be the answer: A biopsychological perspective. *Proceedings of the Royal Society B, 284,* 20162837. https://doi.org/10.1098/rspb.2016.2837

Cooper, A. (1998). Sexuality and the internet: Surfing into the new millennium. *Cyberpsychology and Behavior, 1,* 187–193. https://doi.org/10.1089/cpb.1998.1.187

Crosby, J. M., & Twohig, M. P. (2009). *Acceptance and commitment therapy for the treatment of compulsive pornography use: Treatment manual.* Utah State University.

Crosby, J. M., & Twohig, M. P. (2016). Acceptance and commitment therapy for problematic internet pornography use: A randomized trial. *Behavioral Therapy, 47,* 355–366. https://doi.org/10.1016/j.beth.2016.02.001

Delmonico, D. L., Putney, H. L., & Griffin, E. J. (2017). Sexting and the @ generation: Implications, motivations, and solutions. In K. S. Young, & Nabuco de Abreu, C. (Eds.), *Internet addiction in children and adolescents: Risk factors, assessment, and treatment* (pp. 65–82). Springer Publishing.

DiSabatino, J. (2000). Mattel wins case against cybersquatter. *Computerworld, 34,* 8.

Doidge, N. (2007). *The brain that changes itself: Stories of personal triumph from the frontiers of brain science.* Penguin Group.

Doring, N. M. (2009). The internet's impact on sexuality: A critical review of 15 years of research. *Computers in Human Behavior, 25,* 1089–1101. https://doi.org/10.1016/j.chb.2009.04.003

Doring, N., Daneback, K., Shaughnessy, K., Grov, C., & Byers, E. S. (2017). Online sexual activity experiences among college students: A four-country comparison. *Archives of Sexual Behavior, 46,* 1641–1652. https://doi.org/10.1007/s10508-015-0656-4

Elsey, J. W. B., van Andel, K., Kater, R. B., Reints, I. M., & Spiering, M. (2019). The impact of virtual reality versus 2D pornography on sexual arousal and presence. *Computers in Human Behavior, 97,* 35-43. https://doi.org/10.1016/j.chb.2019.02.031

Fernandez, D. P., & Griffiths, M. D. (2019). Psychometric instruments for problematic pornography use: A systematic review. *Evaluation and the Health Professions.* https://doi.org/10.1177/0163278719861688

Giordano, A. L., & Cashwell, C. S. (2017). Cybersex addiction among college students: A prevalence study. *Sexual Addiction and Compulsivity, 24,* 47–57. https://doi.org/10.1080/10720162.2017.1287612

Goodman, A. (2001). What's in a name? Terminology for designating a syndrome of driven sexual behavior. *Sexual Addiction and Compulsivity, 8*, 191–213. https://doi.org/10.1080/107201601743459919

Griffiths, M. D. (2012). Internet sex addiction: A review of empirical research. *Addiction Research and Theory, 20*, 111–124. https://doi.org/10.3109/16066359.2011.588351

Grubbs, J. B., Kraus, S. W., & Perry, S. L. (2019). Self-reported addiction to pornography in a nationally representative sample: The roles of use habits, religiousness, and moral incongruence. *Journal of Behavioral Addictions, 8*, 88–93. https://doi.org/10.1556/2006.7.2018.134

Hasinoff, A. A. (2015). *Sexting panic: Rethinking criminalization, privacy, and consent*. University of Illinois Press.

Hayes, S. C., & Smith, S. (2005). *Get out of your mind and into your life: The new acceptance and commitment therapy*. New Harbinger Publications.

Hayes, S. C., Strosahl, K. D., & Wilson, K. G. (2012). *Acceptance and commitment therapy: The process and practice of mindful change* (2nd ed.). Guilford Press.

Herbenick, D., Fu, T. C., Wright, P., Paul, B., Gradus, R., Bauer, J., & Jones, R. (2020). Diverse sexual behaviors and pornogprahy use: Findings from a nationally representative probability survey of Americans aged 18 to 60 years. *Journal of Sexual Medicine, 17*, 623–633. https://doi.org/10.1016/j.jsxm.2020.01.013

Hesse, C., & Floyd, K. (2019). Affection substitution: The effect of pornography consumption on close relationships. *Journal of Social and Personal Relationships, 36*, 3887–3907. https://doi.org/10.1177/0265407519841719

Hilton, D. L. (2013). Pornography addiction- A supranormal stimulus considered in the context of neuroplasticity. *Socioaffective Neuroscience and Psychology, 3*, 20767. https://doi.org/10.3402/snp.v3i0.20767

International Service Organization of Sexual Compulsives Anonymous. (n.d.). *The tools that help us get better*. https://sca-recovery.org/WP/recovery-program/tools

Jones, K. E., & Tuttle, A. E. (2012). Clinical and ethical considerations for the treatment of cybersex addiction for marriage and family therapists. *Journal of Couple and Relationship Therapy, 11*, 274–290. https://doi.org/10.1080/15332691.2012.718967

Kafka, M. P. (2010). Hypersexual disorder: A proposed diagnosis for DSM-V. *Archives of Sexual Behavior, 39*, 377–400. https://doi.org/10.1007/s10508-009-9574-7

Kafka, M. P. (2014). What happened to hypersexual disorder? *Archives of Sexual Behavior, 43*, 1259–1261. https://doi.org/10.1007/s10508-014-0326-y

Kor, A., Zilcha-Mano, S., Fogel, Y. A., Mikulncer, M., Reid, R. C., & Potenza, M. N. (2014). Psychometric development of the problematic pornography use scale. *Addictive Behaviors, 39*, 861–868. https://doi.org/10.1016/j.addbeh.2014.01.027

Kraus, S. W., Martino, S., & Potenza, M. N. (2016). Examining correlates of problematic internet pornography use among university students. *Journal of Behavioral Addictions, 5*, 179–191. https://doi.org/10.1556/2006.5.2016.022

Kraus, S., & Rosenberg, H. (2014). The pornography craving questionnaire: Psychometric properties. *Archives of Sexual Behavior, 43*, 451–462. https://doi.org/10.1007/s10508-013-0229-3

Kuhn, S., & Gallinat, J. (2014). Brain structure and functional connectivity associated with pornography consumption: The brain on born. *Journal of the American Medical Association Psychiatry, 71*, 827–834. https://doi.org/10.1001/jamapsychiatry.2014.93

Lee, J. R., & Darcy, K. M. (2020). Sexting: What's law got to do with it? *Archives of Sexual Behavior*. https://doi.org/10.1007/s10508-020-01727-6

Lorang, M. R., McNiel, D. E., & Binder, R. L. (2016). Minors and sexting: Legal implications. *The Journal of the American Academy of Psychiatry and the Law, 44,* 73–81.

Love, T., Laier, C., Brand, M., Hatch, L., & Hajela, R. (2015). Neuroscience of internet pornography addiction: A review and update. *Behavioral Sciences, 5,* 388–433. https://doi.org/10.3390/bs5030388

Luoma, J. B., Hayes, S. C., & Walsler, R. D. (2017). *Learning ACT: An acceptance & commitment therapy skills training manual for therapists* (2nd ed.). Context Press.

Madigan, S., Ly, A., Rash, C. L., Van Ouytsel, J., & Temple, J. R. (2018). Prevalence of multiple forms of sexting behavior among youth: A systematic review and meta-analysis. *Journal of the American Medical Association Pediatrics, 172,* 327–335. https://doi.org/10.1001/jamapediatrics.2017.5314

Maltz, W., & Maltz, L. (2008). *The porn trap: The essential guide to overcoming problems caused by pornography.* HarperCollins Publishers.

Menegas, W., Babayan, B. M., Uchida, N., & Watabe-Uchida, M. (2017). Opposite initialization to novel cues in dopamine signaling in ventral and posterior striatum in mice. *eLife, 6,* e21886. https://doi.org/10.7554/eLife.21886

Miller, D. J., Kidd, G., & Hald, G. M. (2019). Measuring self-perceived effects of pornography: A short-form version of the pornography consumption effects scale. *Archives of Sexual Behavior, 48,* 753–761. https://doi.org/10.1007/s10508-018-1327-z

Money, J. (1984). Paraphilias: Phenomenology and classification. *American Journal of Psychotherapy, 38,* 164–179. https://doi.org/10.1176/appi.psychotherapy.1984.38.2.164

Nelson, K. M., & Rothman, E. F. (2020). Should public health professionals consider pornography a public health crisis? *American Journal of Public Health, 110,* 151–153. https://doi.org/10.2105/AJPH.2019.305498

Park, B. Y., Wilson, G., Berger, J., Christman, M., Reina, B., Bishop, F., Klam, W. P., & Doan, A. P. (2016). Is internet pornography causing sexual dysfunctions? A review with clinical reports. *Behavioral Sciences, 6,* 17. https://doi.org/10.3390/bs6030017

Pornhub Insights. (2018). *2018 year in review.* https://pornhub.com/insights/2018-year-in-review

Regnerus, M., Gordon, D., & Price, J. (2016). Documenting pornography use in America: A comparative analysis of methodological approaches. *The Journal of Sex Research, 53,* 873–881. https://doi.org/10.1080/00224499.2015.1096886

Riemersma, J., & Sytsma, M. (2013). A new generation of sexual addiction. *Sexual Addiction and Compulsivity, 20,* 306–322. https://doi.org/10.1080/10720162.2013.843067

Schwartz, R. C. (2013). Moving from acceptance toward transformation with internal family systems therapy (IFS). *Journal of Clinical Psychology, 69,* 805–816. https://doi.org/10.1002/jclp.22016

Schwartz, R. C., & Sweezy, M. (2020). *Internal family systems therapy* (2nd ed.). Guilford.

Sexaholics Anonymous Inc. (2020). *How do we define sobriety?* https://www.sa.org

Shaughnessy, K., & Byers, E. S. (2014). Contextualizing cybersex experience: Heterosexually identified men and women's desire for and experiences with cybersex with three types of partners. *Computers in Human Behavior, 32,* 178–185. https://doi.org/10.1016/j.chb.2013.12.005

Twohig, M. P., & Crosby, J. M. (2010). Acceptance and commitment therapy as a treatment for problematic internet pornography viewing. *Behavior Therapy, 41,* 285–295. https://doi.org/10.1016/j.beth.2009.06.002

Wery, A., & Billieux, J. (2017). Problematic cybersex: Conceptualization, assessment, and treatment. *Addictive Behaviors, 64,* 238–246. https://doi.org/10.1016/j.addbeh.2015.11.007

Wilson, G. (2014). *Your brain on porn: Internet pornography and the emerging science of addiction.* Commonwealth.

Wonder, N. (2013). Treating pornography addiction with IFS. In M. Sweezy & E. L. Ziskind (Eds.), *Internal family systems therapy: New dimensions* (pp. 159–165). Routledge.

World Health Organization. (2018). *International statistical classification of diseases and related health problems* (11th Rev.). https://icd.who.int/browse11/l-m/en

Wright, P. J., Herbenick, D., & Paul, B. (2020). Adolescent condom use, parent-adolescent sexual health communication, and pornography: Findings from a U. S. probability sample. *Health Communication, 35,* 1576–1582. https://doi.org/10.1080/10410236.2019.1652392

YouPorn. (2020). *YouPorn 2018 year in retrospect.* https://www.youporn.com/world/youporn-2018-year-in-retrospect

Zhang, X. (2010). Charging children with child pornography- using the legal system to handle the problem of "sexting." *Computer Law and Security Review, 26,* 251–259. https://doi.org/10.1016/j.clsr.2010.03.005

7

Love Addiction

HOW DO I CONCEPTUALIZE IT?

Fisher (1998) described three distinct yet interdependent emotional systems that contribute to mammalian mating and reproduction: the sex drive, attraction, and attachment. While sex drive and attachment are important components of romantic pairings, the emotional system of *attraction*, or *romantic love*, is most closely linked to the construct of love addiction and thus is the focus of this chapter (to learn more about sex addiction, see Chapter 5). Romantic love is a universal phenomenon that exists across cultures and time periods (Fisher, 1998; Fletcher et al., 2015). The experience of falling in love is common, as researchers found that among a sample of adults, men reported an average of 4.44 different loves (SD = 4.44) and women reported an average of 4.57 (SD = 3.43; Galperin & Haselton, 2010). Additionally, among a list of reasons for getting married, 90% of American adults identified love as a major reason, outranking companionship (identified as a major reason to get married by 66%), having children (31%), financial reasons (13%), or convenience (10%; Horowitz et al., 2019). Furthermore, it appears that the experience of being in love adds to life satisfaction. Among over 4,000 adults in the United States, researchers found that those with higher life-satisfaction scores identified finding meaning in four key areas: (a) friends, (b) career, (c), romantic partners, and (d) health (Kessel & Hughes, 2018).

Given the universality of love and associated benefits, how then could it be a behavioral addiction? The experience of being in love is naturally rewarding (involving neurotransmitters and hormones related to pleasure and bonding). Thus individuals who are highly sensitive to rewards or who are biologically susceptible to addiction may be at risk of relying on love to regulate their emotions. Reynaud et al. (2010) noted, "As with substance dependence, 'love addiction' requires the convergence of a vulnerable individual with a rewarding (desired) object" (p. 263). Love addiction can be expressed in different ways, depending on the object of the addiction. For example, an individual with love addiction could be compulsively obsessed with: (a) a specific person, (b) the experience of being in a romantic relationship, (c) the feelings associated with romance, or (d) some combination of the three (Peabody, 2005).

Although all experiences of being in love may have addiction-like qualities (e.g., preoccupation with loved one, craving/yearning for loved one, loved one becomes most salient feature of one's life, desiring increased amounts of time with loved one, feeling restless, irritable, and depressed if loved one is unavailable, feeling euphoric when thinking about or in the presence of loved one; Fisher et al., 2016; Frascella et al., 2010), some individuals may exhibit pathological love behaviors that exceed the typical experience of being "lovestruck." Rather, these individuals may experience a loss of control over their behaviors, continue to engage despite a range of negative consequences, and rely solely on love experiences to manage emotions (Sanches & John, 2019). As with other naturally rewarding processes, love behaviors can be conceptualized on a continuum spanning from unhealthy to healthy or immature to mature (Mellody et al., 1992; Sophia et al., 2009; Sussman, 2010). For the majority of individuals, love is a beneficial, adaptive, and pleasurable experience. For a small portion of people, however, love patterns and behaviors can become compulsive, out of control, continue despite negative consequences, and foster cravings or mental preoccupation, which are characteristics of love addiction.

Love addiction is not widely understood among the general public or even among many clinicians. One reason for this confusion is the fact that love addiction can present in varied ways. To best conceptualize love addiction, counselors must assess the object of clients' unhealthy preoccupation, such as an individual (on whom the client projects their fantasies of the perfect partner), the experience of being in a relationship (in which the specific partners are not as important as the emotional bond), or the thrill of passion in early romance (the experience of falling in love; Peabody, 2005). Clients may present to counseling with varied symptoms, all of which may indicate love addiction. For example, a client with love addiction may present with an unhealthy, obsessive preoccupation with a particular person (regardless of whether or not the love is reciprocated), leading to detrimental or risky behaviors. Alternatively, a client may describe quickly shifting from one relationship to another in order to experience the excitement and thrill that comes from the early stages of love, ending each relationship once the passion begins to fade. Finally, a client may report a compulsive need to have a romantic partner at all times, and even when the client is in a relationship, they are fostering relationships with other potential romantic partners in case the current relationship ends. Each of these clients may have love addiction, although the object of the addiction is different in each scenario.

Furthermore, it is important to note that love addiction is distinct from sex addiction. Sexual activity may occur in the romantic relationships of those with love addiction, yet the object of the addictive behavior is the person or the relationship, rather than the pleasure of sex (Reynaud et al., 2010). It is possible, however, for clients to have both sex and love addiction; so clinicians should be familiar with both sets of symptoms and assess clients appropriately. Reviewing the proposed diagnostic criteria for hypersexual disorder (Kafka, 2010, 2014) and compulsive sexual behavior (World Health Organization, 2018; see Chapter 5) can help counselors determine if sex addiction also may be an issue for clients with love addiction. In sum, counselors should be aware of the various manifestations of love addiction (e.g., addiction to a person, to romantic relationships, or to the euphoria of falling in love) and be able to differentiate between love addiction and sex addiction, while noting that the two conditions could co-occur.

LIMERENCE

In addition to becoming addicted to a particular person or the emotional bonds of a relationship, those with love addiction may become dependent on the euphoric sensations associated with falling in love (Peabody, 2005). The early stage of romantic love that is marked by a strong rush of pleasurable emotions is called *limerence* (Tennov, 1979). Money (1997) defined limerence as "the personal experience of having fallen in love and of being irrationally and fixatedly love stricken or love smitten, irrespective of the degree to which one's love is requited or unrequited" (p. 119). The focus of one's affection (i.e., the desired person), referred to as the *limerent object* (Tennov, 1979; Willmott & Bentley, 2015), triggers the activation of reward circuitry in the brain. The high energy and alertness of limerence is associated with phenylethylamine, which can act as a neurotransmitter to increase arousal and alertness (Money, 1997; Schaeffer, 2009) as well as the release of dopamine, a neurotransmitter implicated in reward (Willmott & Bentley, 2015). In addition to euphoric feelings, limerence involves cognitions. Tennov (1979) noted, "limerence is, above all else, a mental activity. It is an interpretation of events, rather than the events themselves" (p. 18). Thus, individuals in limerence find themselves energized, ruminating about the limerent object, fantasizing about meaningful encounters, and attending to actions that may denote reciprocation of love while minimizing actions that suggest rejection (Tennov, 1979).

The experience of limerence appears to be marked by common characteristics. In a qualitative study of men and women in limerence, researchers noted several shared themes: (a) rumination of the limerent object (i.e., obsessive thoughts), (b) anxiety and depression cultivated by the uncertainty of reciprocation from the limerent object, (c) experience of a disintegrated sense of self marked by vacillating emotions, (d) reintegration of previous life events and relationships (e.g., relationships with early caregivers, fantasies about ideal relationships, negative relational experiences), and (e) opportunity for authenticity (i.e., disclosure of feelings to limerent object moves individual toward authenticity; Willmott & Bentley, 2015). It is important to note that the limerence stage of romantic love does not last indefinitely; instead, if the limerent object reciprocates feelings and a relationship ensues, it transforms into other stages of love marked by less intense emotions (e.g., companionate love; Ortigue et al., 2010). If the limerent object does not reciprocate feelings of love, an individual's attention may be directed toward a new limerent object (Tennov, 1979).

Some individuals with love addiction may indeed be addicted to the experience of limerence, specifically the rush and excitement of falling in love and euphoria of being "lovestruck." Thus, they repeatedly seek out the experience of limerence and shift from one limerent object to the next. Cyclical limerence is described as:

> A reiterative dependency on the elated high of multiple new love affairs. The fixation is on repeatedly going through the cycle of a broken heart, a period of debilitating misery, and a return of elation generated in a new love affair (Money, 1997, p. 136).

Counselors can assess clients' romantic histories and the function of romantic relationships to identify whether they may be dependent on the rewarding nature of limerence.

CODEPENDENCE AND LOVE ADDICTION

A closely related construct to love addiction is *codependence*—a concept that is contested among clinicians and scholars alike. Some professionals conceptualize codependency as an addiction (Whitfield, 1991), and 12-step programs exist to address codependence in a manner similar to other behavioral addictions (e.g., Co-Dependents Anonymous). Others, however, believe the concept of codependence lacks validity (Calderwood & Rajesparam, 2014) or is a harmful way of conceptualizing those in challenging relationships (Weiss, 2019).

CLINICAL NOTE 7.1

The 12-step fellowship Co-Dependents Anonymous (CoDA) is a program for individuals seeking to develop healthy relationships and abstain from codependent behaviors (Co-Dependents Anonymous, Inc., 2018). Step one of CoDA is, "We admitted we were powerless over others—that our lives had become unmanageable" (Co-Dependents Anonymous, Inc., 1998, p. 18). To learn more about CoDA, visit their website at coda.org.

Despite the controversy, understanding proposed definitions of codependence and its relationship with love addiction may be helpful for counselors in their work with clients, some of whom may self-identify as codependent.

Whitfield (1991) defined codependency as "any suffering or dysfunction that is associated with or results from focusing on the needs and behaviors of others" (p. 3). The concept emerged from the addiction field as a way to understand relationships between those with substance use disorders and their nonaddicted partners (Calderwood & Rajesparam, 2014; Mellody et al., 1992; Whitfield, 1991). Since then, the definition has broadened to refer to many types of relationships, not only those involving an individual with addiction. Indeed, Wright and Wright (1991) noted:

> It is becoming increasingly clear, however, that similar patterns can occur in any relationship in which it is possible for one person, out of an inordinate concern for the status or well being of her or his partner, to assume an excessive degree of responsibility for that partner (p. 440).

Codependency is thought to stem from early childhood trauma or family dysfunction (Mellody et al., 1985). Specifically, proponents of the codependency construct postulate that children in traumatic or dysfunctional environments develop into adults who choose partners that resemble the attachment figures of their early childhood experiences, "thereby mirroring to some degree their past relationships, losses, and trauma" (Weiss, 2019, p. 179). Thus, a woman whose father had an alcohol use disorder may be attracted to men with substance use disorders, given that these relationships are familiar and reinforce the role she assumed as a child.

Although diverse descriptions of codependency exist, Mellody et al. (1985, 1992) described individuals with codependency as experiencing difficulty in five key areas: (a) self-esteem (self-esteem may be very low or grandiose), (b) boundaries (physical, sexual, emotional, and psychological), (c) sense of self and sense of reality (clear understanding of one's identity and experiences), (d) attending to needs and wants (difficulty identifying and meeting one's needs and wants), and (e) moderate expressions of self and reality (existing in extremes rather than moderation). These areas of difficulty in codependency manifest in all types of relationships, including romantic. Therefore, codependence is perceived to be a broader construct than love addiction. While codependency can be reflected in any type of relationship, love addiction entails maladaptive behavioral patterns only in the sphere or romantic relationships (Hayes, 1989). Specifically, Mellody et al. (1992) wrote, "Although being a codependent can lead some people into love addiction, not all codependents are love addicts" (p. 2). Thus, along with addressing symptoms of love addiction among clients, it may be helpful for counselors to examine characteristics of clients' nonromantic relationships with the five key features of codependency in mind (Mellody et al., 1985, 1992).

Whether or not counselors subscribe to the concept of codependence, there appears to be wide agreement that love addiction is linked to attachment issues and childhood trauma (Schaeffer, 2009; Sussman, 2010). Mellody et al. (1992) noted, "love addicts usually didn't have enough appropriate bonding with their caregivers, and probably experienced serious abandonment (or sense of abandonment) in childhood" (p. 15). Indeed, in the study of 50 adults with pathological love and 39 nonpathological controls, researchers found that those in the pathological love group had more anxious-ambivalent attachment styles, while the nonpathological controls had more secure attachment styles (Sophia et al., 2009). Additionally, in her groundbreaking work on pathological love, Norwood (1985) wrote, "For the woman who loves too much, her primary disease is her addiction to the pain and familiarity of an unrewarding relationship" (p. 225). Accordingly, counselors can assess the attachment styles of clients with love addiction and incorporate attachment work into their treatment plans.

PREVALENCE OF LOVE ADDICTION

There is limited information related to the prevalence of love addiction given the lack of uniform diagnostic criteria. Sussman et al. (2011) surmised that 3% of adults in the United States have love addiction; however, this frequency is speculative. Eisenman et al. (2004) surveyed over 9,000 college students who rated their level of dependence or addiction to a variety of behaviors and drugs of abuse on a scale from 0 to 100. The highest addiction rating was to being in love (mean rating = 49.49, SD = 35.02), followed by food (mean rating = 39.80, SD = 33.20) and having sex (mean rating = 33.90, SD = 33.65). Although these are self-reported ratings, it appears that college students resonate with the idea of being addicted to love and that this form of addiction is more prevalent than an addiction to other naturally rewarding behaviors (e.g., food, sex) or drugs of abuse (e.g., alcohol, cigarettes); see Eisenman et al. (2004). Finally, Sussman et al. (2014) surveyed 717 young adults (mean age = 19.8) and found that 23.2% reported experiencing love addiction in the previous 30 days and 34.3% experiencing love addiction at some point in their lives. Again, these results were self-report responses to one item in which a description of addiction was provided followed by the prompt, "Have you ever been addicted to the following things?" (Sussman et al., 2014, p. 35). More research regarding the prevalence of love addiction is needed, particularly with the use of standardized assessments.

NEUROSCIENCE RELATED TO LOVE ADDICTION

There are many neurological similarities between the experience of being in love and addiction to drugs of abuse. Indeed, Burkett and Young (2012) noted, "virtually every neurochemical system implicated in addiction also participates in social attachment processes" (pp. 18–19). The experience of being in love is naturally rewarding, involving the activation of neurotransmitters such as dopamine and endogenous opioids (Burkett & Young, 2012; Earp et al., 2017; Reynaud et al., 2010) as well as neuropeptides, including oxytocin and vasopressin (Burkett & Young, 2012; Frascella et al., 2010). Additionally, some evidence suggests that the neurotransmitter serotonin may be suppressed in early love, which contributes to the experience of obsessive thoughts about the loved one (Reynaud et al., 2010). When in love, contact with the love object (e.g., seeing one's romantic partner) provides positive reinforcement (caused by reward circuitry activation) as well as negative reinforcement (eliminating negative mood states associated with withdrawal and craving for the loved one; Earp et al., 2017). Thus, the romantic partner can become a means of emotion regulation. If romantic love experiences are an individual's only means of modulating emotions, however, the behaviors can become problematic and potentially addictive. Schaeffer (2009) wrote, "In addictive love, we unconsciously use the objects of love, sex, or romance to stimulate the chemicals in our neuropathways to provide the high" (p. 26).

Researchers have found an association between being in love and activation of the mesolimbic dopamine system (Burkett & Young, 2012; Reynaud et al., 2010; Sussman, 2010; Zou et al., 2016), similar to the activation caused by drugs of abuse. Indeed, romantic love activates the ventral tegmental area, nucleus accumbens, caudate, and insula (among other regions)—all areas also associated with drug addiction (Aron et al., 2005; Fisher et al., 2016; Zou et al., 2016). In a meta-analysis of functional magnetic resonance imaging (fMRI) studies, researchers found that when shown a picture of their loved ones, individuals in romantic love demonstrated increased activation in their dopaminergic system and decreased activation in brain areas implicated in fear and anxiety (Ortigue et al., 2010). Additionally, researchers studied 10 women and 7 men who were intensely in love and, using fMRI methods, found that brain regions implicated in reward and motivation were activated when participants viewed a picture of their romantic partners while amygdala activity (implicated in fear responses) decreased (Aron et al., 2005). The researchers concluded, "romantic love is better characterized as a motivation or goal-oriented state that *leads to* various specific emotions such as euphoria or anxiety" (Aron et al., 2005, p. 335). Consequently, research indicates that being in love activates brain regions associated with motivation and reward, and decreases activation of regions associated with fear and anxiety.

It is important to note that dopamine release is associated with behaviors that are necessary for survival (e.g., eating, sexual activity; Christensen, 2017; Doidge, 2007). Thus, the dopamine-induced state of reward associated with being in love is thought to have a unique purpose for propagating the species. Specifically, it is believed that the experience of romantic love developed as a means to facilitate pair-bonding to strengthen the process of child rearing, thus ensuring the survival of the next generation (Fisher et al., 2016; Fletcher et al., 2015; Frascella et al., 2010). Scholars have proposed that romantic love, or the attraction system (which is distinct from the sex drive), specifically evolved as a means to facilitate mate selection and focus the individual's attention on a preferred partner (Fisher, 1998). Therefore, dopamine release during the early stages of romantic love may be adaptive, serving to motivate individuals toward pair-bonding.

In addition to neurotransmitter stimulation within the reward system (e.g., dopamine, opioids), romantic love includes the release of two neuropeptides: *oxytocin* and *vasopressin* (Earp et al., 2017). Oxytocin is released in both men and women during sexual activity and while gazing into another person's eyes, and in women during labor and when nursing their infants (Burkett & Young, 2012; Carter, 2017; Doidge, 2007; Fletcher et al., 2015). It is clear that oxytocin plays a substantial role in attachment and social bonding given the results of groundbreaking research conducted on prairie voles. Specifically, researchers studied monogamous prairie voles and polygamous montane voles and found differences in the number of oxytocin receptors (Insel & Shapiro, 1992). Higher densities of oxytocin receptors were found in specific brain areas of the prairie voles (who mate for life and raise young together), but not in the montane voles (Insel & Shapiro, 1992; Lewis et al., 2000). Thus, these findings implicate oxytocin in the experience of attachment and pair-bonding. Furthermore, the club drug methylenedioxymethamphetamine (known as MDMA or ecstasy) is colloquially called the "love drug," as it is known to trigger oxytocin release and foster feelings of relational closeness and trust among users (Thompson et al., 2007).

Oxytocin often works in conjunction with vasopressin, a similar neuropeptide that is particularly relevant to attachment and bonding processes in men (Burkett & Young, 2012; Carter, 2017; Doidge, 2007). Specifically, vasopressin is released when men become fathers (Doidge, 2007) and also is implicated in protective or possessive attachment behaviors (Carter, 2017). Both oxytocin and vasopressin are released during social encounters (Burkett & Young, 2012) and are implicated in activating the dopaminergic system, further inducing rewards (Reynaud et al., 2010).

Therefore, neurotransmitter and neuropeptide activation during romantic love is responsible for the feelings of pleasure and social bonding associated with the experience. However, the fact that being in love is rewarding does not mean that all love constitutes an addictive behavior (defined by compulsivity, a lack of control, continued engagement despite negative consequences, and cravings or mental preoccupation). Instead, for a small portion of individuals who are genetically predisposed toward abnormally strong and chronic feelings of reward, the experience of being in love may become the primary means of regulating emotions, which can lead to addiction (Earp et al., 2017).

HOW DO I IDENTIFY IT?

Although love or relationship addiction is not included in the fifth edition of the *Diagnostic and Statistical Manual of Mental Disorders* (5th ed.; *DSM-5*; American Psychiatric Association [APA], 2013), scholars have proposed criteria for identifying the condition. For example, Reynaud et al. (2010) proposed six criteria for love addiction: (a) withdrawal symptomology when the loved one is unavailable, (b) substantial time devoted to the relationship (via thoughts or behaviors), (c) decreased activity in other important areas (e.g., professional, social, leisure activities) due to the relationship, (d) unsuccessful attempts to cut back, control, or decrease contact with the loved one, (e) continuing to pursue the relationship in spite of negative consequences, and (f) attachment difficulties evidenced by frequent, short-lived romantic relationships or recurrent distressing relationships marked by insecure attachment. According to Reynaud et al. (2010), endorsing three or more criteria in a 12-month period is indicative of love addiction.

In addition, based on a thorough literature review, Redcay and Simonetti (2018) developed 11 criteria of love addiction categorized into four factors: (a) impaired control, (b) life impairment, (c) disregard of partner's behavior, and (d) prevention or reduction of undesirable emotions. The criteria comprising these categories include: (a) the desire to stop engaging with the desired person, (b) unsuccessful attempts to stop engaging with the desired person, (c) frequent contact with or thoughts about the desired person, (d) intense urges to continue contact with the desired person, (e) engagement with the desired person that interferes with one's ability to fulfill important obligations, (f) engagement with the desired person that continues despite problems, (g) withdraw from other activities in order to engage with the desired person, (h) exhibition of maladaptive or unusual behaviors to maintain engagement with the desired person (e.g., lying, self-injury), (i) continued engagement despite maladaptive behavior by the desired person (e.g., physical abuse, manipulation), (j) engagement (or reengagement) with the desired person to prevent negative emotional experiences (initially engagement is euphoric, yet later, engagement is needed to prevent negative mood states), and (k) engagement (or reengagement) with the desired person to decrease negative emotional experiences (engagement utilized as a means of reducing loneliness, depression, distress, or anxiety; Redcay & Simonetti, 2018). The four factors of these proposed criteria reflect the common features of addiction (e.g., loss of control, compulsivity, continued engagement despite negative consequences, and craving or mental preoccupation).

Finally, it may be helpful for counselors to consider Mellody et al.'s (1992) three characteristics of love addiction: (a) disproportionate or obsessive amounts of time, attention, focus, and value placed on the person whom the individual loves; (b) unrealistic expectations of the person whom the individual loves, such as providing constant unconditional positive regard; and (c) diminished valuing and caring for themselves while in a romantic relationship. In addition, those with love addiction often display a profound fear of abandonment (stemming from childhood attachment wounds) as well as a fear of healthy intimacy (stemming from a lack of exposure to healthy intimacy in childhood). Specifically, "love addicts consciously want intimacy but can't tolerate healthy closeness, so they must unconsciously choose a partner who cannot be intimate in a healthy way" (Mellody et al., 1992, p. 10). These sets of criteria may assist counselors in identifying whether their clients need further assessment related to love addiction.

NEGATIVE CONSEQUENCES OF LOVE ADDICTION

Unlike ingesting a drug of abuse that can cause bodily harm, being in love is not physically harmful, in and of itself. Instead, pathological or addictive love can lead to risky or detrimental behaviors. Fisher et al. (2016) noted, "even when romantic love can't be regarded as harmful, it is associated with intense craving and can compel the lover to believe, say, and do dangerous and inappropriate things" (p. 2). These "dangerous and inappropriate things" can include self-injury, suicidal behavior, or criminal acts. One specific criminal act that has been linked to love addiction is stalking (Schaeffer, 2009). Although many individuals with love addiction do not engage in stalking, some individuals who stalk others may have love addiction. According to the U.S. Department of Justice, stalking is, "a course of conduct directed at a specific person that would cause a reasonable person to feel fear" (Catalano, 2012, p. 1). Among the three neurological systems associated with mating (sex, attraction, and attachment; Fisher, 1998), stalking is most associated with the attraction system, also known as romantic love (Meloy & Fisher, 2005). When love is unrequited, most individuals grieve the loss and focus their attraction on another potential romantic partner. Those who engage in stalking behaviors, however, become fixated on the object of their attraction and continue trying to secure contact despite their rejection. It is hypothesized that these individuals may be caught in a "negative feedback loop" in which elevated levels of dopamine and suppressed levels of serotonin reinforce each other, leading to high energy and motivation coupled with and obsessive thoughts and dysphoria (Meloy & Fisher, 2005, p. 1476). Therefore, when working with love addiction, counselors should assess clients' responses to rejection or unrequited love and address stalking behaviors if they are present.

> **CLINICAL NOTE 7.2**
>
> According to the National Intimate Partner and Sexual Violence Survey, 16% of women and 5.8% of men in the United States experienced stalking at some point in their lives (Smith et al., 2018). Stalking tactics may include unwanted phone calls, texts, emails, social media messages, gifts, or visits, watching the victim from a distance, following the victim, spying, unwanted visits, or breaking into the victim's home (Smith et al., 2018). It is important for counselors to distinguish between stalking behaviors and symptoms of love addiction. Although some individuals with love addiction may engage in stalking, there are many other motives for stalking behaviors (e.g., revenge, intimidation, harassment, predatory, delusional, and mental illness; Miller, 2012).

HOW DO I ASSESS IT?

There is a dearth of published assessments specific to love addiction. Therefore, in what follows, you will find the descriptions of a love addiction scale and a codependency scale. Both measures may be useful in your work with clients who present with symptoms of love addiction.

LOVE ADDICTION INVENTORY

The 24-item Love Addiction Inventory (LAI; Costa et al., 2019) and six-item Love Addiction Inventory Short Form (LAI-SF; Costa et al., 2019) are self-report measures of addictive love. The 24-item LAI is composed of four items representing each of the six components of addiction proposed by Brown (1993) and Griffiths (1996, 2005): salience, tolerance, mood modification, relapse, withdrawal, and conflict. Items of the LAI correspond to five-point Likert-type scales ranging from *never* (1) to *very often* (5) with higher summed scores indicating more love addiction symptoms. Example LAI items include: *How often do you feel anxious when you are not in the company of your partner* and *How often do you neglect time studying or working to be in relationship with your partner*. Scores on the six subscales of the LAI have demonstrated acceptable reliability with Cronbach's alpha levels ranging from .77 to .95 among an Italian sample (Costa et al., 2019). The LAI-SF includes one item corresponding to each of the six components of addiction in which higher summed scores indicate more love addiction symptomology. Scores on the LAI-SF also demonstrated acceptable reliability (Cronbach's alpha = .82). Items of the LAI are listed in the table of the original Costa et al. (2019) article.

COMPOSITE CODEPENDENCY SCALE

The 19-item Composite Codependency Scale (CCS; Marks et al., 2012) was developed as a means to revise and improve existing codependency measures. The authors reviewed previously published scales and developed the CCS to address their limitations and provide a holistic assessment of codependency. Using a sample of adults from the general community as well as members of Co-Dependents Anonymous, the authors identified 19 items that provided an acceptable three-factor structure for the scale. Thus, the CCS provides a total score and three subscale scores: (a) interpersonal control, (b) self-sacrifice, and (c) emotional suppression. Each item corresponds with a five-point Likert-type scale ranging from *strongly disagree* (1) to *strongly agree* (5). Example items of the CCS include: *What I feel isn't important as long as those I love are okay* and *I try to control events and how other people should behave*. Scores on the CCS demonstrated good reliability with the following Cronbach's alpha scores: total scale (.83), interpersonal control subscale (.80), self-sacrifice subscale (.77), and emotional suppression subscale (.83). All items of the CCS can be found in the original Marks et al. (2012) article.

HOW DO I TREAT IT?

Individuals with love addiction often have low levels of self-esteem, histories of trauma or dysfunctional attachments, fear of abandonment, and poor boundaries. They use romance as a means to meet unmet needs of love and attachment and escape uncomfortable or distressing emotions (Norwood, 1985). Therefore, counseling clients with love addiction is multifaceted and includes addressing both intrapersonal and interpersonal issues, which may take substantial amounts of time. Indeed, "recovery from addictive love is not one single event but a very gradual process" (Hayes, 1989, p. 36). Providing psychoeducation related to the features of mature, independent love (as opposed to pathological, dependent love) can be an important component of counseling (Sussman, 2010). In addition, given that feelings of romance or romantic partners are utilized as a primary means of emotion regulation, clients with love addiction can benefit from learning and developing alternative methods of mood management and self-soothing techniques (Sussman, 2010). Although seeking support from caring individuals often can be a healthy form of emotion regulation, the complete dependence on one person or the euphoria of romance to stabilize one's mood can be detrimental.

It also is common for those with love addiction to have incomplete, fragmented, or unclear views of themselves (as they typically define themselves within the context of a romantic relationship). Therefore, counselors can work with clients to help them gain clear, complete, and comprehensive self-identities, independent of romantic partners (Hayes, 1989). A value-sort activity or assessment of personal goals may be helpful tools to assist clients in identifying and appreciating their own unique ways of being in the world. Additionally, Fisher et al. (2016) suggested that clients with love addiction can benefit by engaging in "self-expanding activities" (p. 6) such as new personal hobbies, novel interesting experiences, rewarding or challenging activities, or spiritual practices. Along with promoting clients' self-discovery, novel self-expanding activities can trigger activation of the dopaminergic system, thereby creating replacement rewards for addictive love (Fisher et al., 2016).

Finally, it is likely that clients with love addiction have histories of unhealthy attachment with caregivers or significant figures in their lives; thus trauma work and attachment work may be essential components of treatment. Specifically, modeling secure attachment in counseling with appropriate boundaries and unconditional positive regard can be a corrective experience for those with love addiction. As clients experience secure attachments in counseling, they will be able to foster healthy relationships with appropriate boundaries outside of the counseling room.

VOICES FROM THE FIELD: Clinical Work With Love Addiction

I enjoy working with clients with love addiction because when clients are motivated, there is a high potential for change and recovery. I believe it is imperative for clients struggling with love addiction to understand the origins of their love addicted responses and behavioral patterns. Understanding the profound impact of neglect and/or abandonment helps clients move from judgment of self to curiosity about their reactions and behaviors. This understanding occurs through both education and experiential trauma work such as inner child work and eye movement desensitization and reprocessing. With this understanding, the client is increasingly able to move to self-compassion, which is critical for recovery.

Another important component of treatment is helping the client to understand theirr love addiction cycle and recognize when they are either in or moving into the cycle. Working on emotional regulation skills and self-soothing is also an important part of treatment. These skills are essential for the client to manage their emotional dysregulation, particularly when in the withdrawal phase of the cycle.

As a clinician, it is important to maintain a nonjudgmental attitude, especially when the client returns to maladaptive behaviors and patterns and/or returns to a dysfunctional relationship. Moving into healthier responses and behaviors tends to be a gradual process; therefore, as a clinician, it is important to be patient with the client's change process. Love addiction, because it is connected to early attachment and therefore, survival, can be one of the most difficult addictions from which to recover. In fact, sometimes love addiction is the primary addiction underneath other addictive processes such as compulsive overeating and substance abuse, which are used to regulate the client's abandonment distress from love addiction.

Sarah Bridge LCSW; LLC; Senior Clinical Advisor for The Meadows Behavioral Health

EYE MOVEMENT DESENSITIZATION AND REPROCESSING

For clients with love addiction who have histories of trauma, eye movement desensitization and reprocessing (EMDR) may be a useful intervention. Indeed, Schaeffer (2009) noted, "Healing trauma is probably the single most important factor for the successful long-term recovery from sex, romance, and love addiction" (p. 52). Developed by Francine Shapiro in the 1980s, EMDR is a therapeutic intervention to resolve distressing memories of both big "T" trauma (events meeting the clinical definition of trauma) and small "t" trauma (events that do not meet the clinical definition of trauma, yet are painful and troubling; Shapiro & Forrest, 1997). The tenets of EMDR stem from a mind–body connection described in the Adaptive Information Processing (AIP) model (Shapiro, 2018). Specifically, the AIP model proposes that traumatic events often become stuck in an individual's nervous system and affect the way in which they engage with the world (Shapiro, 2018; Shapiro & Forrest, 1997). Traumatic experiences disrupt the functioning of an individual's natural information processing system, resulting in a lack of integration or assimilation of distressing events. Instead, the sensations, cognitions, feelings, and reactions to the traumatic events are stored in their distressing forms as unresolved experiences. Using an eight-phase protocol, trained EMDR clinicians activate the brain's information processing system to work through the traumatic memories so that they are diffused, resolved, and integrated in a way that does not affect the individual's daily experiences. The activation of the information processing system occurs through bilateral dual stimulation, often in the form of eye movements in which a client tracks a clinician's fingers in diagonal movements (Shapiro, 2018; Shapiro & Forrest, 1997).

The eight phases of EMDR include: (a) developing a treatment plan (after taking a client's history and determining the target traumatic event to be addressed by the intervention), (b) preparation (building a strong therapeutic alliance with the client, describing the theory and process of EMDR, and equipping the client with relaxation strategies), (c) assessment (selecting a scene or image that represents the target event, identifying the negative self-belief and negative emotion associated with the event, choosing a positive self-statement that the client would like to believe instead of the negative self-statement, and identifying the subjective units of distress rating associated with the target event), (d) desensitization (leading clients through eye movement sets to activate the information processing system), (e) installation (strengthening the client's belief in the positive self-statement, which must be endorsed both intellectually and affectively), (f) body scan (asking the client to consider the original target event and assess whether tension remains in the body; if so, the counselor and client reprocess the residual tension), (g) closure (ensuring the client is in a calm state of equilibrium at the end of the session and equipping the client with calming techniques), and (h) reevaluation (at the start of each subsequent session, checking in with the client to assess whether the gains made in the previous session were sustained and identify new target events on which to focus; Shapiro, 2018; Shapiro & Forrest, 1997).

Scholars have described the appropriateness of EMDR with unrequited love and codependence (Knipe, 2005) as well as attachment issues in couples (Moses, 2007). Specifically, Moses (2007) noted, "EMDR's promise lies in its uniquely rapid processing of attachment injuries that are often at the core of relational issues" (p. 162). In light of the prevalence of childhood trauma and family dysfunction among those with love addiction, EMDR may be a useful intervention among those with both big "T" or small "t" trauma histories. Importantly, clinicians should not practice EMDR without proper training and certification, so interested readers should review the websites of the EMDR International Association (emdria.org) and EMDR Institute (emdr.com) to learn more about EMDR and training opportunities.

PYSCHODRAMA

Lorena et al. (2008) examined the impact of a psychodrama therapy group to treat pathological love. The researchers classified pathological love as an obsessive, manic style of love in which one's personal interests are neglected in order to care for a romantic partner. Eight participants who demonstrated signs of pathological love were recruited and participated in 18 weeks of group therapy based on psychodramatic analysis. Group topics included: recognizing oneself, decreasing illusions related to one's partner, working through negative feelings, assessing the function of the relationship, exploring family-of-origin relationships, and working through inner conflict. At the conclusion of the group therapy, participants' dependency on their romantic relationship improved as well as their predominant love style. The researchers concluded that group psychodrama holds promise for treating pathological love (Lorena et al., 2008).

12-STEP SUPPORT

Sex and Love Addicts Anonymous (SLAA) is a 12-step fellowship that emerged in the late 1970s as a support group for those addicted to sex, love, or both. Modeled after Alcoholics Anonymous, SLAA endorses the 12 steps, with the first step stating, "We admitted we were powerless over sex and love addiction—that our lives had become unmanageable" (The Augustine Fellowship, Sex and Love Addicts Anonymous, 1986, p. 67). According to SLAA, sex and love addiction manifests as, "a compulsive need for sex, extreme dependency on one person (or many), and/or chronic preoccupation with romance, intrigue or fantasy" (The Augustine Fellowship, Sex and Love Addicts Anonymous, 2004, p. 2). SLAA offers a recovery community for those with love and/or sex addiction, with the only requirement for membership being the desire to stop addictive sexual and/or emotional behaviors. Like other 12-step programs, members of SLAA attend meetings, work with sponsors, read literature and a common text, work the 12 steps, rely on a Higher Power, and strive to carry the message of SLAA to others with sex or love addiction. SLAA provides a 40-question assessment to help individuals determine if they may have sex or love addiction. Example items include: *Do you find yourself unable to stop seeing a specific person even though you know that seeing this person is destructive to you* and *Do you make promises to yourself or rules for yourself concerning your sexual or romantic behavior that you find you cannot follow* (The Augustine Fellowship, Sex and Love Addicts Anonymous, 1985).

According to SLAA, sobriety from sex and love addiction entails remaining abstinent from compulsive pursuits of sex and romance, hyperdependency on others, and obsession with sexual or emotional intrigue or fantasy. Like other behavioral addictions, the goal is not to remain abstinent from sex or love, but instead, to abstain from the compulsive, out-of-control, obsessive behaviors that foster negative consequences. Members of SLAA work with sponsors to identify and name their bottom lines—or behaviors from which they are choosing to abstain. These bottom line behaviors are detrimental to the individual's "physical, mental, emotional, sexual, and spiritual wholeness" (The Augustine Fellowship, Sex and Love Addicts Anonymous, 1997). It is important to note that bottom line behaviors are unique to each individual and are determined with their sponsor in a state of sobriety. Bottom line behaviors could include: pursuing an unavailable romantic partner, compulsive fantasy that interferes with other responsibilities, anonymous sexual encounters, pursuing multiple romantic partners simultaneously, lying to others about sexual or romantic pursuits, using pornography, or using sex to earn other's affection. SLAA is a free program that is widely available and may be a helpful resource to clients with love addiction. Learn more about SLAA by visiting their website (slaafws.org).

DIAGNOSTIC CONSIDERATIONS

Currently, there is no formal diagnosis for love addiction or pathological love in the *DSM*. Therefore, counselors working with clients with love addiction may choose to diagnose co-occurring disorders (e.g., depression, anxiety) or coaddictions (e.g., substance use disorder, gambling disorder) when appropriate. Additionally, it is important for counselors to rule out other diagnoses that could manifest as symptoms of love addiction. Specifically, differential diagnoses could include mania, borderline personality disorder, or dependent personality disorder (Sanches & John, 2019). According to the *DSM-5*, dependent personality disorder is marked by an individual's excessive need to be cared for and pervasive fear of being alone (APA, 2013). Although some of the criteria for this disorder reflect symptoms of love addiction, the motivation of those with dependent personality disorder is to be nurtured and avoid the extreme discomfort felt when alone, rather than securing positive and negative reinforcement through the euphoria of romance or a romantic partner. Additionally, the erotomanic type of delusional disorder may have overlapping symptoms with love addiction (specifically, fantasy and persistent desires to procure contact with the object of one's attraction), yet in erotomania, the relationship (which often is with someone of higher status, such as a celebrity) is not grounded in reality (APA, 2013). Thus, love addiction involves actual contact with a potential romantic partner while erotomania is marked by delusions.

HOW CAN I LEARN MORE?

If you are working with clients with love addiction or would like to learn more about the condition, consider the following resources.

BOOKS

- Mellody, P., Miller, A. W., & Miller, J. K. (1992). *Facing love addiction: Giving yourself the power to change the way you love*. HarperCollins Publishers.
- Peabody, S. (2005). *Addiction to love: Overcoming obsession and dependency in relationships* (3rd ed.). Celestial Arts.
- Schaeffer, B. (2009). *Is it love or is it addiction?* (3rd ed.). Hazelden.

PEER-REVIEWED ARTICLES

- Burkett, J. P., & Young, L. J. (2012). The behavioral, anatomical and pharmacological parallels between social attachment, love and addiction. *Psychopharmacology, 224*, 1–26. https://doi.org/10.1007/s00213-012-2794-x

- Reynaud, M., Karila, L., Blechai, L., & Benyamina, A. (2010). Is love passion an addictive disorder? *The American Journal of Drug & Alcohol Abuse, 36,* 261–267. https://doi.org/10.3109/00952990.2010.495183
- Sussman, S. (2010). Love addiction: Definition, etiology, treatment. *Sexual Addiction & Compulsivity, 17,* 31–45. https://doi.org/10.1080/10720161003604095

WEBSITES

- Co-Dependents Anonymous: coda.org
- Sex and Love Addicts Anonymous: slaafws.org

REFERENCES

American Psychiatric Association. (2013). *Diagnostic and statistical manual of mental disorders* (5th ed.).

Author.Aron, A., Fisher, H., Mashek, D. J., Strong, G., Li, H., & Brown, L. L. (2005). Reward, motivation and emotion systems associated with early-stage intense romantic love. *Journal of Neurophysiology, 94,* 327–337. https://doi.org/10.1152/jn.00838.2004

The Augustine Fellowship, Sex and Love Addicts Anonymous. (1985). *40 questions for self diagnosis.* https://slaafws.org/download/core-files/The_40_Questions_of_SLAA.pdf

The Augustine Fellowship, Sex and Love Addicts Anonymous. (1986). *Sex and love addicts anonymous.* Author.

The Augustine Fellowship, Sex and Love Addicts Anonymous. (1997). *The welcome pamphlet.* https://slaafws.org/slaaterms

The Augustine Fellowship, Sex and Love Addicts Anonymous. (2004). *Addicted to sex? Addicted to love?* slaafws.org/pamphlets/addicted.pdf

Brown, R. I. F. (1993). Some contributions of the study of gambling to the study of other addictions. In W. R. Eadington & J. A. Cornelius (Eds.), *Gambling behaviour and problem gambling* (pp. 341–272). University of Nevada Press.

Burkett, J. P., & Young, L. J. (2012). The behavioral, anatomical and pharmacological parallels between social attachment, love and addiction. *Psychopharmacology, 224,* 1–26. https://doi.org/10.1007/s00213-012-2794-x

Calderwood, K. A., & Rajesparam, A. (2014). A critique of the codependency concept considering the best interests of the child. *Families in Society: The Journal of Contemporary Social Services, 95,* 171–178. https://doi.org/10.1606/1044-3894.2014.95.22

Carter, C. S. (2017). The role of oxytocin and vasopressin in attachment. *Psychodynamic Psychiatry, 45,* 499–518. https://doi.org/10.1521/pdps.2017.45.4.499

Catalano, S. (2012). *Stalking victims in the United States-revised.* https://www.bjs.gov/content/pub/pdf/svus_rev.pdf

Christensen, J. F. (2017). Pleasure junkies all around! Why it matters and why 'the arts' might be the answer: A biopsychological perspective. *Proceedings of the Royal Society B, 284,* 20162837. https://doi.org/10.1098/rspb.2016.2837

Co-Dependents Anonymous, Inc. (1998). *The fellowship service manual of Co-Dependents Anonymous*. https://coda.org/wp-content/uploads/2020/01/FSM-Part-2-Meeting-Handbook.pdf

Co-Dependents Anonymous, Inc. (2018). *Welcome to co-dependents anonymous*. https://coda.org/newcomers

Costa, S., Barberis, N., Griffiths, M. D., Benedetto, L., & Ingrassia, M. (2019). The love addiction inventory: Preliminary findings of the development process and psychometric characteristics. *International Journal of Mental Health and Addiction*. https://doi.org/10.1007/s11469-019-00097-y

Doidge, N. (2007). *The brain that changes itself: Stories of personal triumph from the frontiers of brain science*. Penguin Group.

Earp, B. D., Wudarczyk, O. A., Foddy, B., & Savulescu, J. (2017). Addicted to love: What is love addiction and when should it be treated. *Philosophy, Psychiatry, and Psychology, 24*, 77–92.

Eisenman, R., Dantzker, M. L., & Ellis, L. (2004). Self ratings of dependency/addiction regarding drugs, sex, love, and food: Male and female college students. *Sexual Addiction and Compulsivity, 11*, 115–127. https://doi.org/10.1080/10720160490521219

Fisher, H. E. (1998). Lust, attraction, and attachment in mammalian reproduction. *Human Nature, 9*, 23–52. https://doi.org/10.1007/s12110-998-1010-5

Fisher, H. E., Xu, X., Aron, A., & Brown, L. L. (2016). Intense, passionate, romantic love: A natural addiction? How the fields that investigate romance and substance abuse can inform each other. *Frontiers in Psychology, 7*, 687. https://doi.org/10.3389/fpsyg.2016.00687

Fletcher, G. J. O., Simpson, J. A., Campbell, L., & Overall, N. C. (2015). Pair-bonding, romantic love, and evolution: The curious case of homo sapiens. *Perspectives on Psychological Science, 10*, 20–36. https://doi.org/10.1177/1745691614561683

Frascella, J., Potenza, M. N., Brown, L. L., & Childress, A. R. (2010). Shared brain vulnerabilities open the way for nonsubstance addictions: Carving addiction at a new joint? *Annals of the New York Academy of Science, 1187*, 294–315. https://doi.org/10.1111/j.1749-6632.2009.05420.x

Galperin, A., & Haselon, M. (2010). Predictors of how often and when people fall in love. *Evolutionary Psychology, 8*, 5–28. https://doi.org/10.1177/147470491000800102

Griffiths, M. D. (1996). Behavioural addiction: An issue for everybody? *Journal of Workplace Learning, 8*, 19–25.

Griffiths, M. (2005). A 'components' model of addiction within a biopsychosocial framework. *Journal of Substance Use, 10*, 191–197. https://doi.org/10.1080/14659890500114359

Hayes, J. (1989). *Smart love: A codependence recovery program based on relationship addiction support groups*. Jeremy P. Tarcher Inc.

Horowitz, J. M., Graf, N., & Livingston, G. (2019). *Marriage and cohabitation in the U.S.* pewsocialtrends.org/2019/11/06/marriage-and-cohabitation-in-the-U-S

Insel, T. R., & Shapiro, L. E. (1992). Oxytocin receptor distribution reflects social organization in monogamous and polygamous voles. *Proceedings of the National Academy of Sciences of the United States of America, 89*, 5981–5985.

Kafka, M. P. (2010). Hypersexual disorder: A proposed diagnosis for DSM-V. *Archives of Sexual Behavior, 39*, 377–400. https://doi.org/10.1007/s10508-009-9574-7

Kafka, M. P. (2014). What happened to hypersexual disorder? *Archives of Sexual Behavior, 43*, 1259–1261. https://doi.org/10.1007/s10508-014-0326-y

Kessel, P. V., & Hughes, A. (2018). *Americans who find meaning in these four areas have higher life satisfaction.* pewresearch.org/fact-tank/2018/11/20/americans-who-find-meaning-in-these-four-areas-have-higher-life-satisfaction

Knipe, J. (2005). Targeting positive affect to clear the pain of unrequited love, codependence, avoidance, and procrastination. In R. Shapiro (Ed.), *EMDR solution: Pathways to ealing* (pp. 189–212). W. W. North & Company.

Lewis, T., Amini, F., & Lannon, R. (2000). *A general theory of love.* Vintage Books.

Lorena, A., Sophia, E. C., Mello, C., Tavares, H., & Zilberman, M. (2008). Group therapy for pathological love. *Brazilian Journal of Psychiatry, 30,* 292–293. https://doi.org/10.1590/S1516-44462008000300019

Marks, A. D. G., Blore, R. L., Hine, D. W., & Dear, G. E. (2012). Development and validation of a revised measure of codependency. *Australian Journal of Psychology, 64,* 119–127. https://doi.org/10.1111/j.1742-9536.2011.00034.x

Mellody, P., Miller, A. W., & Miller, J. K. (1989). *Facing codependence: Where it is, where it comes from, how it sabotages our lives.* Harper Collins Publishers.

Mellody, P., Miller, A. W., & Miller, J. K. (1992). *Facing love addiction: Giving yourself the power to change the way you love.* Harper Collins Publishers.

Meloy, J. R., & Fisher, H. (2005). Some thoughts on the neurobiology of stalking. *Journal of Forensic Sciences, 50,* 1472–1480.

Miller, L. (2012). Stalking: Patterns, motives, and intervention strategies. *Aggression and Violent Behavior, 17,* 495–506. https://doi.org/10.1016/j.avb.2012.07.001

Money, J. (1997). *Principles of developmental sexology.* The Continuum Publishing Company.

Moses, M. D. (2007). Enhancing attachments: Conjoint couple therapy. In F. Shapiro, F. W. Kaslow, & L. Maxfield (Eds.), *Handbook of EMDR and family therapy processes* (pp. 146–166). John Wiley & Sons Inc.

Norwood, R. C. (1985). *Women who love too much: When you keep wishing and hoping he'll change.* Pocket Books.

Ortigue, S., Bianchi-Demicheli, F., Patel, N., Frum, C., & Lewis, J. W. (2010). Neuroimaging of love: fMRI meta-analysis evidence toward new perspectives in sexual medicine. *Journal of Sexual Medicine, 7,* 3541–3552. https://doi.org/10.1111/j.1743-6109.2010.01999.x

Peabody, S. (2005). *Addiction to love: Overcoming obsession and dependency in relationships* (3rd ed.). Celestial Arts.

Redcay, A., & Simonetti, C. (2018). Criteria for love and relationship addiction: Distinguishing love addiction from other substance and behavioral addictions. *Sexual Addiction and Compulsivity, 25,* 80–95. https://doi.org/10.1080/10720162.2017.1403984

Reynaud, M., Karila, L., Blechai, L., & Benyamina, A. (2010). Is love passion an addictive disorder? *The American Journal of Drug and Alcohol Abuse, 36,* 261–267. https://doi.org/10.3109/00952990.2010.495183

Sanches, M., & John, V. P. (2019). Treatment of love addiction: Current status and perspectives. *The European Journal of Psychiatry, 33,* 38–44. https://doi.org/10.1016/j.ejpsy.2018.07.002

Schaeffer, B. (2009). *Is it love or is it addiction?* (3rd ed.). Hazelden.

Shapiro, F. (2018). *Eye movement desensitization and reprocessing (EMDR) therapy* (3rd ed.). Guilford Press.

Shapiro, F., & Forrest, M. S. (1997). *EMDR: A breakthrough therapy for overcoming anxiety, stress, and trauma.* BasicBooks.

Smith, S. G., Zhang, X., Basile, K. C., Merrick, M. T., Wang, J., Kresnow, M., & Chen, J. (2018). *The National Intimate Partner and Sexual Violence Survey (NISVS): 2015 data brief—Updated release*. National Center for Injury Prevention and Control, Centers for Disease Control and Prevention.

Sophia, E. C., Tavares, H., Berti, M. P., Pereira, A. P., Lorena, A., Mello, C., Gorenstein, C., & Zilbreman, M. L. (2009). Pathological love: Impulsivity, personality, and romantic relationship. *CNS Spectrums, 14,* 268–274.

Sussman, S. (2010). Love addiction: Definition, etiology, treatment. *Sexual Addiction and Compulsivity, 17,* 31–45. https://doi.org/10.1080/10720161003604095

Sussman, S., Arpawong, T. E., Sun, P., Tsai, J., Rohrbach, L. A., & Spruijt-Metz, D. (2014). Prevalence and co-occurrence of addictive behaviors among former alternative high school youth. *Journal of Behavioral Addictions, 3,* 33–40. https://doi.org/10.1556/JBA.3.2014.005

Sussman, S., Lisha, N., & Griffiths, M. (2011). Prevalence of the addictions: A problem of the majority or the minority? *Evaluation and the Health Professions, 34,* 3–56. https://doi.org/10.1177/0163278710380124

Tennov, D. (1979). *Love and limerence: The experience of being in love*. Scarborough House.

Thompson, M. R., Callaghan, P. D., Hunt, G. E., Cornish, J. L., & McGregor, I. S. (2007). A role for oxytocin and 5-HT$_{1A}$ receptors in the prosocial effects of 3,4 methylenedioxymethamphetamine ("ecstasy"). *Neuroscience, 146,* 509–515. https://doi.org/10.1016/j.neuroscience.2007.02.032

Weiss, R. (2019). Prodependence vs. codependency: Would a new model (prodependence) for treating loved ones of sex addicts be more effective than the model we've got (codependency)? *Sexual Addiction and Compulsivity, 26,* 177–190. https://doi.org/10.1080/10720162.2019.1653239

Whitfield, C. L. (1991). *Co-dependence: Healing the human condition*. Health Communications.

Willmott, L., & Bentley, E. (2015). Exploring the lived experience of limerence: A journey toward authenticity. *The Qualitative Report, 20,* 20–38.

World Health Organization. (2018). *International statistical classification of diseases and related health problems* (11th Rev.). https://icd.who.int/browse11/l-m/en

Wright, P. H., & Wright, K. D. (1991). Codependency: Addictive love, adjustive relating, or both? *Contemporary Family Therapy, 13,* 435–454.

Zou, Z., Song, H., Zhang, Y., & Zhang, X. (2016). Romantic love vs. drug addiction may inspire a new treatment for addiction. *Frontiers in Psychology, 7,* 1436. https://doi.org/10.3389/fpsyg.2016.011436

8

Gambling Addiction

HOW DO I CONCEPTUALIZE IT?

Gambling refers to wagering something of value to win something more valuable in an activity determined to some degree by chance (American Psychiatric Association [APA], 2013; Hunt & Blaszczynski, 2019). Many forms of gambling exist, such as land-based casino games (e.g., poker, roulette, blackjack), lotteries, scratch-off tickets, bingo, horse racing, dog racing, live sports betting, fantasy sports (FS) betting, electronic gambling machines (EGMs), and, more recently, internet gambling. Gambling is a popular activity in the United States. According to the American Gaming Association (AGA), there are 979 casinos spread throughout 43 states (AGA, 2019a) and 44% of U.S. adults visited a casino in the previous 12 months (AGA, 2019b). Many individuals gamble recreationally without experiencing negative consequences (except, perhaps, a decrease in their bank accounts). For a small portion of individuals, however, gambling becomes compulsive, they experience a loss of control over their gambling activities, they continue to gamble despite negative consequences, and they crave or are mentally preoccupied with gambling when they are not engaging in the behavior. These individuals likely have gambling addiction.

Addiction is a complex phenomenon that is best conceptualized as the result of a relationship between a susceptible individual (host) and a rewarding activity or substance (agent; Ahrens et al., 2014; Centers for Disease Control and Prevention, 2012; Schüll, 2012; see Chapter 1). Although genetic predispositions and biological vulnerability contribute to the development of addiction, so too do the *properties of the addictive behaviors* or substances themselves. For example, in chemical addiction, certain individuals are more susceptible to substance use disorders (based on their genetic makeup; Blum et al., 1996; Leshner, 2001), yet the substances themselves also have properties that contribute to the development of addiction (specifically, the way in which the substances interfere with neurotransmission and affect reward circuitry in the brain; see Chapter 2). Thus, addiction is the result of the unique relationship between the individual and the addictive behavior (Giovino, 2000; Miller et al., 2019; Rasmussen, 2000), and this also is true for gambling. Schüll (2012) wrote, "Just as certain individuals are more vulnerable to addiction than others, it is also the case that some objects, by virtue of their unique pharmacological or structural characteristics, are more likely than others to trigger or accelerate addiction" (p. 17). Gambling behaviors are uniquely appealing and activate reward circuitry in ways that are distinct from other activities (e.g., driving to work, brushing one's teeth, watching television). Additionally, there are diverse forms of gambling that can influence susceptible individuals in various ways. For example, playing the lottery is distinctively different from playing EGMs, just like heroin is distinctively different from marijuana. Therefore, it is important for counselors to consider both their clients' unique traits and propensities as well as the characteristics of the specific gambling activity when working with gambling addiction.

TYPES OF GAMBLING ACTIVITIES

Clients with gambling addiction often engage in multiple forms of gambling. Among participants with both gambling disorders and substance use disorders, researchers found that 83.3% gambled in casinos, 70.5% played the lottery, and 48.1% engaged in sports betting (Rennert et al., 2014). Additionally, clients in treatment for pathological gambling in the United Kingdom reported playing the lottery (78.5%), betting on sports (66.3%), using betting terminals (64.7%), internet gambling (64.4%), using EGMs (57.3%), and playing casino games (41.7%; Ronzitti et al., 2017). Although many forms of gambling have existed for hundreds of years, some activities are relatively new, such as internet gambling and EGMs.

Internet gambling websites emerged in the early 1990s at offshore locations (e.g., the Caribbean) and changed the landscape of gambling behavior (Sulkunen et al., 2019). Instead of traveling to a casino, individuals could now engage in a variety of gambling activities (e.g., poker, bingo, sports betting, casino games) using their home computers, smartphones, or other devices at any time—day or night (Gainsbury, 2012). Additionally, with low overhead costs (i.e., a website domain versus a land-based casino building), internet gambling sites can offer more payouts to players (Gainsbury, 2012). The ease of access and low regulations of internet gambling make it a particularly important consideration for treating gambling addiction. Indeed, among participants who met criteria for problem gambling, 48.7% participated in internet gambling in the previous month (Petry & Gonzalez-Ibanez, 2015). Moreover, those who engaged in internet gambling wagered larger amounts of money, gambled more frequently, incurred more gambling-related debt, and experienced more anxiety and gambling-related problems (Petry & Gonzalez-Ibanez, 2015). The internet offers constant access to gambling; therefore, one necessary aspect of gambling addiction treatment is to help clients construct plans for how to engage with the internet without utilizing gambling sites.

EGMs are another newer form of gambling. Rather than the previous version of slot machines with pull handles and gears, EGMs are computer-operated with buttons and touch screens. These machines are becoming a major source of revenue in the gambling industry and are replacing table games in casinos (Schüll, 2012). EGMs stimulate the senses with colors and sounds and offer the opportunity for rapid play (using EGMs, individuals can play a new game every 3–4 seconds; Schüll, 2012). Rather than a social activity, EGMs offer a "solitary, absorptive activity" that can "suspend time, space, monetary value, social roles, and sometimes even one's very sense of existence" (Schüll, 2012, p. 12). Schüll (2012) recounted players' experience of playing EGMs and described entering *the zone*—a trancelike state in which nothing else exists other than the machine. This zone experience can provide an escape from negative emotional states by producing a rhythmic, rewarding, calming experience. Thus, rather than becoming addicted to winning, those with a gambling disorder become addicted to staying in the zone and continuing in the state of play (Schüll, 2012). Counselors should explore the function of EGM play with their clients to identify the purpose of the behavior. This information can help with treatment planning as counselors and clients devise new coping and emotion regulation strategies other than relying on the zone facilitated by EGM play.

CLINICAL NOTE 8.1

Another proposed form of gambling, which is deemed to be more socially acceptable than other activities, is stock market investing (Granero et al., 2012). Among a sample of 1,470 clients in treatment for pathological gambling, 5.2% of the sample reported stock market investments as a secondary gambling problem and 1.2% identified stock market investments as their primary gambling problem. Researchers found that higher levels of education significantly predicted stock market investments as a gambling problem among participants (Granero et al., 2012).

PREVALENCE OF GAMBLING ADDICTION

Prevalence rates of gambling addiction vary considerably depending on whether researchers are investigating the general population, samples of gamblers, or specific subgroups of the population. For example, a meta-analysis of problem gambling among college students from seven different countries revealed prevalence rates ranging from 3% to 32% (Nowak & Aloe, 2014). Subramaniam et al. (2015) reviewed 25 studies of pathological gambling among older adults in various countries and found rates ranging from 0.01% (in Denmark) to 10.6% (in the United States). Furthermore, a recent review of problem gambling among adolescent samples revealed rates ranging from 0.9% (Norway) to 7.9% (Finland), with varying frequencies in between (e.g., 5.6% Greece, 4.8% New Zealand, 4.0% Italy, 3.2% Croatia; Floros, 2018). Researchers also have investigated the prevalence of gambling problems among veteran populations. Amid a nationally representative sample of 3,157 veterans, 2.2% were classified as problem gamblers and 35.1% gambled recreationally (Stefanovics et al., 2017). Within populations with mental illnesses, researchers found that 5.3% were at-risk gamblers (Bergamini et al., 2018). Despite the variability in these prevalence rates, scholars consistently find that gambling disorder is more prevalent among men compared to women (Black & Shaw, 2019; Moghaddam et al., 2015). Additionally, researchers have reported the age of first gambling experience among those who met criteria for problem gambling to be approximately 14 years old (Petry & Gonzalez-Ibanez, 2015).

GAMBLING-RELATED COGNITIVE DISTORTIONS

Common features of gambling addiction include cognitive distortions related to chance, probability, randomness, control, and skill (APA, 2013; Clark et al., 2013; Hunt & Blaszczynski, 2019; Shaffer & Shaffer, 2014). Those with gambling addiction may erroneously believe they can somehow influence the outcome of games of chance by using a certain machine, choosing particular numbers, or engaging in specific rituals or behaviors while playing (i.e., *illusions of control*; Clark et al., 2013). Additionally, those with gambling addiction often develop distorted beliefs about chance, assuming that cards, dice, or slot machines "remember" previous outcomes and adapt accordingly so that a payout is "due" after a string of losses (i.e., the *gambler's fallacy*; Lepley, 1963). Finally, gamblers often have distorted thoughts about near misses. In games of chance (such as EGMs, bingo, the lottery, and scratch-off tickets), a near miss (e.g., getting four of the five lottery numbers) is still a loss, yet may be erroneously perceived to be "close" to winning (Parke & Griffiths, 2004). Near misses can cause a spike of excitement, arousal, and anticipation as the gambler interprets them as signs that they are nearing a win. However, logic tells us that in games of chance, a near miss has no bearing on future outcomes (Parke & Griffiths, 2004). These distorted beliefs about chance, random play, skill, and control are powerful motivators to keep individuals gambling. Indeed, among a sample of video lottery terminal players in Canada, researchers found that gambling-related cognitive distortions mediated the relationship between personality traits and problem gambling (MacLaren et al., 2015).

In light of the prevalence of cognitive distortions among those with gambling addiction, cognitive work often is an important component of treatment (e.g., identifying distorted beliefs, using Socratic questioning, disputing, engaging in cognitive restructuring, providing psychoeducation). For instance, among 125 Canadian clients in treatment for moderate-to-severe gambling disorder, researchers identified common distortions including the belief that clients were unable to stop gambling, belief in the ability to control gambling, and the ability to predict gambling outcomes (Ledgerwood et al., 2019). After the completion of residential treatment, researchers found significant reductions in all cognitive distortion scores among participants (Ledgerwood et al., 2019).

NEUROSCIENCE RELATED TO GAMBLING ADDICTION

Gambling addiction develops from a convergence of genetic, psychological, social, and cultural characteristics (Shaffer & Shaffer, 2014). Rather than conceptualizing those who gamble as a homogeneous group, Blaszczynski and Nower (2002) proposed a pathway model describing three subgroups of problem gamblers. The first pathway to problem gambling transpires through *behavioral conditioning*. When individuals engage in gambling activities, they are aware of the possibility of a reward (the percentage of land-based gambling machine payouts is regulated), yet do not know when that reward is coming. This type of reinforcement schedule is called *variable ratio*, meaning that the reward is unpredictable and occurs after an unknown number of engagements in a behavior (Skinner, 1969, 1976). Variable ratio reinforcement schedules differ from *fixed ratio reinforcement schedules* in which a reward follows an identified, predictable number of engagements in a behavior. (Consider a teenager who gets to use his tablet after completing five chores. In this scenario, the reward comes after the fifth response.) Although fixed ratio reinforcement schedules increase the likelihood that a behavior will be repeated, they do not induce the same excitement and motivation as variable ratio reinforcement schedules (Skinner, 1969, 1976). Indeed, unexpected schedules of rewards tend to be the most reinforcing (Platt et al., 2010) and if an outcome is better than one expected (e.g., winning the jackpot rather than winning $2), dopamine release (the neurotransmitter implicated in the experience of reward) in the reward system of the brain is much greater (Shultz et al., 1997). Thus, the excitement and anticipation caused by the variable ratio reinforcement schedule of gambling activities motivates individuals to continue playing, anxiously waiting to see if *this* round will be the winning round.

It is important to note that after repeated engagement in a behavior, *learning* occurs and dopamine gets released upon exposure to the reward *cue* (Shultz et al., 1997). Once particular stimuli (e.g., gambling machines, casinos, cards, football games) are paired with rewards, dopamine is activated by exposure to the stimuli itself (i.e., cue), rather than the actual reward (Shultz et al., 1997). Thus, even without a monetary payout, those with gambling addiction find the experience of being in a casino, placing bets, or staying in action rewarding due to the activation of the dopaminergic system.

According to Blaszczynski and Nower (2002), the behaviorally conditioned subgroup of problem gamblers initiates gambling for social or recreational purposes (in regions where gambling is available and accessible). These gamblers do not have any preexisting mental health disorders, but are especially susceptible to the effects of operant conditioning (i.e., variable ratio reinforcement schedules) and gambling-related cognitive distortions. Treatment for this subgroup of gamblers can be brief and focused on psychoeducation about gambling, behavioral interventions, and cognitive restructuring (Blaszczynski & Nower, 2002).

The second pathway to problem gambling described in the model is emotional vulnerability (Blaszczynski & Nower, 2002). Although the same principles of operant conditioning affect this group, the motivation for gambling is different from those in the behaviorally conditioned subgroup. Emotionally vulnerable gamblers have preexisting mental health concerns (e.g., anxiety, depression, phobias, a history of trauma, substance use disorders), and gambling is sought as a means of regulating negative emotional experiences. Gambling activities (particularly solitary games such as online gambling or EGMs) can produce a type of dissociative state in which the gambler focuses solely on the game, thereby escaping the troubles, stresses, and discomforts of life (i.e., what Schüll [2012] described as *the zone*). Consequently, for those who are emotionally vulnerable, gambling can be an effective, albeit potentially detrimental, means of escape and mood modification. Treatment for this subgroup includes a focus on problem gambling as well as addressing preexisting mental health concerns (Blaszczynski & Nower, 2002).

Finally, Blaszczynski and Nower (2002) described the third pathway to problem gambling as antisocial, impulsivist characteristics. This subgroup of problem gamblers is characterized by impulsivity, which manifests in other problem behaviors beyond gambling (e.g., substance misuse, hypersexuality, criminal activity). Like the previous subgroup, these individuals have psychological and biological vulnerabilities and are affected by operant conditioning principles, yet they demonstrate features of antisocial personality disorder including a disregard for social norms, narcissistic tendencies, reckless behavior, and irresponsibility (APA, 2013). Gamblers in this subgroup tend to have poorer treatment prognoses and may be disinclined to seek help for gambling or other addictions (Blaszczynski & Nower, 2002). Counselors may need to work on increasing motivation (see the section on motivational interviewing) prior to implementing gambling treatment protocols. Overall, the pathway model can help clinicians identify the biological, psychological, and social attributes of gambling addiction among their clients and tailor treatment appropriately.

It also can be helpful for counselors to conceptualize gambling as but one manifestation of an addictive disorder with various potential expressions

(Shaffer & Shaffer, 2014). In support of this notion, researchers have identified neurobiological similarities between chemical addiction and gambling addiction (Fauth-Buhler et al., 2017; Pirritano et al., 2014; Romanczuk-Seiferth et al., 2014). Common neurological traits among those with both chemical and gambling addiction include changes in executive functioning (i.e., operations of the prefrontal cortex), alterations in reward circuitry, and decreased reward sensitivity (Romanczuk-Seiferth et al., 2014). Reduced prefrontal cortex activity (found among those with gambling addiction) has been linked to difficulty predicting potential detrimental consequences of risky behavior, increased impulsivity, and decreased cognitive flexibility (Fauth-Buhler et al., 2017). In the examination of 52 studies of gambling addiction, researchers found that those with gambling disorder exhibited more impulsivity, deficits in inhibition, and impaired decision-making compared to control participants (Loannidis et al., 2019). The authors thus concluded that some individuals have a proclivity toward premature, risky, or hasty actions, which puts them at higher risk for the development of gambling addiction (Loannidis et al., 2019). Therefore, after controlling gambling behavior, it is important for counselors to work with clients on issues related to executive functioning such as decision-making, assessing risk, delay discounting, and problem-solving.

CLINICAL NOTE 8.2

Researchers have found increased gambling problems among a portion of individuals with Parkinson's disease who are being treated with dopamine replacement medications (dopamine agonists; Olley et al., 2015; Pirritano et al., 2014). Although dopamine medication adjustments may be helpful, more research is needed to identify effective treatment strategies among Parkinson's patients who develop gambling disorder.

SPORTS BETTING AND DAILY FANTASY SPORTS

Another form of gambling that counselors should be familiar with is *sports betting*. In the 2018 case, *Murphy vs. National Collegiate Athletic Association*, the Supreme Court ruled that the 1992 Professional and Amateur Sports Protection Act, which prohibited state sanctioning of sports betting, was unconstitutional (Melone, 2018). This ruling gave states the authority to regulate sports betting, and, since then, many states have legalized or are currently considering the legalization of the activity. According to the AGA (2019b), 13 states have legalized sports betting with more states taking steps to legalize it in the near future. With reference to betting on sports, scholars have used the term *gamblification*, which means "expanding the areas of sport susceptible to being gambled upon" (Lopez-Gonzalez & Griffiths, 2018, p. 405). There are many ways to make wagers on sports outcomes (e.g., point spread wagering), and the recent legalization of sports betting creates greater accessibility and availability of gambling activities. Future research will determine whether sports betting legalization correlates with a greater prevalence of gambling disorder, yet, for now, clinicians should explore clients' engagement in sports betting in addition to other gambling activities.

Along with betting on live sports activities, individuals also can bet on FS. FS entail using sports data to assemble virtual teams who earn FS users points based on real-time players' performances (Nower et al., 2018). According to the Fantasy Sports and Gaming Association (FSGA, 2020a), 19% of American adults play FS, the most popular of which is fantasy football. FS participation is rising exponentially with 15.2 million participants in 2003 and 59.3 million in 2017 (FSGA, 2020a).

Betting on traditional FS spans the duration of an athletic sport's season as virtual teams are created and points are distributed after every game. At the end of the season, money is exchanged based on the total number of FS users' points. This type of FS betting differs from *daily fantasy sports* (DFS) betting, which allows participants to bet on the outcomes of specific games and players' performances happening the day the game is played. Draftkings and Fanduels are two prominent servers that organize DFS. Users pay to enter contests and create their fantasy player lineups in hopes of winning a daily contest (Nelson et al., 2019). Using data from Draftkings, researchers found that users' average age was 34 years old and they spent a median of $87 on contest entry fees during a professional football season (Nelson et al., 2019).

DFS betting seems to be a distinct form of gambling. Researchers found that DFS players (compared to those who gambled without betting on DFS) were more likely to be male, use drugs, have mental health problems, contemplate suicide, and use pornography (Nower et al., 2018). Additionally, 97.7% of DFS players engaged in other forms of gambling (Nower et al., 2018). Moreover, another study of DFS players revealed that 14% were at high risk for problem gambling and 24% were at moderate risk (Dwyer et al., 2018). Therefore, counselors should assess whether their clients participate in DFS betting and assess the frequency of the activity, the amount of money wagered, time spent on the activity, the function of the activity, the experience of negative consequences, and involvement in other addictive behaviors.

CLINICAL NOTE 8.3

According to the Fantasy Sports and Gaming Association (2020b), each state determines whether paid fantasy sports contests are games of skill or considered forms of gambling. The organization offers details related to each state's legislation concerning fantasy sports (thefsga.org/current-u-s-state-by-state-regulations). Counselors should stay up to date related to gambling laws and regulations in their states.

HOW DO I IDENTIFY IT?

The authors of the fifth edition of the *Diagnostic and Statistical Manual of Mental Disorders* (*DSM-5*; APA, 2013) made important changes related to the diagnosis for gambling addiction. First introduced in the third edition of the *Diagnostic and Statistical Manual of Mental Disorders* (*DSM-III*; APA, 1980), Pathological Gambling was included in the section for impulse-control disorders and this classification remained consistent in the fourth edition of the *Diagnostic and Statistical Manual of Mental Disorders* (*DSM-IV*; APA, 1994). In the *DSM-5*, however, Pathological Gambling was renamed Gambling Disorder and reclassified from an impulse-control disorder to a nonsubstance-related addictive disorder in the section "Substance-Related and Addictive Disorders" (APA, 2013). This change denotes the similarities between behavioral and chemical addictions.

To meet diagnostic criteria for gambling disorder in the *DSM-5*, individuals must experience impairing problematic gambling with at least four of the following nine symptoms within a 12-month period: (a) gambling with increasing quantities of money to experience desired excitement; (b) feelings of restlessness associated with the cessation or decrease of gambling activity; (c) inability to control or cut back gambling behaviors despite numerous attempts; (d) mental preoccupation with gambling; (e) engaging in gambling behaviors to relieve dysphoric mood; (f) chasing losses (i.e., trying to win back lost money); (g) lying to hide the truth about gambling behaviors; (h) experiencing the loss of important jobs, relationships, or opportunities due to gambling behaviors; and (i) experiencing financial difficulty from gambling and seeking help via bailouts from others (APA, 2013). Gambling disorder can be episodic (i.e., when symptoms discontinue for several months in between periods of meeting diagnostic criteria), persistent (i.e., uninterrupted symptoms meeting diagnostic criteria), in early remission (i.e., no symptoms meeting diagnostic criteria for at least 3 months but less than 1 year), or sustained remission (i.e., no symptoms meeting diagnostic criteria for at least 12 months), and is not better explained by mania. The severity of the diagnosis is represented by mild (four or five criteria met), moderate (six or seven criteria met), or severe (eight or nine criteria met; APA, 2013).

Gambling disorder also is listed as a "Disorder due to Addictive Behaviours" in the *International Classification of Diseases*, 11th revision (*ICD-11*; World Health Organization [WHO], 2018) with many similarities to the description in the *DSM-5*. Specifically, the criteria in the *ICD-11* refer to online or offline gambling in which an individual experiences the loss of control, prioritizes gambling above other life activities and responsibilities, continues to gamble despite negative consequences, and has impaired functioning due to gambling (WHO, 2018). Researchers have confirmed that the criteria in both the *DSM* and *ICD* are prevalent among those with gambling addiction. Among over 500 individuals who met criteria for both the fourth and fifth editions of the *DSM* diagnoses of Pathological Gambling and Gambling Disorder respectively, the most endorsed symptoms were preoccupation with gambling (98.6%), chasing losses (89.3%), relying on others for financial bailouts (85.6%), a need to gamble increasing amounts of money (83.1%), and lying about gambling behaviors (78.7%; Rennert et al., 2014). Indeed, the act of chasing losses, or continuing to gamble in hopes of regaining money lost in previous gambling ventures, is a unique hallmark of gambling addiction and can serve as a signal to counselors to assess further for gambling disorder.

RISK FACTORS FOR GAMBLING ADDICTION

Researchers have identified several risk factors and correlates of gambling addiction. In a review of longitudinal studies, scholars reported that male gender, greater degrees of impulsivity, and inadequate academic performance predicted problematic gambling with medium or small-to-medium effect sizes (Dowling et al., 2017). Additionally, among gamblers in a psychiatric unit, researchers identified the following predictors of problem gambling: drug abuse, having two or more psychiatric disorders, and a family history of gambling (Bergamini et al., 2018). Interestingly, 55.9% of participants in the study reported that they engaged in gambling prior to the onset of the psychiatric disorder (Bergamini et al., 2018). With regard to correlates reported in cross-sectional studies, researchers found relationships between problem gambling and a variety of characteristics and experiences. For example, in an exploration of veterans, those in the problem gambler group had greater odds of physical and sexual trauma histories, suicidal ideation or attempts, poorer sleep, mood disorders, and substance use disorders than nonproblem gamblers (Stefanovics et al., 2017). Moreover, researchers found that older adults with gambling disorder were more likely to abuse alcohol, have medical illnesses, and have a psychiatric diagnosis (Subramaniam et al., 2015). Clients may come to counseling with a variety of presenting concerns (e.g., substance misuse, depression, anxiety, sleep problems, financial issues), yet it is important for counselors to assess whether the client engages in gambling activities as well. The shame associated with gambling addiction may hinder some clients from being forthcoming with their gambling behavior, yet knowing risk factors and correlates can help counselors assess appropriately.

GAMBLING ADDICTION AND CRIMINAL BEHAVIOR

Although no longer a criterion for gambling disorder in the *DSM-5*, a correlation exists between gambling addiction and criminal behavior (Hunt & Blaszczynski, 2019; Sulkunen et al., 2019). Those with gambling addiction may engage in criminal activity to secure money for gambling, engage in illegal gambling practices, or violate gambling regulations (Sulkunen et al., 2019). Indeed, 53.3% of those who met criteria for gambling disorder reported committing illegal acts (Rennert et al., 2014). Moreover, in a meta-analysis of 12 studies of gambling disorder among individuals in prison, researchers found that between 5.9% and 73% of samples met criteria for problem gambling (Banks et al., 2019). Additionally, the authors of the Gamblers Anonymous (GA) text stated, "Obtaining money becomes of paramount importance, often necessitating such devious actions as writing bad checks, stealing money from a child's savings account, cheating on an expense account, or embezzling" (GA, 1984, p. 10). Rather than taking a moralistic perspective of those with gambling addiction, it is important for counselors to consider that these clients may engage in criminal activity as a desperate attempt to fund the addiction they believe they cannot live without. Those with gambling disorder may rationalize that although they are committing a crime, they will win back the money via gambling to make appropriate restitutions.

GAMBLING ADDICTION AND SUICIDE

Gambling addiction differs from other addictive behaviors due to the nature of the negative consequences experienced by those with the disorder. Although all addictive behaviors can indirectly impact one's financial situation (e.g., paying for pornography), gambling by nature directly affects an individual's financial assets. Gambling addiction can bring with it the loss of one's savings account, children's college fund, retirement savings, income needed to pay the mortgage, rent, or electric bills, and financial security. The finality of the loss of thousands, or hundreds of thousands, of dollars in one weekend of gambling can lead to thoughts of suicide. In fact, among a national nonclinical sample in the United States, 49.2% of those who met criteria for problem gambling reported suicidal ideation and 18.3% reported a history of at least one suicide attempt (Moghaddam et al., 2015). Furthermore, in a sample of patients in treatment for pathological gambling in the United Kingdom, 46.77% presented with current suicidal ideation and 62.18% reported at least one experience of suicidal ideation in the past (Ronzitti et al., 2017). Moreover, approximately 23% of those with suicidal ideation attempted suicide (Ronzitti et al., 2017). Additionally, Penfold et al. (2006) assessed individuals upon hospital admission who had attempted suicide and found that 17% met criteria for problematic gambling. Therefore, it is imperative that counselors assess for suicidal ideation and histories of suicide attempts among their clients with gambling addiction and continue this assessment throughout treatment.

HOW DO I ASSESS IT?

Many assessment and screening tools exist to examine gambling behaviors among clients. Along with the criteria outlined in the *DSM-5* and *ICD-11*, the three instruments described in the following text may be helpful tools for your clinical work with gambling addiction.

SOUTH OAKS GAMBLING SCREEN

The South Oaks Gambling Screen (SOGS; Lesieur & Blume, 1987) is a widely utilized instrument to assess problematic gambling. The 20-item screen (with additional nonscored items) is based on the criteria for pathological gambling described in the *DSM-III*. Items on the SOGS assess type and frequency of gambling activities, amount of money wagered, family history of gambling problems, experience of chasing losses, loss of control, deceptive behavior, and borrowing money to pay gambling debts. Example items include *When you gamble, how often do you go back another day to win back money you lost* and *Have you ever felt like you would like to stop gambling but didn't think you could*. Endorsing five or more of the 20 scored items is indicative of problematic gambling. Scores on the SOGS demonstrated excellent reliability with a Cronbach's alpha of .97 and test–retest reliability of .71 and have been utilized in a variety of samples in several different countries (Lesieur & Blume, 1987). The full SOGS and scoring instructions can be found in the appendix of Lesieur and Blume's (1987) original article.

CANADIAN PROBLEM GAMBLING INDEX

The Canadian Problem Gambling Index (CPGI) was created to assess problem gambling in general populations (Ferris & Wynne, 2001). The scale was normed on large samples of Canadian adults and demonstrated acceptable reliability (Cronbach's alpha = .84; test–retest reliability = .78). To score the instrument, the nine items are summed (these nine items [5–13] make up the Problem Gambling Severity Index; the remaining items provide useful information for clinical assessment but are not scored). Scores are interpreted as: 0 = nonproblem gambler, 1 to 2 = low-risk gambler, 3 to 7 = moderate-risk gambler, and 8 or higher = problem gambler. Items on the CPGI examine the frequency of gambling activities, time spent gambling, amount of money spent in gambling ventures, betting more than one can afford, increasing the amount of money wagered, chasing losses, borrowing money to gamble, problems caused by gambling, inability to stop, and deceptive activity (Ferris & Wynne, 2001). The entire CPGI can be found in the original Ferris and Wynne (2001) publication.

BRIEF BIOSOCIAL GAMBLING SCREEN

The Brief Biosocial Gambling Screen (BBGS) was developed to be a short screening instrument to identify members of the general population who may meet criteria for pathological gambling (Gebauer et al., 2010). The three items of the BBGS reflect the domains of neuroadaptations (withdrawal), psychosocial characteristics (lying), and adverse social behavior (borrowing money). An example item includes *During the past 12 months, have you become restless, irritable, or anxious when trying to stop/cut down on gambling.* Using a large nationally representative sample, the BBGS demonstrated strong sensitivity (.96) for identifying those with pathological gambling. The short screen may be particularly helpful in clinical and medical settings. Clients who endorse any of the three items warrant further exploration of gambling disorder (Gebauer et al., 2010). The full BBGS is available in the original article (Gebauer et al., 2010) and on the International Center for Responsible Gaming website (www.icrg.org/resources/brief-biosocial-gambling-screen).

HOW DO I TREAT IT?

Although multiple forms of treatment for gambling addiction exist, a limited number of individuals with gambling disorder seek help for their addiction. Hapuisto (2019) interviewed 12 clients in treatment for problem gambling in Finland and identified the following barriers to help-seeking: shame, pride, anger, denial, and secrecy. Additionally, participants identified mental health professionals as a barrier to gambling treatment by not recognizing, or by minimizing, gambling addiction. Finally, participants reported that gambling culture served as a barrier to treatment due to the fact that gambling establishments normalize gambling behavior and do not differentiate between social and problematic gambling (Hapuisto, 2019).

When clients do present for treatment, it is likely that they are already experiencing legal, financial, or relational difficulties due to prolonged problematic gambling. The client may be in treatment voluntarily, as part of a gambling diversion program, or to appease a loved one or employer. It is important for counselors to empathetically meet clients where they are and work to increase motivation when needed (see the section on motivational interviewing). Additionally, counselors working with gambling addiction should be familiar with referral sources for debt management and financial counseling to help clients improve their financial situation (e.g., development of a financial recovery plan). Counselors also may work with clients' family members or significant others to identify and equip another individual to manage the client's money, which can serve as a trigger for gambling activity. Finally, in conjunction with group or individual counseling, couple or family counseling may be helpful to address the family systems affected by the gambling disorder.

When working with clients with gambling addiction in an individual counseling format, counselors have a variety of approaches to consider, including brief interventions. In a meta-analysis, Quilty et al. (2019) found that brief (one session) interventions composed of psychoeducation to increase awareness, advice, goal setting, increasing motivation, and feedback significantly correlated with short-term decreases in gambling behavior.

Long-term outcomes, however, were not significantly affected (Quilty et al., 2019). Thus, brief interventions may be particularly effective for the behaviorally conditioned subgroup of problem gamblers described in the pathway model (Blaszczynski & Nower, 2002), rather than those with co-occurring disorders or antisocial characteristics. Clients presenting only with gambling disorder may be the minority, however, as co-occurring mental health concerns are common among this population. In a meta-analysis of problem or pathological gamblers, researchers found that 57.5% of participants also had a substance use disorder, 37.9% had a mood disorder, 37.4% had an anxiety disorder, and 28.8% met criteria for antisocial personality disorder (Lorains et al., 2011). In particular, high comorbidity exists between substance use disorders and gambling disorders (Black & Shaw, 2019; Fauth-Buhler et al., 2017). Therefore, counselors working with clients with substance use disorders should assess for gambling activity and counselors working with clients who gamble should assess for substance use as well. Additionally, given the prevalence rates, counselors should routinely assess for suicidal ideation among those who seek treatment for gambling disorder (Ronzitti et al., 2017).

VOICES FROM THE FIELD: Clinical Work With Gambling Addiction

I started working in the drug and alcohol addiction field long before I got involved with the gambling population. The difference is that you can't recognize a gambling client by outward appearances (oftentimes they have good jobs, make good money, are well dressed, and live in affluent areas) and there isn't a test you can give to see if they have been gambling recently. By the time a client comes to me for counseling, they have already hit the bottom—meaning they cannot pay their bills and are in large amounts of debt. They may have many maxed-out credit cards, have exhausted their savings accounts, taken out multiple bank loans, and lost their pensions. The statistics say that one out of five gamblers attempts suicide.

What contributes to the successful treatment of gambling addiction is to help clients replace gambling with something else. I often ask clients to think about what they used to enjoy doing before they started gambling. Some clients tend to be prone to risky behaviors (like bungee jumping), but you can help them find substitutions through exercise/physical activities or learning new hobbies. Some clients explore (or reexplore) spirituality and can benefit from faith communities, meditation, yoga, and relaxation activities. Ultimately, it is important for clients to replace gambling with something in which they find enjoyment. I often say to my clients: "If you stop gambling and never have fun again, why would you want to stop?"

What I have learned over the years is that there is not one type of therapy that works for all gambling clients. Motivational interviewing, cognitive behavioral therapy, and client-centered counseling are all good—but one size does not fit all. For example, Gamblers Anonymous can be extremely important for some clients, but it isn't for everyone. There are great resources out there to support those with gambling addiction; for example, the 1-800-GAMBLER hotline operated by the Council on Compulsive Gambling is a valuable tool.

Counseling those with gambling addiction can be challenging—but also can be the most rewarding and satisfying counseling experiences you'll ever have. Take the gamble!

Pamela Dobbs, LCADC, CCS, SAC, MA, ICGC-II

COGNITIVE BEHAVIORAL APPROACH

In light of the effects of cognitive distortions and operant conditioning on gambling addiction, a cognitive behavioral therapy (CBT) approach can be an effective treatment method. Raylu and Po Oei (2010) created a CBT manual for counselors working with clients who identify problem gambling as their presenting concern. The treatment approach addresses gambling-related cognitive distortions, fosters coping skills, and emphasizes relapse prevention strategies. Specifically, the manual outlines 10 core sessions followed by three elective sessions. The core sessions entail: (a) assessing problem gambling behavior and increasing motivation, (b) providing psychoeducation related to gambling and stabilizing gambling activity, (c) identifying gambling-related cognitive distortions, (d) challenging gambling-related cognitive distortions, (e) addressing additional cognitive distortions related to gambling behaviors, (f) training in relaxation and utilizing imaginal exposure to gambling cues, (g) increasing problem-solving capabilities and goal-setting skills, (h) developing emotion regulation skills and coping strategies, (i) engaging in relapse prevention through attaining life balance, and (j) engaging in relapse prevention by coping with gambling triggers and cues. The three elective sessions address interpersonal relationships and social skills, financial issues, and the impact of gambling addiction on others. The authors of the manual noted that this structure is only a guide and counselors should utilize their own counseling style and clinical judgment to tailor the treatment to individual clients (Raylu & Po Oei, 2010).

MOTIVATIONAL INTERVIEWING

Along with CBT, evidence exists supporting the use of motivational interviewing (MI; Miller & Rollnick, 2013) in the treatment of gambling addiction, particularly in conjunction with other approaches (Di Nicola et al., 2019; Petry et al., 2017). Miller and Rollnick (2013) defined MI as "a person-centered counseling style for addressing the problem of ambivalence about change" (p. 21). As a communication style, MI can be used as a brief primary approach (one to two sessions), a precursor to treatment, or integrated throughout another treatment method. The basic premise of MI is that ambivalence is a natural step in the process of change. For clients caught in a state of ambivalence (i.e., wanting to change while simultaneously not wanting to change), MI works to help clients discover their own reasons for making the change, thereby increasing motivation toward positive outcomes.

MI is defined by both the spirit of the approach as well as the processes involved. Miller and Rollnick (2013) identified four components of the spirit of MI: partnership (it is a collaborative process between counselors and clients), acceptance (counselors affirm clients, recognize their absolute worth, respect their autonomy, and demonstrate accurate empathy), compassion (the use of MI is always to support clients' welfare), and evocation (rather than imparting information to clients, MI counselors seek to draw out clients' own motivations for change). With this spirit in mind, counselors engage in MI using four processes: engaging (developing a strong alliance with the client), focusing (identifying the direction of the work), evoking (drawing out the client's own reasons for change), and planning (developing specific strategies for how to enact the change; Miller & Rollnick, 2013).

Therefore, when working with a client with gambling addiction, the counselor can first work to fully understand the client's experience and communicate empathy (e.g., "I know it is difficult to talk about your internet gambling. I appreciate your honesty and the fact that a part of you does not want to give it up."). Next, the counselor and client would determine the focus of their work (e.g., "You mentioned being concerned about your marriage, feelings of depression, and your alcohol use. During our time together, we can talk about all of those issues, and particularly how gambling may or may not affect them.") and then move into the evoking process. When evoking, the counselor uses particular communication tools to elicit *change talk*, or any client statements supporting change. The counselor may ask questions eliciting change talk (e.g., "What might be the benefits of quitting gambling?," "What troubles you about your gambling?"), examine clients' values and goals (in order to highlight discrepancies between gambling behavior and values/goals), or ask a ruler-type question (e.g., "On a scale from 0 to 10, with 0 being not important and 10 being very important, how important is it for you to change your gambling behavior?" Once a client gives a number, MI counselors follow up with, "Why did you say [given number] and not a [lower number]?" to elicit change talk). Once the client shifts to using mostly change talk and begins considering changing their gambling behavior, the planning process begins. Specifically, counselors work with clients to develop concrete strategies for how change will take place (e.g., "What is the first step you need to do to quit gambling?," "Who can you ask to support you in this?," "What will you do next Friday when you get paid instead of going to the casino?"; Miller & Rollnick, 2013). If you are interested in learning more about MI, visit https://motivationalinterviewing.org and review the Miller and Rollnick (2013) text for great examples and resources.

SELF-EXCLUSION

Another component of recovery from gambling addiction may be *self-exclusion*. This process entails individuals putting themselves on a list barring them from gambling establishments statewide (if this option is available) or from specific gambling venues (and some states offer self-exclusion options for fantasy sports betting and internet gambling, as well). To apply for self-exclusion, individuals must complete an application, which, along with their photo, is sent to gambling facilities in the state. The self-exclusion ban prohibits the individual from entering the property of gambling establishments and precludes them from collecting any winnings. It may be helpful for counselors to discuss the self-exclusion option with their clients to see if it would be a useful component to their recovery plan. For an example of a self-exclusion policy, visit the website of the Responsible Gaming Association of New Mexico at rganm.org/self-exclusion.

12-STEP SUPPORT

Another resource for clients with gambling addiction is involvement in the 12-step program, Gamblers Anonymous. GA began in the 1950s following the format of Alcoholics Anonymous (AA) as a program to help individuals with the desire to stop gambling. According to the GA text, "members of the Fellowship gather to reinforce their efforts, as well as those of other compulsive gamblers, to abstain from gambling and to grow personally and spiritually" (GA, 1984, p. 57). GA follows the 12 steps of AA with Step One stating, "we admitted we were powerless over gambling—that our lives had become unmanageable" (GA, 1984, p. 67). GA created Twenty Questions to help individuals assess their gambling behaviors, including items such as *Have you ever considered self-destruction as a result of your gambling* and *Have you ever gambled to escape worry or trouble* (GA, 1984, p. 62). According to GA, if an individual endorses seven or more items on the Twenty Questions, they likely have a gambling addiction. Like other 12-step programs, GA is predicated on recovery in community and consists of meetings, sponsors, literature, texts, and relying on a Higher Power. Empirical evidence suggests that GA can be a helpful adjunct to counseling for some individuals with gambling addiction (Petry et al., 2017; Schuler et al., 2016). For more information, visit the GA website at gamblersanonymous.org.

HOW CAN I LEARN MORE?

Clinicians who are interested in more training related to gambling addiction should consider pursuing credentialing from the International Gambling Counselor Certification Board at www.igccb.org. If you would like to learn more about working with clients with gambling addiction, the following items are helpful resources.

BOOKS

- Heinz, A., Romanczuk-Seiferth, N., & Potenza, M. N. (Eds.). (2019). *Gambling disorder*. Springer Publishing Company.
- Raylu, N., & Po Oei, T. (2010). *A cognitive behavioural therapy programme for problem gambling: Therapist manual*. Routledge.
- Schüll, N. D. (2012). *Addiction by design: Machine gambling in Las Vegas*. Princeton University Press.

PEER-REVIEWED ARTICLES

- Blaszczynski, A., & Nower, L. (2002). A pathway model of problem and pathological gambling. *Addiction, 97*, 487–499. https://doi.org/10.1046/j.1360-0443.2002.0015.x
- Petry, N. M., Ginley, M. K., & Rash, C. J. (2017). A systematic review of treatments for problem gambling. *Psychology of Addictive Behaviors, 31*, 951–961. https://doi.org/10.1037/abd0000290
- Shaffer, H. J., & Shaffer, P. M. (2014). Psychiatric epidemiology, nosology, and treatment: Considering internet gambling. *Psychiatric Annals, 44*, 371–378. https://doi.org/10.3928/00485713-20140806-04

WEBSITES

- American Gaming Association: americangaming.org
- Gamblers Anonymous: gamblersanonymous.org
- National Council on Problem Gambling: ncpgambling.org
- International Center for Responsible Gaming: icrg.org

REFERENCES

Ahrens, W., Krickeberg, K., & Pigeot, I. (2014). An introduction to epidemiology. In W. Ahrens, & I. Pigeot (Eds.), *Handbook of epidemiology* (2nd ed., pp. 3–41). Springer Publishing Company.

American Gaming Association. (2019a). *State of play.* americangaming.org/state-of-play

American Gaming Association. (2019b). *Record support for casino gaming.* americangaming.org/wp-content/uploads/2019/10/AGA_AmerAtt_Final.pdf

American Psychiatric Association. (2013). *Diagnostic and statistical manual of mental disorders* (5th ed.). Author.

Banks, J., Waters, J., Andersson, C., & Olive, V. (2019). Prevalence of gambling disorder among prisoners: A systematic review. *International Journal of Offender Therapy and Comparative Criminology, 64*(12), 1199–1216. https://doi.org/10.1177/0306624x19862430

Bergamini, A., Turrina, C., Bettini, F., Toccagni, A., Valsecchi, P., Sacchetti, E., & Vita, A. (2018). At-risk gambling in patients with severe mental illness: Prevalence and associated features. *Journal of Behavioral Addictions, 7*, 348–354. https://doi.org/10.1556/2006.7.2018.47

Black, D. W., & Shaw, M. (2019). The epidemiology of gambling disorder. In A. Heinz, N. Romanczuk-Seiferth, & M. N. Potenza (Eds.). *Gambling disorder* (pp. 29-48). Springer Publishing Company.

Blaszczynski, A., & Nower, L. (2002). A pathway model of problem and pathological gambling. *Addiction, 97*, 487–499. https://doi.org/10.1046/j.1360-0443.2002.0015.x

Blum, K., Cull, J. G., Braverman, E. R., & Comings, D. E. (1996). Reward deficiency syndrome. *American Scientist, 84*, 132–146.

Centers for Disease Control and Prevention. (2012). *Principles of epidemiology in public health practice* (3rd ed). Author.

Clark, L., Averbeck, B., Payer, D., Sescousse, G., Winsanley, C. A., & Xue, G. (2013). Pathological choice: The neuroscience of gambling and gambling addiction. *Journal of Neuroscience, 33*, 17617–17623. https://doi.org/10.1523/JNEUROSCI.3231-13.2013

Di Nicola, M., De Crescenzo, F., D'Alo, G. L., Remondi, C., Panaccione, I., Moccia, L., Molinaro, M., Dattoli, L., Lauriola, A., Martinelli, S., Giuseppin, G., Maisto, F., Crosta, M. L., Di Pietro, S., Amato, L., & Janiri, L. (2019). Pharmacological and psychosocial treatment of aduts with gambling disorder: A meta-review. *Journal of Addiction Medicine*, Advanced Online Publication. https://doi.org/10.1097/ADM.0000000000000574

Dowling, N. A., Merkouris, S. S. Greenwood, C. J., Oldenhof, E., Toumbourou, J. W., & Youssef, G. J. (2017). Early risk and protective factors for problem gambling: A systematic review and meta-analysis of longitudinal studies. *Clinical Psychology Review, 51*, 109–124. https://doi.org/10.1016/j.cpr.2016.10.008

Dwyer, B., Shapiro, S. L., & Drayer, J. (2018). Daily fantasy football and self-reported problem behavior in the United States. *Journal of Gambling Studies, 34*, 689–707. https://doi.org/10.1007/s10899-017-9720-4

Fantasy Sports and Gaming Association. (2020a). *Industry demographics.* thefsga.org/industry-demographics

Fantasy Sports and Gaming Association. (2020b). *Distinguishing fantasy sports from sports betting*. https://thefsga.org/distinguishing-fantasy-sports-from-sports-betting

Fauth-Buhler, M., Mann, K., & Potenza, M. N. (2017). Pathological gambling: A review of the neurobiological evidence relevant for its classification as an addictive disorder. *Addiction Biology, 22*, 885-897. https://doi.org/10.1111/adb.12378

Ferris, J., & Wynne, H. (2001). *The Canadian Problem Gambling Index: Final report.* Submitted for the Canadian Centre on Substance Abuse.

Floros, G. D. (2018). Gambling disorder in adolescents: Prevalence, new developments, and treatment challenges. *Adolescent Health, Medicine and Therapeutics, 9*, 43–51. https://doi.org/10.2147/AHMT.S135423

Gainsbury, S. (2012). *Internet gambling: Current research findings and implications.* Springer Publishing Company.

Gamblers Anonymous. (1984). *Sharing recovery through Gamblers Anonymous*. Gamblers Anonymous Publishing Inc.

Gebauer, L., LaBrie, R., & Shaffer, H. J. (2010). Optimizing DSM-IV-TR classification accuracy: A brief biosocial screen for detecting current gambling disorders among gamblers in the general household population. *The Canadian Journal of Psychiatry, 55*, 82–90. https://doi.org/10.1177/070674371005500204

Giovino, G. A. (2002). Epidemiology of tobacco use in the United States. *Oncogene, 21*, 7326–7340. https://doi.org/10.1038/sj.onc.1205808

Granero, R., Tarrega, S., Fernandez-Aranda, F., Aymami, N., Gomez-Pena, M., Moragas, L., Custal, N., Orekhova, L., Savvidou, L. G., Menchón J. M., & Jimenez-Murcia, S. (2012). Gambling on the stock market: An unexplored issue. *Comprehensive Psychiatry, 53*, 666–673. https://doi.org/10.1016/j.comppsych.2011.12.004

Hapuisto, M. (2019). Problem gambler help-seeker types: Barriers to treatment and help-seeking processes. *Journal of Gambling Studies, 35*, 1035–1045. https://doi.org/10.1007/s10899-019-09846-z

Hunt, C. J., & Blaszczynski, A. (2019). Gambling disorder as a clinical phenomenon. In A. Heinz, N. Romanczuk-Seiferth, & M. N. Potenza (Eds.), *Gambling disorder* (pp. 15–27). Springer Publishing Company.

Ledgerwood, D. M., Dyshniku, F., McCarthy, J. E., Ostojic-Aitkens, D., Forfitt, J., & Rumble, S. C. (2019). Gambling-related cognitive distortions in residential treatment for gambling disorder. *Journal of Gambling Studies, 36*(2), 669–683. https://doi.org/10.1007/s10899-019-09895-4

Lepley, W. M. (1963). "The maturity of the chances": A gambler's fallacy. *The Journal of Psychology, 56*, 69–72. https://doi.org/10.1080/00223980.1963.9923

Leshner, A. I. (2001). Addiction is a brain disease. *Issues in Science and Technology, 3*, 75–80.

Lesieur, H. R., & Blume, S. B. (1987). The South Oaks Gambling Screen (SOGS): A new instrument for the identification of pathological gamblers. *American Journal of Psychiatry, 144*, 1184–1188. https://doi.org/10.1176/ajp.144.9.1184

Loannidis, K., Hook, R., Wickham, K., Grant, J. E., & Chamberlain, S. R. (2019). Impulsivity in gambling disorder and problem gambling: A meta-analysis. *Neuropsychopharmacology, 44*, 1354–1361. https://doi.org/10.1038/s41386-019-0393-9

Lopez-Gonzalez, H., & Griffiths, M. D. (2018). Betting, forex trading, and fantasy gaming sponsorships – a responsible marketing inquiry into the 'gamblification' of English football. *International Journal of Mental Health and Addiction, 16*, 404–419. https://doi.org/10.1007/s11469-017-9788-1

Lorains, F. K., Cowlishaw, S., & Thomas, S. A. (2011). Prevalence of comorbid disorders in problem and pathological gambling: Systematic review and meta-analysis of population surveys. *Addiction, 106*, 490–498. https://doi.org/10.1111/j.1360-0443.2010.03300.x

MacLaren, V., Ellery, M., & Knoll, T. (2015). Personality, gambling motives and cognitive distortions in electronic gambling machine players. *Personality and Individual Differences, 73*, 24–28. https://doi.org/10.1016/j.paid.2014.09.019

Melone, M. A. (2018). New Jersey beat the spread: Murphy V. National Collegiate Athletic Association and the demise of PASPA allows for states to experiment in regulating the rapidly evolving sports gambling industry. *University of Pittsburgh Law Review, 80*, 35–367. https://doi.org/10.5195/lawreview.2018.604

Miller, W. R., Forcehimes, A. A., & Zweben, A. (2019). *Treating addiction: A guide for professionals* (2nd ed.). The Guilford Press.

Miller, W. R., & Rollnick, S. (2013). *Motivational interviewing: Helping people change* (3rd ed.). Guilford Press.

Moghaddam, J. F., Yoon, G., Dickerson, D. L., Kim, S. W. & Westermeyer, J. (2015). Suicidal ideation and suicide attempts in five groups with different severities of gambling: Findings from the National Epidemiologic Survey on Alcohol and Related Concerns. *The American Journal on Addictions, 24*, 292–298. https://doi.org/10.1111/ajad.12197

Nelson, S. E., Edson, T. C., Singh, P., Tom, M., Martin, R. J., LaPlante, D. A., Gray, H. M., & Shaffer, H. J. (2019). Patterns of daily fantasy sport play: Tackling the issues. *Journal of Gambling Studies, 35*, 181–204. https://doi.org/10.1007/s10899-018-09817-w

Nowak, D., & Aloe, A. (2014). The prevalence of pathological gambling among college students: A meta-analytic synthesis, 2005–2013. *Journal of Gambling Studies, 30*, 819–843. https://doi.org/10.1007/s10899-013-9399-0

Nower, L., Caler, K. R., Pickering, D., & Blaszczynski, A. (2018). Daily fantasy sports players: Gambling addiction, and mental health problems. *Journal of Gambling Studies, 34*, 727–737. https://doi.org/10.1007/s10899-018-9744-4

Olley, J., Blaszczynski, A., & Lewis, S. (2015). Dopaminergic medication in Parkinson's disease and problem gambling. *Journal of Gambling Studies, 31*, 1085–1106. https://doi.org/10.1007/s10899-014-9503-0

Parke, J., & Griffiths, M. (2004). Gambling addiction and the evolution of the 'near miss'. *Addiction Research & Theory, 12*, 407–411. https://doi.org/10.1080/16066350410001728118

Penfold, A., Hatcher, S., Sullivan, S., & Collins, N. (2006). Gambling problems and attempted suicide. Part 1. High prevalence amongst hospital admissions. *International Journal of Mental Health and Addiction, 3*, 265–272. https://doi.org/10.1007/s11469-006-9025-9

Petry, N. M., Ginley, M. K., & Rash, C. J. (2017). A systematic review of treatments for problem gambling. *Psychology of Addictive Behaviors, 31*, 951–961. https://doi.org/10.1037/abd0000290

Petry, N. M., Gonzalez-Ibanez, A. (2015). Internet gambling in problem gambling college students. *Journal of Gambling Studies, 31*, 397–408. https://doi.org/10.1007/s10899-013-9432-3

Pirritano, D., Plastino, M., Bosco, D., Gallelli, L., Siniscalchi, A., & De Sarro, G. (2014). Gambling disorder during dopamine replacement treatment in Parkinson's disease: A comprehensive review. *BioMed Research International, 2014*, 728038. https://doi.org/10.1155/2014/728038

Platt, M. L., Watson, K. K., Hayden, B. Y., Shepherd, S. V., & Klein, J. T. (2010). Neuroeconomics: Implications for understanding the neurobiology of addiction. In C. M. Kuhn & G. F. Koob (Eds.), *Advances in the neurobiology of addiction* (pp. 193–227). Taylor & Francis Group.

Quilty, L. C., Wardell, J. D., Thiruchselvam, T., Keough, M. T., & Hendershot, C. S. (2019). Brief interventions for problem gambling: A meta-analysis. *PLoS One, 14,* 1–7. https://doi.org/10.1371/journal.pone.0214502

Rasmussen, S. (2000). *Addiction treatment: Theory and practice.* Sage.

Raylu, N., & Po Oei, T. (2010). *A cognitive behavioural therapy programme for problem gambling: Therapist manual.* Routledge.

Rennert, L., Denis, C., Peer, K., Lynch, K. G., Gelernter, J., & Kranzler, H. R. (2014). DSM-5 gambling disorder: Prevalence and characteristics in a substance use disorder sample. *Experimental and Clinical Psychopharmacology, 22,* 50–56. https://doi.org/10.1037/a0034518

Romanczuk-Seiferth, N., van den Brink, W., & Goudriann, A. E. (2014). From symptoms to neurobiology: Pathological gambling in light of the new classification in DSM-5. *Neuropsychobiology, 72,* 95–102. https://doi.org/10.1159/000362839

Ronzitti, S., Soldini, E., Smith, N., Potenza, M. N., Clerici, M., & Bowden-Jones, H. (2017). Current suicidal ideation in treatment seeking individuals in the United Kingdom with gambling problems. *Addictive Behaviors, 74,* 33–40. https://doi.org/10.1016/j.addbeh.2017.05.032

Shaffer, H. J., & Shaffer, P. M. (2014). Psychiatric epidemiology, nosology, and treatment: Considering internet gambling. *Psychiatric Annals, 44,* 371–378. https://doi.org/10.3928/00485713-20140806-04

Schüll, N. D. (2012). *Addiction by design: Machine gambling in Las Vegas.* Princeton University Press.

Schuler, A., Ferentzy, P., Turner, N. E., Skinner, W., McIsaac, K. E., Ziegler, C. P., & Matheson, F. I. (2016). Gamblers Anonymous as a recovery pathway: A scoping review. *Journal of Gambling Studies, 32,* 1261–1278. https://doi.org/10.1007/s10899-016-9596-8

Shultz, W., Dayan, P., & Montague, P. R. (1997). A neural substrate of prediction and reward. *Science, 275,* 1593–1599. https://doi.org/10.1126/science.275.5306.1593

Skinner, B. F. (1969). *Contingencies of reinforcement: A theoretical analysis.* Meredith Corporation.

Skinner, B. F. (1976). *About behaviorism.* Vintage Books.

Stefanovics, E. A., Potenza, M. N., & Pietrzak, R. H. (2017). Gambling in a national U. S. veteran population: Prevalence, socio-demographics, and psychiatric comorbidities. *Journal of Gambling Studies, 33,* 1099–1120. https://doi.org/10.1007/s10899-017-9678-2

Subramaniam, M., Wang, P., Soh, P., Vaingankar, J. A., Chong, S. A., Browning, C. J., & Thomas, S. A. (2015). Prevalence and determinants of gambling disorder among older adults: A systematic review. *Addictive Behaviors, 41,* 199–209. https://doi.org/10.1016/j.addbeh.2014.10.007

Sulkunen, P., Babor, T. F., Ornberg, J. C., Egerer, M., Hellman, M., Livingstone, C., Marionneau, V., Nikkinen, J., Orford, J., Room, R., & Rossow, I. (2019). *Setting limits: Gambling, science, and public policy.* Oxford.

World Health Organization. (2018). *International statistical classification of diseases and related health problems* (11th Rev.). https://icd.who.int/browse11/l-m/en

9

Nonsuicidal Self-Injury

HOW DO I CONCEPTUALIZE IT?

Nonsuicidal self-injury (NSSI) refers to intentional acts of bodily harm without the intent to die (Favazza, 2011). NSSI behaviors can include cutting, burning, scratching, interfering with wound healing, head banging, skin carving, skin pricking, biting, hitting oneself, punching oneself, and other injurious acts. Self-injury typically begins in adolescence and may increase in intensity, severity, frequency, or number of self-harming methods over time. Rather than an attempt to end one's life, NSSI often is used as a means of mood modification to cope with life's adversities.

Intentional acts of harm to oneself without the desire to die can be difficult to understand. Specifically, it seems counterintuitive that NSSI could be a form of coping. How does drawing blood with a razor blade on one's arm cause relief from anxiety? How does physical pain affect psychological pain? In addition to the puzzling effects of the behavior, treatment for NSSI is complicated by the fact that not all forms of self-injury constitute behavioral addictions. In the same way that not everyone who gambles has a gambling addiction, not everyone who engages in NSSI is addicted to self-injury. Instead, those who engage in NSSI compulsively, lose control of the behavior, continue to engage in NSSI despite negative consequences, and experience cravings or are mentally preoccupied with NSSI likely have a behavioral addiction. Although all forms of NSSI often warrant clinical treatment, counselors should differentiate between the various types of self-injury (of which some may be an addiction) and tailor treatment accordingly.

TYPES OF NONSUICIDAL SELF-INJURY

Armando Favazza (2011), one of the leading researchers in NSSI, described self-harm behaviors on a continuum. One end includes "culturally sanctioned body modification" such as religious rituals or socially acceptable forms of body alterations, while the other end of the continuum contains pathological NSSI (Favazza, 2011, p. 199). There are several classifications within pathological NSSI: *major* self-injury (significant destruction of body tissue that occurs infrequently, such as castration), *stereotypic* self-injury (repetitive or monotonous actions such as head banging, often associated with conditions like autism or intellectual disabilities), *compulsive* self-injury (repetitive behavior often associated with a compulsive disorder such as trichotillomania or excoriation), and *impulsive* self-injury (behaviors such as cutting, burning, excessive rubbing, and pin sticking driven by an impulse to relieve tension followed by relief and/or pleasure; Favazza, 2011).

Impulsive NSSI is the type most likely to be an addictive behavior. Individuals who engage in impulsive NSSI often are mentally preoccupied with the behavior and experience cravings to self-injure (Favazza, 2011). Indeed, for some individuals, impulsive NSSI provides both negative and positive reinforcement: negative reinforcement because it causes relief from distressing emotions and positive reinforcement because it induces feelings of calm (caused by the activation of the body's endogenous opioid system [Walsh, 2012], which will be discussed later). Further delineating types of self-injury is the fact that impulsive NSSI can be *episodic* (typically associated with a mental health concern such as borderline personality disorder [BPD]) or *repetitive* (a separate, independent condition; Favazza, 2011). Favazza (2011) described impulsive, repetitive NSSI as, "when the behavior becomes an overwhelming preoccupation in those persons who may adopt an identity as a 'cutter' or 'burner,' who describe themselves as addicted to their self-harm, and whose NSSI seems to assume an autonomous course" (p. 215). This type of NSSI reflects the characteristics of addiction.

MOTIVES FOR NONSUICIDAL SELF-INJURY

Like other addictive behaviors, a primary motive for NSSI is *emotion regulation*. Specifically, some individuals engage in self-injury to change the way that they feel. In their study of adolescents in an inpatient unit, Nock and Prinstein (2004) found that 52.9% of the sample reported engaging in NSSI to stop bad feelings. Moreover, 79% of the adolescents in Doyle et al.'s (2017) study reported engaging in NSSI to experience relief from a terrible state of mind. Self-injury can be a means of coping with emotional distress by (a) transferring deep emotional pain into more manageable physical pain, (b) releasing blood, which is perceived as a release of "badness" within, and (c) providing a sense of control over one's pain (Favazza, 2011; Strong, 1998; Wester & Trepal, 2017). As an example, Strong (1998) documented the following statement from an individual who engaged in NSSI: "Cutting substitutes the pain inside with a physical pain that I can control, which is easier to handle. The pain is now real, tangible. It can be seen" (p. 43).

NSSI also can be motivated by the desire to punish oneself. Researchers explored NSSI among male adolescents in a residential correctional facility and found that among those with high rates of NSSI (seven or more incidents), the most frequently endorsed function of the behavior was emotion regulation, followed by self-punishment (Silverman et al., 2018). Additionally, 31.8% of the adolescents in the Nock and Prinstein study (2004) and 38% in the Doyle et al. (2017) study endorsed self-punishment as a motive for their NSSI behavior. Thus, anger or disgust toward one's self or one's body, or an overwhelming sense of guilt or shame, could lead some individuals to self-injure.

Another possible motive for NSSI is to induce a sensation, even a painful one, to jolt an individual out of a state of numbness (Nock & Prinstein, 2004). Indeed, dissociation, or the discontinuity between one's conscious awareness, perception, experience, behavior, and memory (American Psychiatric Association [APA], 2013), is a predictor of NSSI. Dissociative symptoms often occur during traumatic or overwhelming events and are listed in the criteria for posttraumatic stress disorder and acute stress disorder (APA, 2013). Franzke et al. (2015) investigated women in inpatient treatment with and without a history of NSSI and found that those with a history of NSSI experienced more trauma and abuse than those without NSSI. Importantly, Franzke and colleagues found that dissociative symptoms had a direct, significant, effect on NSSI, meaning that higher dissociative scores were related to more self-injury. This relationship between dissociation and NSSI makes intuitive sense. Consider a client who frequently dissociated as a means of surviving chronic childhood sexual abuse. Those dissociative tendencies may persist even after the trauma stops, particularly when the individual experiences stress, anxiety, or fear. The infliction of pain through NSSI can jar clients back into the present moment and thus end dissociative states.

It is important for counselors to create strong therapeutic alliances with clients who self-injure, devoid of judgment or evaluation, in order to assess the function of self-injury. Clients may engage in NSSI as a means of emotion regulation (i.e., seeking positive and negative reinforcement), self-punishment, or to ward off dissociation. Furthermore, NSSI can vary considerably in terms of frequency, type, severity, and the circumstances in which self-harm takes place (e.g., under the influence of alcohol or another drug of abuse). Thus, a thorough assessment of clients' history of NSSI, in conjunction with a trauma history, can help counselors develop effective treatment plans.

PREVALENCE OF NONSUICIDAL SELF-INJURY

Determining prevalence rates of NSSI can be difficult due to the use of different instruments, differing "doses" of NSSI (e.g., one incident verses multiple incidents), the time period under study (e.g., lifetime prevalence versus the past 30 days), and variance among subsets of the population. For example, Whitlock et al. (2014) found 15.4% of over 11,000 university students reported engaging in NSSI at least one time in their lives. Among military members, researchers found past year rates of NSSI to be 1.2% for active duty soldiers and 1.3% for new soldiers (Turner et al., 2019). Finally, among 131 women who met criteria for bulimia nervosa, researchers found that 14.5% engaged in NSSI within a 2-week period (Muehlenkamp et al., 2009). Thus, prevalence rates vary substantially among subgroups.

Researchers frequently report that the first NSSI experience occurs during the adolescent years. Indeed, among 111 undergraduates with a history of NSSI, researchers found the average age of the first NSSI act to be 12.16 (O'Loughlin et al., 2020). Additionally, among adolescents in psychiatric treatment, researchers found the average age of the first NSSI behavior to be 12.29 (Zhu et al., 2016). With regard to gender, a meta-analysis of 116 articles (N = 245,506 participants) revealed that women were 1.5 times more likely to report NSSI then men, representing a small effect size (Bresin & Schoenleber, 2015).

Finally, researchers also have found evidence indicating that NSSI prevalence is increasing. Specifically, Wester et al. (2018) found that current NSSI rates (past 90 days) among university freshmen increased from 2.6% in 2008 to 19.4% in 2015. In addition, clinicians are reporting more clients presenting with NSSI. In 2007, Trepal and Wester surveyed 74 practitioners and found that 81% (n = 60) had at least one client reporting NSSI. Later, Giordano et al. (2020) surveyed 94 licensed clinicians and found that 97.9% reported working with NSSI at some point during their careers.

CLINICAL NOTE 9.1

Researchers have examined gender differences in NSSI methods among participants in a treatment program for self-injury (Victor et al., 2018). The data revealed that no gender differences existed among prevalence of cutting as a method for NSSI, yet scratching, rubbing, and pinching were more common methods among female participants, and burning and branding were more common methods among males (Victor et al., 2018). NSSI methods can vary considerably; therefore, counselors should assess for a range of self-harm behaviors beyond cutting.

NEUROSCIENCE RELATED TO NONSUICIDAL SELF-INJURY

Research is burgeoning related to the neuroscience of NSSI. To understand the body's response to self-injury, it is important to examine the brain's response to pain. The *pain pathway* is activated when a signal of pain is sent from the sensory system to the spinal cord, then to the brainstem (lower brain region regulating automatic functions), then to the thalamus (receives and processes sensory input), and then to the cortex (responsible for higher order functioning), specifically, the cingulate cortex (Simpkins & Simpkins, 2013). Once the pain signal is received, the brain responds by releasing natural *opioids* (e.g., endorphins, enkephalins, dynorphins) to inhibit and soothe the pain. Indeed, the body's endogenous opioids are responsible for pain reduction and varying degrees of euphoric feelings with receptors located throughout the brain and along the spinal cord (Simpkins & Simpkins, 2013). Scholars have posited that some individuals intentionally trigger the body's natural response to physical pain (i.e., endogenous opioid release) in an effort to soothe emotional pain. Specifically, Lewis et al. (2000) noted that when some individuals experience psychological distress:

> Then follows an episode of self-harm—a prick, a burn, an incision into the skin. Beneath and within the abused epidermis, palpitating pain fibers send their drumbeat signal to the brain, warning of damage. These messages release pain's counterweight: the blessed, calming flow of opiates, and thus, surcease of sorrow. Chronic self-mutilators provoke the lesser pain to trick their nervous systems into numbing the unendurable one (pp. 95–96).

Therefore, self-injurious behaviors activate the pain pathway, culminating in the release of natural opioids, which can be used to soothe both physical and psychological pain. For some clients, endogenous opioid release serves as both positive and negative reinforcement (i.e., increasing feelings of calm and decreasing psychological distress), which increases the likelihood of repeating the behavior.

In addition to the pain pathway, it is important to understand the brain's emotional regulation system when conceptualizing NSSI. Specifically, the *amygdala* is a small structure located in the limbic region of the brain that is implicated in emotion regulation processes (Simpkins & Simpkins, 2013). There are two emotion regulation processes that transpire within the brain: (a) the *bottom-up process* in which the thalamus communicates with the amygdala without engaging the cortex (remember, the cortex is the part of the brain related to higher order functioning such as reason, logic, and planning) and (b) the *top-down process* in which the thalamus communicates with the cortex and then the amygdala and limbic system. The bottom-up process is fast and does not involve cognitive interpretation and rationalization. The top-down process is slower, yet includes cognitive interpretation of emotional experiences. Although important in both processes, the amygdala is central to the bottom-up process of emotional response. Specifically, the amygdala processes emotional experiences (both positive and negative) and is implicated in creating emotional memories (i.e., it remembers associations between emotions and past experiences; Simpkins & Simpkins, 2013).

Researchers have found that clients who self-injure have reduced connectivity between the amygdala and the cortex when compared to individuals who do not engage in NSSI (Schreiner et al., 2017). Specifically, Schreiner and colleagues found a deficit in communication between the amygdala and the frontal lobe region of the brain among those who self-injured. Thus, it is possible that clients with NSSI respond to emotions quickly and automatically, relying heavily on the bottom-up process of emotion regulation and bypassing the cognitive processes and executive functioning of the frontal cortex (De Stefano & Atkins, 2017). Among these individuals, the amygdala may rapidly process emotions (e.g., fear, anxiety, threat) and initiate a response without waiting for the reasoned, regulatory functions of the frontal cortex (De Stefano & Atkins, 2017; Schreiner et al., 2017). For these reasons, enhancing emotion regulation skills (including identifying, labeling, expressing, and tolerating emotions) is an important part of treatment for NSSI.

SOCIAL CONTAGION AND THE ROLE OF THE INTERNET

When conceptualizing NSSI it also is important to understand *social contagion*. Scholars have described contagion as a series of events in which a behavior is imitated by others within the immediate environment (Walsh & Rosen, 1985). Thus, NSSI contagion occurs when an individual engages in self-injury and the incident is repeated by others in the same community (consider NSSI behaviors spreading through a peer group in a middle school). Walsh and Rosen (1985) studied the behavior of 25 adolescents receiving treatment for mental health concerns and found significant clustering of NSSI incidents among the group, providing empirical evidence for NSSI contagion. Thus, treatment facilities may serve as grounds for learning NSSI and imitating the behavior among those who previously did not self-injure (Walsh, 2012). Although contagion initially referred to imitation among those in one's immediate environment, the internet has created new avenues for exposure to NSSI.

Rather than exposure via a person in their community or school, individuals can be exposed to NSSI online. Zhu et al. (2016) interviewed 90 adolescents in an inpatient treatment program who currently or previously engaged in NSSI. Eighty-seven percent reported being exposed to NSSI prior to their first engagement in self-injury (average age of exposure = 10.85). The researchers found a significant association between frequency of self-injurious behavior and exposure to NSSI on social media (e.g., online social networking platforms) as well as traditional media sources (e.g., TV, movies). Additionally, 37.5% of the adolescents disclosed seeking out NSSI content via social/traditional media and those who sought out NSSI content engaged in the behavior more frequently (Zhu et al., 2016).

Exposure to NSSI via media outlets is common in light of the prevalence of NSSI on social networking and other internet sites. Researchers explored the 100 most viewed YouTube videos related to NSSI in 2009 and found that they were viewed over 2.3 million times with 64% of the videos revealing images of NSSI (Lewis et al., 2011). Moreover, Miguel et al. (2017) examined a sample of NSSI posts on three social media sites (Instagram, Twitter, and Tumblr) and

CLINICAL NOTE 9.2

Giordano et al. (2020) surveyed licensed clinicians and found that 35.1% of the sample never asked their clients with NSSI about their use of the internet to share or view NSSI content. Approximately 28% of clinicians said they asked about internet use *sometimes* and 7.4% said they asked *about half the time*. With the growing prevalence of NSSI content online, it is important for counselors to ask clients who self-injure about their use of the internet and whether they view, share, comment on, or upload images related to NSSI.

classified 59.5% of the posts as graphic (depicting blood, scars, injuries, or paraphernalia). Additionally, webpages (e.g., psyke.org) include photo galleries of NSSI wounds, Google image searches can quickly retrieve NSSI pictures, and online message boards (e.g., quora.com) can be used to discuss methods of NSSI. Thus, NSSI treatment may include monitoring clients' online behaviors and encouraging those with a history of viewing and sharing NSSI online content to discontinue (either temporarily or permanently) their social media use.

HOW DO I IDENTIFY IT?

The current edition of the *Diagnostic and Statistical Manual of Mental Disorders* (5th ed.; *DSM-5*; APA, 2013) includes proposed criteria for NSSI disorder in Section III, Conditions for Further Study. These criteria provide a uniform means of conceptualizing and identifying NSSI. The proposed criteria specify engaging in NSSI on five or more days within the previous year with one or more of the following expectations: (a) to gain relief from negative emotions or thoughts, (b) to resolve relational conflict or difficulty, and (c) to experience positive feelings or sensations. In addition, the criteria require one or more of the following associations with NSSI: (a) negative emotions or interpersonal conflict prior to self-injury, (b) mental preoccupation with NSSI prior to self-injury, and (c) frequent NSSI-related thoughts even when not engaging in the behavior. Andover (2014) surveyed a community sample of 548 adults and found that 2.6% met the proposed criteria for NSSI disorder.

Like other diagnoses in the *DSM*, NSSI must cause significant distress and interfere with an individual's functioning to substantiate a diagnosis. Additionally, the self-injurious behavior must be distinct from socially sanctioned forms of self-injury (e.g., piercings, tattoos, religious rituals, cultural rituals). Finally, the proposed criteria specify that the diagnosis is not appropriate for self-injury that occurs only during states of psychosis, delirium, substance intoxication, or substance withdrawal. For example, when intoxicated on methamphetamines, some individuals have sensations of insects crawling on or under their skin (commonly referred to as "crank bugs" or "meth mites"), which may lead individuals to scratch, pick, or even carve into their skin to get rid of the imagined creatures (see methproject.org for more details about crank bugs). Although this behavior is deliberate, self-inflicted harm to the body, it would not constitute NSSI disorder because it occurs exclusively during drug intoxication. Therefore, identifying NSSI disorder requires a thorough assessment of both substance use and mental health conditions.

DISTINGUISHING BETWEEN NONSUICIDAL SELF-INJURY AND A SUICIDE ATTEMPT

It is imperative for counselors to understand the complex relationship between NSSI and suicide attempts and also recognize differences between the behaviors. Although both NSSI and suicide attempts involve harming the body, the motives are very different. Suicide attempts reflect an intent to die, while NSSI is an attempt to cope with overwhelming distress, thereby reflective of an intent to continue living. Given that those who engage in NSSI often are enduring very difficult emotions and circumstances, as well as potential trauma histories, it makes sense that there is a correlation between suicide and NSSI (Wester & Trepal, 2017). Indeed, several research studies indicate that NSSI is a significant predictor of suicide attempts and suicidal ideation (Hamza et al., 2012; O'Loughlin et al., 2020). The reason for this association, however, is debated. Hamza et al. (2012) summarized three theories explaining the relationship between suicide and NSSI: (a) the gateway theory (in which NSSI progresses into suicide); (b) the third variable theory (in which a third variable such as psychological distress, mental illness, or trauma increases both the probability of NSSI and suicide); and (c) Joiner's theory of acquired capability of suicide (in which NSSI familiarizes the individual to pain and fear, thus causing desensitization to suicide; see Joiner, 2005). According to Hamza et al. (2012), aspects of all of the theories may help explain the association between suicide and NSSI.

Given the relationship between suicidal behaviors and NSSI, it is important for clinicians to regularly assess suicidal ideation among clients who self-injure. At the same time, clinicians should recognize that engaging in a behavior such as skin cutting does not automatically reflect an intent to die, but rather, could be a client's best attempt to survive. Thus, regularly dialoguing with clients about the function of self-injury can help distinguish between NSSI and a suicide attempt.

Another practical way to help differentiate between suicide and NSSI is to clearly distinguish the two behaviors on clinical intake forms. Many clinicians have an item related to self-harm on their intake paperwork, yet, this item often is written in conjunction with suicide (e.g., "Have you ever tried to harm or kill yourself?"). Indeed, among a sample of 94 licensed clinicians, 23.4% stated that the self-harm item on their intake form was combined with suicide and 17% reported that they did not have an item related to NSSI on their intake form at all (Giordano et al., 2020). Thus, one way to identify self-injury among clients is to have a separate item on intake paperwork that clearly inquires about NSSI ("Have you ever deliberately hurt yourself [e.g., cutting, excessive rubbing, scratching, sticking needles in skin, banging head] without the desire to die?"). This item gives clients permission to disclose NSSI without fear that it will immediately be perceived as a suicide attempt.

> **CLINICAL NOTE 9.3**
>
> In the study of college students with histories of both NSSI and a suicide attempt, researchers found the average amount of time between the first NSSI act and the first suicide attempt to be 3.09 years (O'Loughlin et al., 2020). Of note, engaging in NSSI as a means of antidissociation was found to be significantly associated with shorter durations of time between the first NSSI act and the first suicide attempt, as did the NSSI methods of cutting and burning (O'Loughlin et al., 2020).

NONSUICIDAL SELF-INJURY WITH AND WITHOUT BORDERLINE PERSONALITY DISORDER

Finally, although recurrent self-mutilating behavior is listed as one potential criterion for BPD (APA, 2013), not all acts of self-harm are indicative of this mental health concern. In the past, clinicians conceptualized NSSI only as a symptom of BPD, yet scholars now propose that NSSI can be an independent disorder (Favazza, 2011; Muehlenkamp, 2005). In fact, researchers have found significant differences in symptomology and co-occurring disorders among clients who self-injure and meet criteria for BPD and those who self-injure yet do not meet criteria for BPD (Turner et al., 2015). Specifically, compared to adult participants who engaged in NSSI without BPD (NSSI only), those who engaged in NSSI and met criteria for BPD demonstrated more frequent and severe NSSI, more co-occurring disorders, more severe depression symptoms, higher suicidal ideation rates, and more emotion regulation difficulties. It is important to note that participants in the NSSI-only group endorsed, on average, less than one BPD criterion (excluding the item related to self-injury; Turner et al., 2015). Therefore, clinicians should carefully assess whether their clients' NSSI is a symptom of BPD or a stand-alone condition. Treatment protocols for clients who engage in NSSI with BPD may differ from the treatment of NSSI as an independent condition, such as a behavioral addiction.

HOW DO I ASSESS IT?

There are many excellent screening and assessment measures for NSSI in the literature, several of which are in the public domain. The following text describes three instruments that may be helpful for you to incorporate into your practice.

DELIBERATE SELF-HARM INVENTORY

The Deliberate Self-Harm Inventory (DSHI; Gratz, 2001) is a popular self-report instrument examining the frequency, age of onset, duration, and severity of 16 different NSSI behaviors (e.g., burning, carving words in skin, dripping acid on skin, broken bones, preventing wounds from healing). Clients also have the opportunity to report any unlisted NSSI behaviors (item 17). Gratz (2001) developed the 17-item scale from clinical experience, a review of NSSI literature, and reports from those who self-injured. She normed the DSHI on undergraduate students, and scores on the instrument demonstrated good internal consistency (Cronbach's alpha = .82), test–retest reliability, and convergent, construct, and divergent validity (Gratz, 2001). Practitioners can use the measure to gain substantial information related to their clients' NSSI history. Specifically, the sum of the frequency questions related to each of the 17 items provides a total lifetime NSSI frequency score. Additionally, endorsing "yes" to any of the 17 items could serve as a dichotomous variable separating those who have self-injured from those who have not (Gratz, 2001). The full DSHI is printed in the appendix of Gratz's original (2001) article.

NONSUICIDAL SELF-INJURY DISORDER SCALE

The Non-Suicidal Self-Injury Disorder Scale (NSSIDS; Victor et al., 2017) reflects the proposed criteria for NSSI disorder in the *DSM-5*. The brief, self-report scale assesses criteria A to F, including NSSI frequency, expectations, associated experiences, socially sanctioned behavior, distress and impairment, substance intoxication, withdrawal, psychosis, delirium, and mental disorders. Example items include: *Do you think about self-harm even when you aren't engaging in it* and *Do you have negative feelings or thoughts right before you engage in self harm*. The majority of the items correspond with seven-point Likert-type scales ranging from *never* (1) to *always* (7). Scoring procedures are unique for each of the five criteria (the full scale and scoring instructions can be found on the author's website at https://www.sarahevictor.com/publications). Victor et al. (2017) tested the NSSIDS on two samples of undergraduate students at universities located in Canada and the United States. The NSSIDS demonstrated adequate internal consistency (α = .87 and .76) and construct validity. This measure can help clinicians determine whether clients meet the proposed criteria for NSSI disorder.

ALEXIAN BROTHERS URGE TO SELF-INJURE SCALE

The Alexian Brothers Urge to Self-Injure Scale (ABUSI; Washburn et al., 2010) measures a client's urge to self-injure. While many assessments investigate the frequency, duration, and type of NSSI, the ABUSI is unique in its assessment of cravings or urges for NSSI. The authors created the tool by adapting a measure assessing alcohol craving and piloting the instrument on a sample of clients in a self-injury recovery program (Washburn et al., 2010). Example items include: *How difficult was it to resist injuring yourself in the last week* and *How much time have you spent thinking about injuring yourself or about how you want to injure yourself.* Scoring for the scale is a simple sum of the five items (with answer choices ranging from 0 to 6), with higher scores indicating stronger urges to self-injure. Washburn et al. (2010) found evidence of internal consistency (Cronbach's alpha = .83), test–retest reliability, and convergent validity for the instrument among a sample of college students. The full ABUSI can be found in the appendix of the original Washburn et al. (2010) article.

HOW DO I TREAT IT?

There are common therapeutic factors associated with the treatment of NSSI. First, it is important to identify the purpose or function of the self-injury (e.g., emotion regulation, self-punishment, communication, or antidissociation; Choate, 2012). Given that NSSI often is cited as a means of coping with emotional distress, emotion regulation strategies likely will be a key component of counseling with those who self-injure (Muehlenkamp, 2006). According to Gross (2014), there are five categories of emotion regulation strategies: (a) situation selection (making decisions to decrease the likelihood that an individual will be in a situation leading to unwanted emotions), (b) situation modification (adjusting aspects of situations to change their effects on emotions), (c) attentional deployment (choosing to direct one's attention to things that will positively impact emotions, particularly in instances when situations cannot be modified), (d) cognitive change (adjusting one's sense of meaning of a situation or engaging in reappraisal techniques), and (e) response modulation (modifying the experiential aspects of an emotional response such as engaging in relaxation techniques). Emotion regulation enhancement in counseling with clients who self-injure can include strategies within any of these categories. Moreover, Walsh (2012) identified replacement skills that may be effective for those who self-injure including mindful breathing techniques, artistic expression, physical exercise, writing, playing/listening to music, diversion techniques, and visualization techniques.

Functional behavioral analysis also is helpful in identifying triggers and reinforcing factors of NSSI (Linehan, 1993). Many treatment approaches include the use of a chart or log in which clients identify the situations, feelings, and thoughts that occur before and after incidents of NSSI. For example, a client may identify a poor work evaluation, feelings of self-loathing and shame, and the thought "I will never be good enough" as antecedents of their self-injurious behavior (carving letters into their skin). Directly following the NSSI, they record feeling calm, powerful, and in control, having the thought "I am stronger than they think," and watching the wound for several minutes before going outside to smoke a cigarette. By engaging in an analysis of antecedents and consequences of NSSI, counselors and clients can work to come up with new ways to respond to triggering events and decrease the reinforcements of NSSI. Additionally, counselors working with clients who self-injure should assess for co-occurring disorders such as substance use disorders, eating disorders, mood disorders, or personality disorders to create holistic treatment plans.

VOICES FROM THE FIELD: Clinical Work With NSSI

One reoccurring theme I have learned from my clients with NSSI is that despite the diversity of their presenting impairments, these clients end up in two categories: (a) the individuals who want to stop self-injuring but find it difficult to cease these conditioned behaviors and (b) those who will not fathom the idea of stopping since the process of mutilating themselves (from the bleeding to reopening wounds) brings a cathartic experience that they want to continue. Having this in my mind helps me identify which methods of treatment would be most effective based on the tools I have acquired from my education.

In my professional opinion, working with those who engage in self-injury takes a clinically integrated approach. Yes, dialectical behavior therapy is the lead runner in the race of treatment for NSSI. However, I cannot dismiss cognitive behavioral therapy, Motivational Interviewing, trauma-based interventions, family therapy approaches, and psychodynamic treatment. Each client is responsive to a different therapeutic approach based on their biological makeup, trauma history, presenting impairments, personality, and motivation to engage in treatment. It takes cultural competency and intentionality to meet my clients where they are and direct them to a healthier functioning lifestyle.

One important part of treatment for NSSI is the development of healthy, alternative coping behaviors in which clients can engage to reduce the likelihood of acting impulsively on intrusive NSSI urges. Some clients do not know where to start when it comes to developing new coping strategies; so I developed a list of 200 healthy distractions and coping skills to help clients start the process.

Even though this work has its downfalls, stressors, and complicated patients, I cannot help but love what I do. I have always loved challenges of any sort, aimed to learn more about treating the complexities of a client's diagnosis, and thoroughly enjoyed working with some of the most difficult individuals. It is sometimes hard to describe the feelings I get when I see my clients have their "ah ha!" enlightened moments when they once were defeated and hopeless.

For those who want to work with individuals who engage in self-injury, I advise you not to surrender in your pursuit of healing when your clients have given up on healing themselves. We as clinicians are not going to help everyone we work with, yet we choose to join with each of our clients and offer the invitation to move toward greater degrees of wellness. Counseling and psychology are not fields of saving, instead they are fields of guidance and tolerance. Working with NSSI is often challenging, but at the same time enlightening. As soon as we think that we have figured out a diagnosis or maladaptive behavior, it sends us on a loop. The inquisitive nature of being a clinician is that we often thrive on these loops and learning experiences. We add this information into our clinical Rolodex and pull from our psychological tool kit to address the new challenges presented to us. So, I dare you to ride the loops, learn and store information in your clinical lexicon, and use your clinical tools to build a healthy foundation in others' lives.

Lauren Colston, PsyD, Licensed Clinical Psychologist, Registered Health Service Psychologist

DIALECTICAL BEHAVIOR THERAPY

Marsha Linehan developed dialectical behavior therapy (DBT) as an innovative therapeutic approach for working with clients with BPD. Specifically, DBT integrates cognitive behavioral work with mindfulness-based acceptance of feelings and situations (Linehan, 1993). Rather than endorsing rigid extremes, which is common among those with BPD, DBT helps clients come to a place of integration and synthesis, similar to the middle path described in the Buddhist faith tradition. Counselors using DBT address a variety of target maladaptive behaviors, yet Linehan (1993) identified suicide attempts and self-injury as primary behaviors to address first. DBT counselors demonstrate a balance between accepting and validating the client and challenging the client to pursue positive change.

DBT has empirical support for its efficacy in addressing NSSI (Muehlenkamp, 2006). Choate (2012) described a 16-week DBT approach for adolescents engaging in self-injurious behaviors. Counselors begin by developing strong therapeutic relationships with clients marked by both acceptance and a challenge to change. Counselors conduct a thorough assessment of NSSI, which is the target maladaptive behavior. Utilizing chain analysis (Linehan, 1993), counselors help clients identify an incident of NSSI and recount the chain of events leading up to the self-injurious behavior. Linehan (1993) noted, "much of the therapeutic work in DBT is the ceaseless analysis of specific instances of targeted behaviors, each time integrating new information with old information to evolve a definition of patterns and to explore possible new behavioral solutions" (p. 258). Counselors and clients then work to identify ways to interrupt the chain of events leading to NSSI and decrease vulnerabilities for NSSI (e.g., substance use, isolation, boredom, disrupted sleep; Choate, 2012). Choate (2012) also described the incorporation of skills training groups composed of adolescents and parents to aid in the development of alternative coping strategies, emotion regulation skills, and interpersonal skills. DBT is a popular, effective approach for addressing NSSI. Counselors interested in DBT can consider pursuing DBT training and certification. Visit behavioraltech.org for more details.

TREATMENT FOR SELF-INJURIOUS BEHAVIOR

Margaret (Peggy) Andover and her colleagues developed a brief, nine-session intervention for young adults engaging in NSSI called Treatment for Self-Injurious Behavior (T-SIB; Andover et al., 2015). The researchers conducted a randomized control trial to examine the effectiveness of T-SIB compared to treatment as usual (TAU) among young adults with NSSI behaviors or urges in the past month (Andover et al., 2017). Although the sample size was too small to produce acceptable statistical power, the researchers found that NSSI frequency significantly decreased in both groups (T-SIB and TAU) and, beginning in week 6, those in the T-SIB condition demonstrated significantly more decreases in NSSI frequency compared to TAU (Andover et al., 2017). Thus, despite sample size limitations, T-SIB demonstrated promise as a potentially effective intervention for young adults engaging in NSSI.

The manual for T-SIB is available upon request from Peggy Andover. In short, the intervention has the following goals: provide psychoeducation about NSSI and increase motivation to change (week 1), conduct functional analysis of NSSI to identify triggers and reinforcements (weeks 2–3), identify replacement behaviors (week 4), discuss distress tolerance and refine replacement behavior list (weeks 5–6), implement individualized modules related to interpersonal communication, distress tolerance, or cognitive distortions (weeks 7–8), assess gains and terminate (week 9; Andover et al., 2015; Andover et al., 2017). Homework assignments between sessions include functional analysis of NSSI, applying distress tolerance skills, and utilizing replacement behaviors in low stress situations (Andover et al., 2015; Andover et al., 2017).

TRAUMA-FOCUSED COGNITIVE BEHAVIORAL THERAPY

Many individuals who engage in NSSI have histories of trauma (Kaess et al., 2013). Specifically, significant associations exist between childhood sexual abuse and self-injury (Lang & Sharma-Patel, 2011). Additionally, in a study of over 500 adolescents in juvenile detention in the United States, researchers found a significant association between interpersonal trauma and NSSI (Modrowski et al., 2019). Therefore, treatment that focuses on addressing trauma can be a helpful approach to clinical work with NSSI. Trauma-focused cognitive behavioral therapy (TF-CBT; Cohen et al., 2006) may be an effective way to address trauma and NSSI simultaneously in children and adolescents (Lang & Sharma-Patel, 2011). TF-CBT provides multiple modalities of treatment including individual, parent, and conjoint sessions (Cohen et al., 2006). Primary components of TF-CBT include learning relaxation techniques (e.g., breathwork, mindfulness strategies, meditation, progressive muscle relaxation), engaging in affective expression and modulation (e.g., identify and express feelings, positive imagery, increasing social skills), and increasing cognitive coping (e.g., modifying maladaptive thoughts), prior to the development of a trauma narrative (Cohen et al., 2006). These components may provide clients with adaptive replacement strategies for NSSI while simultaneously addressing trauma (Lang & Sharma-Patel, 2011). For more information about TF-CBT, including details related to certification, visit tfcbt.org.

DIAGNOSTIC CONSIDERATIONS

Currently, there is no formal diagnosis in the DSM-5 for NSSI disorder (although criteria have been proposed and included in Section III). Thus, given the high rate of co-occurrence between NSSI and other mental health concerns (e.g., depression, anxiety, BPD, eating disorders, posttraumatic stress disorder, substance use disorders), counselors often diagnose the co-occurring disorder when applicable. If a co-occurring disorder is not present, unspecified obsessive-compulsive and related disorder or unspecified anxiety disorder may be appropriate diagnoses (Wester & Trepal, 2017). Although this chapter focused primarily on impulsive NSSI, other forms of self-injury may warrant different diagnoses. For example, major self-injury may merit consideration of psychotic or personality disorders (e.g., delusional disorder, schizotypal personality disorder), stereotypic self-injury may warrant consideration of stereotypic movement disorder or autism spectrum disorder, and compulsive self-injury may necessitate a diagnosis for trichotillomania or excoriation (APA, 2013; White Kress, 2003).

HOW CAN I LEARN MORE?

If you are working with clients who present with NSSI and desire to know more about the condition, consider the following resources.

BOOKS

- Favazza, A. (2011). *Bodies under siege: Self-mutilation, nonsuicidal self-injury, and body modification in culture and psychiatry* (3rd ed.). Johns Hopkins University Press.
- Strong, M. (1998). *A bright red scream: Self-mutilation and the language of pain*. Penguin Group.
- Walsh, B. W. (2012). *Treating self-injury: A practical guide* (2nd ed.). The Guilford Press.
- Wester, K. L., & Trepal, H. C. (2017). *Non-suicidal self-injury: Wellness perspectives on behaviors, symptoms, and diagnosis*. Routledge.

PEER-REVIEWED ARTICLES

- Flaherty, H. B. (2018). Treating adolescent nonsuicidal self-injury: A review of psychosocial interventions to guide clinical practice. *Child and Adolescent Social Work Journal, 35*, 85–95. https://doi.org/ 10.1007/s10560-017-0505-5
- Hasking, P. A., Heath, N. L., Kaess, M., Lewis, S. P., Plener, P. L., Walsh, B. W., Whitlock, J., & Wilson, M. S. (2016). Position paper for guiding response to non-suicidal self-injury in schools. *School Psychology International, 37*, 644–663. https://doi.org/10.1177/0143034316678656
- Mahdy, J. C., & Lewis, S. P. (2013). Nonsuicidal self-injury on the internet: An overview guide for school mental health professionals. *School Psychology Forum, 7*, 148–160.
- Walsh, B. (2007). Clinical assessment of self-injury: A practical guide. *Journal of Clinical Psychology, 63*, 1057–1068. https://doi.org/10.1002/jclp.20413

WEBSITES

- Cornell University Self-Injury & Recovery Resources (SIRR): www.self-injury.bctr.cornell.edu/index.html
- International Society for the Study of Self-Injury: itriples.org
- Self-Injury Outreach & Support (SiOS): sioutreach.org

REFERENCES

American Psychiatric Association. (2013). *Diagnostic and statistical manual of mental disorders* (5th ed.). Author.

Andover, M. S. (2014). Non-suicidal self-injury disorder in a community sample of adults. *Psychiatry Research, 219,* 305–310. https://doi.org/10.1016/j.psychres.2014.06.001

Andover, M. S., Schatten, H. T., Morris, B. W., Holman, C. S., & Miller, I. W. (2017). An intervention for nonsuicidal self-injury in young adults: A pilot randomized controlled trial. *Journal of Consulting and Clinical Psychology, 85,* 620–631. https://doi.org/10.1037/ccp00000206

Andover, M. S., Schatten, H. T., Morris, B. W., & Miller, I. W. (2015). Development of an intervention for non-suicidal self-injury in young adults: An open pilot trial. *Cognitive and Behavioral Practice, 4,* 491–503. https://doi.org/10.1016/j.cbpra.2014.05.003

Bresin, K., & Schoenleber, M. (2015). Gender differences in the prevalence of nonsuicidal self-injury: A meta-analysis. *Clinical Psychology Review, 38,* 55–64. https://doi.org/10.1016/j.cpr.2015.02.009

Choate, L. H. (2012). Counseling adolescents who engage in nonsuicidal self-injury: A dialectical behavioral therapy approach. *Journal of Mental Health Counseling, 34,* 56–71. https://doi.org/10.17744/mehc.34.1.506780307v16m402

Cohen, J. A., Mannarino, A. P., & Deblinger, E. (2006). *Treating trauma and traumatic grief in children and adolescents.* Guilford.

De Stefano, J., & Atkins, S. (2017). Nonsuicidal self-injury, interpersonal neurobiology, and attachment: Implications for counselors and therapists. *Journal of Mental Health Counseling, 39,* 289–304. https://doi.org/10.17744/mehc.39.4.02

Doyle, L., Sheridan, A., & Treacy, M. P. (2017). Motivations for adolescent self-harm and the implications for mental health nurses. *Journal of Psychiatric and Mental Health Nursing, 24,* 134–142. https://doi.org/10.1111/jpm.12360

Favazza, A. (2011). *Bodies under siege: Self-mutilation, nonsuicidal self-injury, and body modification in culture and psychiatry* (3rd ed.). John Hopkins University Press.

Franzke, L., Wabnitz, P., & Catani, C. (2015). Dissociation as a mediator of the relationship between childhood trauma and nonsuicidal self-injury in females: A path analytic approach. *Journal of Trauma and Dissociation, 16,* 286–302. https://doi.org/10.1080/15299732.2015.989646

Giordano, A. L., Lundeen, L. A., Scoffone, C. M., Kilpatrick, E. P., & Gorritz, F. B. (2020). Clinical work with clients who self-injure: A descriptive study. *The Professional Counselor, 10,* 181–193. https://doi.org/10.15241/ag.10.2.181

Gratz, K. L. (2001). Measurement of deliberate self-harm: Preliminary data on the Deliberate Self-Harm Inventory. *Journal of Psychopathology and Behavioral Assessment, 23,* 253–263. https://doi.org/10.1023/A:1012779403943

Gross, J. J. (2014). Emotion regulation: Conceptual and empirical foundations. In J. J. Gross (Ed.), *Handbook of emotion regulation* (2nd ed., pp. 3–20). Guilford Press.

Hamza, C. A., Stewart, S. L., & Willoughby, T. (2012). Examining the link between nonsuicidal self-injury and suicidal behavior: A review of the literature and an integrated model. *Clinical Psychology Review, 32,* 482–495. https://doi.org/10.1016/j.cpr.2012.05.003

Joiner, T. (2005). *Why people die by suicide*. Harvard University Press.

Kaess, M., Parzer, P., Mattern, M., Plener, P. L., Bifulco, A., Resch, F., & Brunner, R. (2013). Adverse childhood experiences and their impact on frequency, severity, and the individual function of nonsuicidal self-injury in youth. *Psychiatry Research, 206*, 265–272. https://doi.org/10.1016/j.psychres.2012.10.012

Lang, C. M., & Sharma-Patel, K. (2011). The relation between childhood maltreatment and self-injury: A review of the literature on conceptualization and intervention. *Trauma, Violence, and Abuse, 12*, 23–37. https://doi.org/10.1177/1524838010386975

Lewis, T., Amini, F., & Lannon, R. (2000). *A general theory of love*. Vintage Books.

Lewis, S. P., Heath, N. L., St. Denis, J. M., & Noble, R. (2011). The scope of nonsuicidal self-injury on YouTube. *Pediatrics, 127*, e552–e557. https://doi.org/10.1542/peds.2010-2317

Linehan, M. M. (1993). *Cognitive-behavioral treatment of borderline personality disorder*. Guilford Press.

Miguel, E. M., Chou, T., Golik, A., Cornacchio, D., Sanchz, A. L., DeSerisy, M., & Comer, J. S. (2017). Examining the scope and patterns of deliberate self-injurious cutting content on popular social media. *Depression and Anxiety, 34*, 786–793. https://doi.org/10.1002/da.22668

Modrowski, C. A., Chaplo, S. D., Kerig, P. K., & Mozley, M. M. (2019). Trauma exposure, posttraumatic overmodulation and undermodulation, and nonsuicidal self-injury in traumatized justice-involved adolescents. *Psychological Trauma: Theory, Research, Practice, and Policy, 11*, 743–750. https://doi.org/10.1037/tra0000469

Muehlenkamp, J. J. (2005). Self-injurious behavior as a separate clinical syndrome. *American Journal of Orthopsychiatry, 75*, 324–333. https://doi.org/10.1037/0002-9432.75.2.324

Muehlenkamp, J. J. (2006). Empirically supported treatments and general therapy guidelines for non-suicidal self-injury. *Journal of Mental Health Counseling, 28*, 166–185. https://doi.org/10.17744/mehc.28.2.6w61cut21xjdg3m7

Muehlenkamp, J. J., Engel, S. G., Wadeson, A., Crosby, R. D., Wonderlich, S. A., Simonich, H., & Mitchell, J. E. (2009). Emotional states preceding and following acts of non-suicidal self-injury in bulimia nervosa patients. *Behavior Research and Therapy, 47*, 83–87. https://doi.org/10.1016/j.brat.2008.10.011

Nock, M. K., & Prinstein, M. J. (2004). A functional approach to the assessment of self-mutilative behavior. *Journal of Consulting and Clinical Psychology, 72*, 885–890.

O'Loughlin, C., Burke, T. A., & Ammerman, B. A. (2020). Examining the time to transition from nonsuicidal self-injury to suicide attempt: A brief report. *Crisis: The Journal of Crisis Intervention and Suicide Prevention, 42*, 157–161. https://doi.org/10.1027/0227-5910/a000715

Schreiner, M. W., Kimes-Dougan, B., Mueller, B. A., Eberly, L. E., Reigstad, K. M., Carstedt, P. A., Thomas, K. M., Hunt, R. H., Lim, K. O., & Cullen, K. R. (2017). Multimodal neuroimaging of adolescents with non-suicidal self-injury: Amygdala functional connectivity. *Journal of Affective Disorders, 221*, 47–55. https://doi.org/10.1016/j.jad.2017.06.004

Silverman, J. R., Ross, E. H., & Kearney, C. A. (2018). Non-suicidal self-injury among male adjudicated adolescents: Psychosocial concerns, coping responses, diagnoses, and functions. *Journal of Child and Family Studies, 27*, 3564–3571. https://doi.org/10.1007/s10826-018-1172-7

Simpkins, C. A., & Simpkins, A. M. (2013). *Neuroscience for clinicians: Evidence, models, and practice*. Springer Publishing.

Strong, M. (1998). *A bright red scream: Self-mutilation and the language of pain*. Penguin Group.

Trepal, H. C., & Wester, K. L. (2007). Self-injurious behaviors, diagnoses, and treatment methods: What mental health professional are reporting. *Journal of Mental Health Counseling, 29*, 363–375. https://doi.org/10.17744/mehc.29.4.d277t298667q5367

Turner, B. J., Dixon-Gordon, K. L., Austin, S. B., Rodriguez, M. A., Rosenthal, M. Z., & Chapman, A. L. (2015). Nonsuicidal self-injury with and without borderline personality disorder: Differences in self-injury and diagnostic comorbidity. *Psychiatry Research, 230*, 28–35. https://doi.org/10.1016/j.psychres.2015.07.058

Turner, B. J., Kleiman, E. M., & Knock, M. K. (2019). Non-suicidal self-injury prevalence, course, and association with suicidal thoughts and behaviors in two large, representative samples of US army soldiers. *Psychological Medicine, 49*, 1470–1480 https://doi.org/10.1017/S0033291718002015

Victor, S. E., Davis, T., & Klonsky, E. D. (2017). Descriptive characteristics and initial psychometric properties of the Non-Suicidal Self-Injury Disorder Scale. *Archives of Suicide Research, 21*, 265–278. https://doi.org/10.1080/13811118.2016.1193078

Victor, S. E., Muehlenkamp, J. J., Hayes, N. A., Lengel, G. J., Styer, D. M., & Washburn, J. J. (2018). Characterizing gender differences in nonsuicidal self-injury: Evidence from a large clinical sample of adolescents and adults. *Comprehensive Psychiatry, 82*, 53–60. https://doi.org/10.1016/j.comppsych.2018.01.009

Walsh, B. W. (2012). *Treating self-injury: A practical guide* (2nd ed.). The Guilford Press.

Walsh, B. W., & Rosen, P. (1985). Self-mutilation and contagion: An empirical test. *The American Journal of Psychiatry, 142*, 119–120. https://doi.org/10.1176/ajp.142.1.119

Washburn, J. J., Juzwin, K. R., Styer, D. M., & Aldridge, D. (2010). Measuring the urge to self-injure: Preliminary data from a clinical sample. *Psychiatry Research, 178*, 540–544. https://doi.org/10.1016/j.psychres.2010.05.018

Wester, K. L., & Trepal, H. C. (2017). *Non-suicidal self-injury: Wellness perspectives on behaviors, symptoms, and diagnosis*. Routledge.

Wester, K., Trepal, H., & King, K. (2018). Nonsuicidal self-injury: Increased prevalence in engagement. *Suicide and Life-Threatening Behavior, 48*, 690–698. https://doi.org/10.1111/sltb.12389

White Kress, V. E. (2003). Self-injurious behaviors: Assessment and diagnosis. *Journal of Counseling and Development, 81*, 490–496. https://doi.org/10.1002/j.1556-6678.2003.tb00276.x

Whitlock, J., Exner-Cortens, D., & Purington, A. (2014). Assessment of nonsuicidal self-injury: Development and initial validation of the non-suicidal self-injury-assessment tool (NSSI-AT). *Psychological Assessment, 26*, 935–946. https://doi.org/10.1037/a0036611

Zhu, L., Westers, N. J., Horton, S. E., King, J. D., Diederich, A., Stewart, S. M., & Kennard, B. D. (2016). Frequency of exposure to and engagement in nonsuicidal self-injury among inpatient adolescents. *Archives of Suicide Research, 20*, 580–590. https://doi.org/10.1080/13811118.2016.1162240

10

Food Addiction

HOW DO I CONCEPTUALIZE IT?

Some people may find it difficult to understand how an individual can be addicted to food, given that eating is necessary for survival. Proponents of food addiction submit that deficiencies or dysfunctions in individuals' reward circuitry in the brain can contribute to the development of addiction to food. Specifically, eating is a naturally rewarding behavior, stimulating the release of neurotransmitters implicated in reward, such as dopamine and endogenous opioids (Wang et al., 2012; Wise, 2013). For a small number of predisposed individuals, however, eating certain foods (particularly processed foods high in sugar or fat) can activate reward circuitry in a unique way (see more on the neuroscience of food addiction later in the chapter) and become compulsive, out of control, continue despite negative consequences, and induce cravings and mental preoccupation with food (Tarman & Werdell, 2014). These individuals likely have food addiction.

The notion of food addiction emerged in the 1950s and has been the topic of numerous research studies over the past several decades. Although overlapping, food addiction is distinct from obesity and eating disorders. Instead, food addiction is, "a brain disorder caused by the interaction of trigger foods on the brains of humans predisposed to addiction" (Tarman & Werdell, 2014, p. 78). Food addiction represents a maladaptive pattern of eating in which individuals are unable to control their food intake, are unsuccessful in attempts to change their compulsive eating behaviors, experience cravings when food is inaccessible, and experience substantial distress as a result of their incontrollable eating patterns and obsessive thoughts about food (Adams et al., 2019; Coker Ross, 2017; Hauck et al., 2020; Salamone & Correa, 2013). Like other addictive behaviors, eating becomes a primary means of emotion regulation by providing both positive reinforcement (e.g., pleasurable sensations) and negative reinforcement (escape from dysphoric mood states).

Although individuals who are categorized as overweight or obese may present with food addiction, it is important to note that food addiction can occur among individuals of any body shape or size. That said, researchers have highlighted a relationship between food addiction and *obesity* (Yu et al., 2018). Specifically, in the study of 80 adults with obesity and 50 adults at normal weight, researchers found that 23.7% of the obesity group had food addiction compared to 6% in the normal weight group (Lopez-Aguilar et al., 2018). Therefore, obesity is a potential negative consequence of food addiction, and recent data indicated that 42.4% of American adults are obese (i.e., have a body mass index [BMI] of 30 or more; Hales et al., 2020) along with 18.5% of American youth (aged 2–19; Hales et al., 2017). Obesity is associated with an increased risk of negative physical and psychological issues including: type 2 diabetes, stroke, hypertension, heart disease, sleep apnea, respiratory issues, cancer, congestive heart failure, gallstones, social stigma, and discrimination (National Heart, Lung, and Blood Institute, 1998). The rise of obesity is caused by a variety of factors, including the availability, affordability, and powerful marketing of highly processed foods (Gearhardt & Corbin, 2012). For example, consider the cost of fast food or sugary processed foods (e.g., doughnuts, cookies, cakes) compared to the cost of organic fruits, vegetables, or meats. It often is much less expensive to buy processed foods, rather than natural, organic foods. Indeed, scholars posit that *hyperphagia*, or chronic overeating, is influenced by food availability, excessive exposure to high-calorie food stimuli (e.g., commercials, billboards), and stress (triggering the release of cortisol among other hormones; Leigh & Morris, 2018). Thus, obesity can be influenced by conditions such as food addiction, as well as environmental factors, cultural norms, and food accessibility.

CONTROVERSY RELATED TO FOOD ADDICTION

The concept of food addiction is controversial, with the main point of contention related to the addictive potential of particular foods or macronutrients. Some scholars propose that certain foods (particularly processed foods high in fat or sugar) have addictive properties due to their high hedonic value (Lerma-Cabrera et al., 2016; Salamone & Correa, 2013; Smith & Robbins, 2013). Therefore, for some vulnerable individuals, the reward of consuming high-calorie foods may lead to addictive, out-of-control eating behaviors. This view is supported by animal studies that have demonstrated how sugar can create addictive-like behavior in rats, particularly if distributed intermittently (Ahmed, 2012; Smith & Robbins, 2013). For those who endorse the addictive nature of certain foods, treatment for food addiction involves identifying and abstaining from *trigger foods* (Meule, 2019). Others, however, argue that no particular food or macronutrient has been found to be addictive in humans (Costin, 2007; Onaolapo & Onaolapo, 2018). Instead, it is believed that some individuals use food as a maladaptive means of emotion regulation or coping, leading to addictive eating behaviors (Coker Ross, 2017). Rather than targeting particular foods, it is the act of eating any food in a compulsive manner that creates the addictive behavior (thus it has been proposed that *eating addiction* may be a more fitting term than food addiction; Coker Ross, 2017). From this perspective, treatment does not involve restricting certain foods, but instead, adapting one's relationship with food and encouraging mindful, intentional eating patterns to meet energy needs (Coker Ross, 2017). Research in this area continues to progress and will eventually reveal whether particular foods (e.g., processed sugar) can be addictive, or if it is the compulsive overeating of any food that best constitutes food addiction.

CLINICAL NOTE 10.1

Consider the current controversy related to food addiction. Some individuals in recovery from food addiction have noted that they need to abstain from certain foods (e.g., processed sugar) in order to have control over their eating behaviors. In contrast, some clinicians who specialize in eating disorders report that moderation, rather than restricting particular food groups, is the goal of healthy eating. What are your thoughts related to the addictive nature of particular foods?

FOOD ADDICTION AND EATING DISORDERS

In order to provide effective services, it is important for counselors to understand both the similarities and differences between food addiction and *eating disorders*. Feeding and eating disorders as described in the fifth edition of the *Diagnostic and Statistical Manual of Mental Disorders* (*DSM-5*; American Psychiatric Association [APA], 2013) are characterized by patterns of disordered eating that lead to significant distress and impairment. Several of these eating disorders are correlated with food addiction, particularly those that include *binge eating* (Hauck et al., 2020; Lopez-Aguilar et al., 2018; Penzenstadler et al., 2019). According to the *DSM-5*, an episode of binge eating refers to eating more food in a discrete period of time than that which most other people would consume, while simultaneously experiencing a loss of control over eating behaviors (APA, 2013). Thus, an episode of binge eating would entail eating a large quantity of food in a short period of time while feeling unable to control the amount of food being consumed.

Binge eating is a feature of both *bulimia nervosa* (BN) and *binge eating disorder* (BED), yet the two diagnoses have important distinctions. The criteria for BN consist of: (a) frequent binge eating episodes, (b) frequent maladaptive compensatory behaviors after a binge eating episode (e.g., self-induced vomiting, misusing laxatives and diuretics, fasting/restricting, overexercising),

(c) binge eating episodes and compensatory behaviors that occur at least one time per week for three or more months, (d) evaluation of the self that is strongly influenced by weight and body shape, and (e) symptoms do not exist only during periods of anorexia (APA, 2013). Accordingly, BN is marked by both bingeing and maladaptive compensatory behaviors. BED criteria, on the other hand, include: (a) frequent binge eating episodes, (b) binge eating that entails at least three of the following characteristics: eating faster than normal, eating until feeling discomfort, eating large portions of food in the absence of hunger, eating in isolation due to shame or embarrassment, and feeling guilt, disgust, or depression after eating, (c) experiencing significant distress as a result of binge eating patterns, (d) engaging in binge eating weekly for at least 3 months, and (e) binge episodes are not followed by compensatory behaviors (e.g., self-induced vomiting, misusing laxatives). Therefore, BED reflects a persistent pattern of binge episodes without the maladaptive compensatory behaviors of BN.

When working with clients who engage in compulsive overeating, it is important to assess for the presence of food addiction, eating disorders, or both. Indeed, some clients with eating disorders may also have food addiction, and some clients with food addiction may also have an eating disorder. The constructs share similarities, yet are distinct (Hauck et al., 2020). In fact, Tarman and Werdell (2014) noted, "obesity, eating disorders, and chemical dependency on food are three distinct and very different diseases" (p. 77). For example, a client may demonstrate features of food addiction (loss of control over eating, eating compulsively, continuing eating patterns despite negative consequences, and craving or being mentally preoccupied with food), yet fail to meet the criteria of an eating disorder (consider a client who grazes compulsively as a means of emotion regulation and experiences negative consequences, yet never binges; Hauck et al., 2020). Therefore, it is important to note that clients with food addiction represent a heterogeneous group. In fact, Jimenez-Murcia et al. (2019) studied women with both food addiction and obesity or eating disorders to assess participant profiles. The researchers found a three-cluster structure among participants: (a) cluster one (25.6% of the sample) was characterized by those with high food addiction symptomology, severe eating disorder symptomology, and the most psychopathological symptoms, (b) cluster two (38.5%) was characterized by high food addiction symptomology, less severe eating disorder symptomology than cluster one, and moderate psychopathological symptoms, and (c) cluster three (35.9%) was characterized by the lowest food addiction symptomology, less severe eating disorder and psychopathological symptoms, and the highest incidence of obesity without accompanying eating disorders. In light of these findings, researchers suggested that treatment for clients with food addiction will differ in light of co-occurring eating disorders and psychopathology (Jimenez-Murcia et al., 2019). Counselors should be well versed in the criteria of both eating disorders and food addiction in order to appropriately assess their client's presenting concerns and develop appropriate treatment plans.

PREVALENCE OF FOOD ADDICTION

Several researchers have investigated the prevalence of food addiction, yet rates vary due to a lack of uniform criteria for the condition. Reviews of recent literature report prevalence rates ranging from 0% to 25.7% among community (nonclinical) samples and 6.7% to 100% among clinical samples (Hauck et al., 2020; Penzenstadler et al., 2019). Moreover, in a community sample of adults, researchers found that 15% met criteria for food addiction (Schulte & Gearhardt, 2017). Additionally, among over 900 college students, researchers found that 4.6% of males and 12.3% of females had food addiction (Yu et al., 2018). Furthermore, in a study of 146 adults waiting to get bariatric surgery with BMIs of 35 or higher, researchers determined that 16.4% had food addiction (Ouellette et al., 2018). Finally, among a sample of over 1,000 German adults, researchers found that 7.9% met criteria for food addiction (Hauck et al., 2017). Thus, prevalence rates vary considerably by subgroup.

In addition, researchers have found that women present with food addiction more than men (Gearhardt et al., 2016; Hauck et al., 2020; Yu et al., 2018). For example, among 642 college students, researchers found that 14% of men met criteria for food addiction compared to 21.3% of women (Carr et al., 2017). Although gender differences in prevalence rates exist, food addiction is not a condition experienced solely by women. It is important for counselors to be aware of the frequency of food addiction (and eating disorders) among men and assess for addictive eating behaviors among all genders.

CLINICAL NOTE 10.2

Among a sample of 356 adults (of which 154 identified as lesbian, gay, or bisexual [LGB]), researchers found that LGB participants endorsed more food addiction symptoms than their heterosexual counterparts after controlling for age and body mass index (Rainey et al., 2018). Additionally, among LGB participants, those with lower levels of self-compassion and those who faced more discrimination endorsed more food addiction symptoms. The authors posited that food addiction may be associated with attempts to cope with the stress of discrimination (Rainey et al., 2018). Given that many behavioral addictions have an emotion regulation component, it is important for counselors to consider clients' experiences with discrimination and systemic oppression in their work with addictive behaviors.

NEUROSCIENCE RELATED TO FOOD ADDICTION

Eating highly palatable foods is neurologically rewarding as it activates the dopaminergic and opioid systems in the brain (Leigh & Morris, 2018; Wise, 2013).

The cascade of neurotransmitters activated by eating was designed to reinforce feeding behaviors to ensure the survival of our species. Food products, however, have changed substantially over time. Additives that protect the freshness of food or enhance taste (e.g., aspartame, saccharin, glutamate) are now commonplace (Onaolapo & Onaolapo, 2018). High-calorie foods with large amounts of processed sugar and flour are widely available and highly marketed (Salamone & Correa, 2013). In this way, refined foods high in fat or sugar have become *supernormal stimuli* (i.e., artificial exaggerations of a natural stimulus), which activate the reward system more strongly than the foods our ancestors consumed (Barrett, 2010; Tarman & Werdell, 2014). Indeed, Barrett (2010) noted that "salt, fat, sugar, and starch are not harmful in their natural contexts," yet in concentrated or refined forms, these macronutrients "exploit" human beings' natural desire for small doses of high-calorie food, which is necessary for survival (p. 78). Consider the differences between the natural sweetness of a peach and the exaggerated sweetness of processed foods such as doughnuts, sugary cereals, and sodas. Processed or refined foods can be more potent and more concentrated than natural foods, causing more reward circuitry activation. The result of these changes to modern foods may be the out-of-control, compulsive consumption of highly palatable foods, leading to food addiction in susceptible individuals.

Some of the most highly cited research studies in the case for food addiction describe the neurological similarities between compulsive eating and drug use (Leigh & Morris, 2018; Salamone & Correa, 2013; Wise, 2013). In line with chemical dependence models, scholars purport that preexisting hypofunctioning of the dopaminergic system, referred to as *reward deficiency syndrome* (Blum et al., 1996, see Chapter 2), may lead individuals to self-stimulate dopamine release by eating highly palatable foods (Coker Ross, 2017; Smith & Robbins, 2013). Specifically, researchers have posited that genetic vulnerabilities, such as decreased dopamine receptors, may be responsible for the emergence of food addiction (Adams et al., 2019; Coker Ross, 2017; Lerma-Cabrera et al., 2016). Wang et al. (2012) noted, "Deficiency in DA (dopamine) pathways may lead to pathological overeating as a means to compensate for an understimulated reward system" (p. 188). Thus, it is important for counselors to recognize that people respond to food with varying degrees of reward. Coker Ross (2017) stated, "People with food addiction are predisposed to find more pleasure than those without food addiction when they eat highly palatable foods. This predisposition can lead to problems with bingeing, cravings, and weight gain" (p. 45).

Like other addictive behaviors, researchers also suggest that neuroadaptations can occur when the brain's reward system is chronically overstimulated by behaviors such as overeating palatable foods. Specifically, overactivation of dopamine release (such as during compulsive overeating) can lead to the downregulation of the dopaminergic system (Adams et al., 2019; Lerma-Cabrera et al., 2016; Schulte & Gearhardt, 2017; Smith & Robbins, 2013; Wang et al., 2012). This neuroadaptation creates tolerance, meaning that more highly palatable foods are required to achieve the same hedonic response. The overactivation of the dopamine system triggered by chronic, compulsive consumption of highly rewarding food, and the subsequent downregulation of dopamine receptors and functioning, creates the cycle of craving and compulsive overeating characteristic of food addiction.

FOOD ADDICTION AND TRAUMA

Another important consideration for counselors working with food addiction is the potential relationship with trauma. Researchers using national data of over 42,000 youth (aged 10–17) found a significant predictive relationship between adverse childhood experiences (ACEs) and childhood obesity (Ahn et al., 2019). Additionally, in the study of almost 3,500 college students, researchers found that higher ACE scores predicted higher BMI scores and less fruit and vegetable consumption (Windle et al., 2018). Moreover, among Black women with type 2 diabetes, researchers found that those who met criteria for food addiction (48% of the sample) had higher BMI and ACE scores than those without food addiction (Stojek et al., 2019). Finally, Imperatori et al. (2016) found that higher childhood trauma scores significantly, positively predicted higher food addiction scores among Italian women with BMIs greater than 25.

One potential explanation for the relationship between early trauma and food addiction is the effect of a dysregulated stress response system. In high stress situations, the hypothalamic–pituitary–adrenal axis triggers the release of the stress hormone, cortisol. Cortisol is linked to eating behaviors as the hormone, "stimulates fat accumulation and also triggers the body to crave high-sugar, high-fat foods" (Burke Harris, 2018, p. 51). Indeed, in the study of 22 overweight women with and without BED, researchers found that participants with BED had higher levels of morning basal cortisol than those without BED (Gluck et al., 2004). Thus, individuals who experienced persistent childhood trauma, and thereby had chronically dysregulated stress responses and elevated cortisol levels, may have felt chronic hunger or cravings for high-calorie foods. In fact, Leigh and Morris (2018) noted, "food addiction may be understood as a disorder involving a dysregulated stress response where compulsive overeating functions as a coping mechanism" (p. 38). Therefore, treatment for food addiction may include the assessment of childhood trauma and the implementation of trauma-informed treatment strategies.

> **CLINICAL NOTE 10.3**
>
> In the original adverse childhood experiences (ACEs) study, researchers found that 12.0% of participants with four or more ACEs had severe obesity (body mass index greater than or equal to 35), compared to 5.4% of those with no ACEs, representing an odds ratio of 1.6 (Felitti et al., 1998).

HOW DO I IDENTIFY IT?

Food addiction cannot be identified only by an individual's body shape or pattern of eating. Instead, counselors must assess clients' relationship with food to correctly determine whether food addiction is present. One sign of food addiction is utilizing food (particularly high-calorie foods) as a primary means of coping and emotion regulation. Food addiction is associated with *hedonic eating*, or eating for pleasure in the absence of hunger or the physiological need for energy (Leigh & Morris, 2018). Thus, it is important for counselors to assess clients' relationship with eating, including their motivation for eating, triggers and consequences of food consumption, and accompanying emotions during and after eating episodes.

Although food addiction does not have official criteria in the *DSM-5*, the Yale Food Addiction Scale (YFAS; Gearhardt et al., 2009) and subsequent revision (YFAS 2.0; Gearhardt et al., 2016) have been frequently utilized to identify food addiction. Using the criteria for substance-related and addictive disorders in the *DSM-5*, the YFAS 2.0 assesses 11 criteria related to food addiction: (a) consuming food in larger amounts and over longer durations of time than intended; (b) unsuccessful attempts to control the intake of particular foods; (c) substantial time spent acquiring, consuming, or recovering from eating behaviors; (d) strong cravings for certain foods; (e) eating patterns that contribute to the failure to fulfill obligations and responsibilities; (f) eating patterns that continue despite social problems; (g) meaningful activities given up due to eating patterns; (h) eating in physically hazardous situations; (i) eating patterns that continue despite physical or psychological problems; (j) evidence of tolerance; and (k) evidence of withdrawal (Carr et al., 2017). Like the current substance-related and addictive disorders in the *DSM-5*, endorsing two or three symptoms is indicative of mild food addiction, four or five symptoms is indicative of moderate food addiction, and six or more is indicative of severe food addiction, when accompanied by distress and impairment (Schulte & Gearhardt, 2017). These criteria can be helpful for counselors seeking to identify food addiction among clients.

FOOD ADDICTION AND MENTAL HEALTH

Along with negative physical consequences of food addiction, researchers have linked food addiction with a variety of mental health concerns including depression, anxiety, posttraumatic stress disorder, and emotion dysregulation (Penzenstadler et al., 2019). In a systematic review of food addiction literature, Burrows et al. (2018) examined 51 research studies and found moderate relationships between food addiction, depression, and anxiety. In addition, Sanlier et al. (2016) studied 793 Turkish university students and found a positive correlation between food addiction scores and depression scores among participants. Therefore, counselors should assess for co-occurring mental health disorders among clients presenting with food addiction. It may be that the mental health symptomology existed prior to the food addiction and eating became the primary means of coping with psychological distress. On the other hand, mental health symptoms may have developed as a result of the progression of food addiction including neuroadaptations in dopaminergic functioning. A third option could be that both food addiction and mental health concerns developed simultaneously with each condition interacting with and reinforcing the other. More longitudinal research studies are needed to understand the relationship between mental health symptomology and food addiction, yet counselors should assess for co-occurring disorders to create holistic treatment plans.

HOW DO I ASSESS IT?

Various assessment instruments exist that can be helpful in your work with clients presenting with food addiction. In what follows are descriptions of two instruments that you may consider utilizing in your clinical practice.

YALE FOOD ADDICTION SCALE

By far, the most commonly utilized assessment instrument for food addiction is the YFAS (Gearhardt et al., 2009). The YFAS was developed from the diagnostic criteria for substance dependence in the *Diagnostic and Statistical Manual of Mental Disorders* (4th ed., text rev.; *DSM-IV-TR*; APA, 2000) in conjunction with behavioral addiction instruments. The researchers conceptualized high-fat and high-sugar foods as the addictive substances and created a corresponding 25-item measure (Gearhardt et al., 2009). Upon release of the *DSM-5*, the authors updated the YFAS to the YFAS 2.0, a 35-item measure assessing the new criteria for substance-related and addictive disorders (Gearhardt et al., 2016). The YFAS 2.0 invites clients to consider eating patterns (particularly related to sweets, salty foods, fatty foods, or starches) over the previous 12 months. Items correspond with eight-point Likert-type scales ranging from *never* (0) to *everyday* (7). Example items include: *I ate to the point where I felt physically ill* and *When I cut down or stopped eating certain foods, I had strong cravings for them*. The YFAS 2.0 provides a continuous score (composed of the number of symptoms endorsed) or a dichotomous score (using thresholds for each question to assess whether the 11 symptoms of substance-related and addictive disorders are met). The YFAS 2.0 has demonstrated strong reliability (Kuder–Richardson = .92) and has been translated to multiple languages (Gearhardt et al., 2016). Additionally, a brief version of the YFAS 2.0 has been created, the modified YFAS 2.0 (Schulte & Gearhardt, 2017). This 13-item brief version demonstrated good reliability (Kuder–Richardson = .86) and performed similarly to the YFAS 2.0 (Schulte

& Gearhardt, 2017). The full YFAS 2.0 and scoring instructions are available in the online supplementary material of the Gearhardt et al. (2016) article.

ADDICTION-LIKE EATING BEHAVIOR SCALE

The authors of the Addiction-like Eating Behaviour Scale (AEBS; Ruddock et al., 2017) sought to create an instrument distinct from the YFAS. Specifically, Ruddock et al. (2017) aimed to focus on observable behavioral symptoms of food addiction beyond the criteria for substance-related and addictive disorders listed in the *DSM-5*. Using results from a qualitative study in which participants described behaviors associated with food addiction, the authors created a 15-item, two-factor scale to assess addiction-like eating patterns. The two factors include appetite drive (nine items) and low dietary control (six items). Each item on the AEBS corresponds with a five-point Likert-type scale ranging from *never or strongly disagree* (1) to *always or strongly agree* (5). Example items include: *I continue to eat despite feeling full* and *Once I start eating certain foods, I can't stop until there is nothing left*. The scale produces a total score or two subscale scores, which have demonstrated strong reliability (Cronbach's alpha = .90 for appetite drive and .85 for low dietary control). The full scale and scoring instructions can be found in the online supplementary materials accompanying the original Ruddock et al. (2017) article.

HOW DO I TREAT IT?

Treatment for clients with food addiction likely will entail psychoeducation related to the characteristics of food addiction, the differences between hedonic eating and eating for energy, and features of healthy, mindful eating patterns. Initially, clients may benefit from understanding the progression of food addiction to validate and normalize their experiences. Tarman and Werdell (2014) proposed four stages of food addiction: (a) *early stage* in which clients begin to lose control over their eating behaviors (which may include binge episodes or overeating through constant grazing), (b) *middle stage* in which clients' overeating leads to weight gain followed by attempts to diet, restrict, or control weight, (c) *late stage* in which clients recognize their loss of control over eating behaviors and begin experiencing negative consequences such as medical concerns and psychological symptoms, and (d) *final stage* in which food addiction has severely, adversely impacted clients' lives by impairing their functioning, leading to extreme obesity, and/or contributing to isolation and shame. Tarman and Werdell (2014) noted that throughout these stages, clients with food addiction engage in behaviors that parallel other addictions, such as stealing money to buy food, stealing food, hoarding food, lying about eating behaviors, and underestimating the extent of their food intake. It is important for counselors and clients to explore the purpose of clients' eating behaviors, including whether clients eat due to hunger and energy depletion or to modify their mood. Examining the function of clients' eating behaviors can help identify whether emotion regulation enhancement may be a viable component of treatment.

Additionally, treating clients with food addiction often entails psychoeducation about the effects of highly palatable foods on reward circuitry in the brain. From an addiction model, treatment includes helping clients identify trigger foods and developing an eating plan in which they abstain from compulsive, out-of-control eating. Indeed, Meule (2019) wrote, "the food addiction concept implies that abstinence (i.e., avoiding certain foods) may be a helpful treatment element for individuals with addiction-like eating behavior" (p. 14). As described in the following section, the 12-step support group, Food Addicts in Recovery Anonymous (FA), recognizes processed sugar and flour as trigger foods. Thus, according to FA, abstinence entails avoiding all foods with these ingredients. Some research exists, albeit with a small sample (three women with obesity, binge eating, and food addiction), that a low-carbohydrate, ketogenic diet (60% fat, 10% carbohydrates, 30% protein) significantly reduced both binge eating and food addiction symptoms (Carmen et al., 2020).

Finally, distinguishing between food addiction, an eating disorder, or co-occurring food addiction and an eating disorder (particularly BN and BED), is an important component of treatment. Specifically, treatment for clients with food addiction and an eating disorder will differ from treatment for clients with food addiction in the absence of an eating disorder. If clients present with eating disorders, counselors should ensure they have the proper training and competency to provide effective treatment. In addition, regardless of whether or not eating disorders are present, counselors working with clients with food addiction should partner with registered dietitians and primary care physicians to help clients create healthy, informed meal plans.

VOICES FROM THE FIELD: Clinical Work With Food Addiction

As an eating disorder specialist, it is part of my daily job to help those struggling with food addiction. Overeating or binge eating can function similarly to other types of eating disorders in that the client's relationship with food, in whatever form it takes, is helping them deal with emotional discomfort.

Like other addictions, we know that individuals do not choose to have an eating disorder or food addiction. The patterns of behavior start as very successful coping mechanisms, but the frequency of eating and quantity of food must often increase for the individual to continue to get the same relief. By the time it becomes clear that the consequences outweigh the benefits, the addiction has already taken hold.

Successful treatment of food addiction and eating disorders must start with clients knowing they are not being judged. A nonevaluative, supportive therapeutic relationship is crucial. Next, food addiction and eating disorder treatment often requires a team approach. I would not be able to do my job, in many cases, if I did not have a strong, non–weight-loss-focused registered dietitian on the team. You cannot stop overeating by restricting—the opposite is actually true. The best way not to binge or overeat is to eat intuitively. Finally, many people with food addiction will benefit from working with a psychiatrist. When a client's unhealthy coping skill is taken away, the emotional discomfort that it was helping manage will increase. Medication may be needed to manage symptoms of depression, anxiety, or other mood disorders.

Working with eating disorders and food addiction is not something I would recommend without training. Clinicians can do a lot of damage unintentionally. Practicing within one's scope of competence and training is important here. If counselors are interested in becoming trained in eating disorders, I would recommend joining their local International Association of Eating Disorders Professionals chapter. That said, this is a very rewarding population with which to work. Counselors interested in pursuing this specialty should first be aware of their own food, shape, and weight beliefs and biases. Having a healthy relationship with food does not mean you never use food to self-soothe (that is normal). Having a healthy body image does not mean you always feel like you look amazing. Rather, understanding how it feels to function under this pressure is a great source of empathy for your clients. "Healthy" can look like a lot of different things (I love the Health At Every Size movement)—and we can help our clients accept that reality and themselves.

Kiersten Rapstine, LPC-S, CEDS-S

MINDFULNESS-BASED INTERVENTIONS

Like other addictive behaviors, those with food addiction engage in eating compulsively, often without pausing to access their cognitive appraisal and goal-directed reasoning skills. Instead, eating becomes an out-of-control, chronic means of changing one's emotional state (consider a man who, after each argument with his romantic partner, consistently finds himself eating high-sugar foods to increase comfort and reduce distress). Therefore, enhancing clients' mindfulness may be a helpful treatment strategy to interrupt the cycle of food addiction (i.e., challenging situation → negative emotions → compulsive eating → positive and negative reinforcement).

Kabat-Zinn (2003) defined mindfulness as "the awareness that emerges through paying attention on purpose, in the present moment, and nonjudgmentally to the unfolding of experience moment by moment" (p. 145). Specifically, mindfulness is a meditation practice involving both attention and awareness, which is common in Buddhist traditions (Kabat-Zinn, 2003). In recent years, clinicians have adopted numerous mindfulness-based interventions (MBIs) into their clinical work such as mindfulness-based stress reduction, mindfulness-based cognitive therapy, and mindfulness-based relapse prevention, among other clinical approaches that incorporate mindfulness strategies (e.g., Acceptance and Commitment Therapy, Dialectical Behavior Therapy; Baer, 2003).

Recently, Kristeller and Wolever (2014), developed Mindfulness-Based Eating Awareness Training (MB-EAT) for compulsive overeating (specifically for individuals with BED and/or obesity). The goal of MB-EAT is to "develop the capacity for self-directed attention to both internal and external stimuli and to cultivate stable and nonreactive awareness of experience" (Kristeller & Wolever, 2014, p. 119). MB-EAT programs aim to develop clients' awareness related to hunger, taste, and fullness, increase self-acceptance, introduce guided meditations, and promote reliance on both inner wisdom (using internal awareness to direct food choices) and outer wisdom (using external knowledge to direct food choices). Kristeller and Wolever (2014) described a 10-session MB-EAT group counseling intervention including mindfulness meditation practices, guided meditations related to satiety and hunger, cultivating inner wisdom (e.g., mindful eating, body scan, taste awareness), cultivating outer wisdom (e.g., nutritional information, knowledge related to calories, knowledge related to physical activity and exercise), loving-kindness sitting practices, forgiveness meditation, wisdom meditation, values exercises, and activities such as the 500 Calorie Challenge in which participants identify 500 calories to eliminate (or reduce) indefinitely from their daily eating habits. MB-EAT has garnered empirical support as an effective intervention for clients with BED and/or obesity (Kristeller & Wolever, 2014). To learn more about MB-EAT, visit mb-eat.com.

Furthermore, O'Reilly et al. (2014) conducted a meta-analysis of 21 studies examining the effects of MBIs on eating behaviors related to obesity (e.g., binge eating, emotional eating, external eating). Although food addiction was not specifically studied, the meta-analysis involved constructs overlapping with or related to addictive eating behaviors such as binge eating and emotional eating. The researchers found that 86% of the studies demonstrated a decrease in obesity-related eating behaviors as a result of the MBI. Specifically, effect sizes for changes in binge eating ranged from small to large (yet the majority were large), effect sizes for changes in emotional eating ranged from moderate to large, and effect sizes for changes in external eating ranged from moderate to large (O'Reilly et al., 2014). In sum, the authors provided empirical support for the role of MBIs in the reduction of obesity-related eating behaviors, which may include or be associated with food addiction. Therefore, counselors working with food addiction may benefit from employing MBIs into their clinical work, yet Kabat-Zinn (2003) cautioned that in order to effectively utilize MBIs, counselors should have histories of practicing mindfulness in their own lives. Specifically:

> Mindfulness meditation is not simply a method that one encounters for a brief time at a professional seminar and then passes on to others for use as needed when they find themselves tense or stressed. It is a way of being that takes ongoing effort to develop and refine (Kabat-Zinn, 2003, p. 149).

For more information related to mindfulness and professional training opportunities, visit mbpti.org, mbct.com, or mindfulrp.com.

COGNITIVE BEHAVIORAL THERAPY

In light of the overlap between food addiction and BED (Burrows et al., 2018), it is helpful to assess treatment modalities that have been successful in reducing binge eating episodes. Hilbert et al. (2019) conducted a meta-analysis of 81 randomized controlled trials of treatment strategies with clients with BED. The authors found that psychotherapy interventions (the majority of which utilized cognitive behavioral therapy [CBT]) significantly decreased binge eating episodes with large effect sizes (Hilbert et al., 2019). Therefore, empirical support exists for the efficacy of CBT among those with BED. Mitchell et al. (2008) developed a treatment manual for providing CBT to clients who engage in binge eating. The empirically supported protocol consists of three phases: (a) *Phase I*: provide information about binge eating, identify cues and triggers, identify clients' chain of responses and consequences, restructure maladaptive beliefs, and develop behavioral strategies to interrupt the response chain; (b) *Phase II*: utilize behavioral and cognitive strategies to address issues related to body image, stress management, self-esteem, assertive communication, and weight management; and (c) *Phase III*: engage in long-term planning and relapse prevention strategies. The treatment typically entails 15 sessions. A primary component of CBT for BED is to help clients identify cues (triggering situations or stimuli), responses (beliefs, emotions, or actions), and subsequent consequences (which can be positive or negative). For example, consider an adult client who had a distressing conversation with her mother in which she felt shamed and humiliated (cue), leading to the beliefs, "I am inadequate," "Eating a piece of dessert will make me feel better," "I can just have one," and "It will be different this time, I can stop when I want to" (response), followed by the consumption of so much food that the client feels ill, disgusted, and hopeless (consequence). Once clients are aware of the sequence between cues, responses, and consequences, they can develop ways to respond to cues differently (e.g., through cognitive restructuring and behavioral techniques) and experience more positive consequences (Mitchell et al., 2008).

Some empirical evidence exists to support the importance of cognitive restructuring in the treatment of food addiction, specifically. Nolan and Jenkins (2019) examined irrational beliefs, emotional eating, and food addiction among 239 adults and found a significant relationship between irrational beliefs and food addiction, mediated by emotional eating (Nolan & Jenkins, 2019). Therefore, preliminary evidence suggests that utilizing a CBT approach to address irrational beliefs and accompanying maladaptive behaviors may be an effective treatment strategy for clients with food addiction.

12-STEP SUPPORT

FA is a fellowship modeled after Alcoholics Anonymous that utilizes the 12 steps to help members overcome food addiction. Step one of FA states, "we admitted we were powerless over food—that our lives had become unmanageable" (FA, 2015, p. 430). The belief endorsed by members of FA is that certain foods (specifically those made with processed flour and sugar) affect those with food addiction in ways that parallel how drugs of abuse affect those with substance use disorders. Like other 12-step fellowships, FA is a spiritual program consisting of meetings, sponsors, a text, literature, traditions, and working the steps. The FA program provides regular, free, in-person or virtual meetings, available to anyone who desires to stop addictive eating behaviors. Comparable to other behavioral addictions (e.g., sex addiction), the goal of FA is not abstinence from food. Instead, abstinence includes the elimination of specific patterns of eating, namely the compulsive, out-of-control consumption of particular foods. According to FA, abstinence entails, "simple, weighed and measured meals, with nothing eaten between mealtimes" in which individuals abstain from processed sugar and flour of any kind (FA, 2015, p. 11). Thus, working with a sponsor, FA members learn the practice of measuring and weighing their food (to prevent overeating) and abstaining from foods that contain addictive macronutrients (e.g., flour and sugar). FA is a highly structured recovery program (not a diet plan) that helps members control the types and quantities of food they eat to experience liberation from food addiction (FA, 2015). You can learn more about FA by visiting their website at foodaddicts.org.

DIAGNOSTIC CONSIDERATIONS

Currently there is no diagnostic code for food addiction in the *DSM-5*. Given the overlap between eating disorders and food addiction, it is important for counselors to thoroughly assess whether their clients meet criteria for an eating disorder, particularly BN or BED, in addition to food addiction. Both the

DSM-5 and *International Classification of Diseases*, 11th Revision (World Health Organization, 2018) have diagnoses and codes for feeding or eating disorders. If clients do not meet criteria for an eating disorder, the diagnostic code for other specified feeding or eating disorder (OSFED) may be appropriate. The OSFED code is fitting for clients with eating disorder symptomology and distress or impairment, yet fail to meet all criteria of an existing eating disorder diagnosis (APA, 2013). Therefore, counselors may diagnose a client with food addiction with OSFED and specify what aspects of an existing eating disorder are not being met (e.g., BED not met due to low frequency of binge episodes). As with other addictions, food addiction often coexists with other mental health concerns such as depression, anxiety, and posttraumatic stress disorder (Burrows et al., 2018; Penzenstadler et al., 2019). Thus clinicians also may diagnose the co-occurring condition, if appropriate.

HOW CAN I LEARN MORE?

If you are working with clients with food addiction or would like to learn more about the condition, consider the following resources.

BOOKS

- Brownell, K. D., & Gold, M. S. (Eds.). (2012). *Food and addiction: A comprehensive handbook.* Oxford University Press.
- Coker Ross, C. (2017). *The food addiction recovery workbook: How to manage cravings, reduce stress, and stop hating your body.* New Harbinger Publications, Inc.
- Tarman, V., & Werdell, P. (2014). *Food junkies: The truth about food addiction.* Dundurn.

PEER-REVIEWED ARTICLES

- Hauck, C., Cook, B., & Ellrott, T. (2020). Food addiction, eating addiction and eating disorders. *Proceedings of the Nutrition Society, 79,* 103–112. https://doi.org/10.1017/S0029665119001162
- Leigh, S. J., & Morris, M. J. (2018). The role of reward circuitry and food addiction in the obesity epidemic: An update. *Biological Psychiatry, 131,* 31–42. https://doi.org/10.1016/j.biopsycho.2016.12.013
- Meule, A. (2019). A critical examination of the practical implication derived from the food addiction concept. *Current Obesity Reports, 8,* 11–17. https://doi.org/10.1007/s13679-019-0326-2

WEBSITES

- Food Addiction Institute: foodaddictioninstitute.org
- Food Addicts in Recovery Anonymous: www.foodaddicts.org
- International Association of Eating Disorders Professionals Foundation: www.iaedp.com
- Overeaters Anonymous: oa.org

REFERENCES

Adams, R. C., Sedgmond, J., Maizey, L., Chambers, C. D., & Lawrence, N. S. (2019). Food addiction: Implications for the diagnosis and treatment of overeating. *Nutrients, 11,* 2086. https://doi.org/10.3390/u11092086

Ahmed, S. H. (2012). Is sugar as addictive as cocaine? In K. D. Brownell & M. S. Gold (Eds.), *Food and addiction: A comprehensive handbook* (pp. 231–237). Oxford University Press.

Ahn, S., Zhang, H., Berlin, K. S., Levy, M., & Kabra, R. (2019). Adverse childhood experiences and childhood obesity: A path analysis approach. *Children's Health Care, 49,* 247–266. https://doi.org/10.1080/02739615.2019.1697928

American Psychiatric Association. (2013). *Diagnostic and statistical manual of mental disorders* (5th ed.). Author.

Baer, R. A. (2003). Mindfulness training as a clinical intervention: A conceptual and empirical review. *Clinical Psychology: Science and Practice, 10,* 125–143. https://doi.org/10.1093/clipsy/bpg015

Barrett, D. (2010). *Supernormal stimuli: How primal urges overran their evolutionary purpose.* W. W. Norton & Company.

Blum, K., Cull, J. G., Braverman, E. R., & Comings, D. E. (1996). Reward deficiency syndrome. *American Scientist, 84,* 132–146.

Burke Harris, N. (2018). *The deepest well: Healing the long-term effects of childhood adversity.* Bluebird.

Burrows, T., Kay-Lambkin, F., Pursey, K., Skinner, J., & Dayas, C. (2018). Food addiction and associations with mental health symptoms: A systematic review with meta-analysis. *Journal of Human Nutrition and Dietetics, 31,* 544–572. https://doi.org/10.111/jhn.12532

Carmen, M., Safer, D. L., Saslow, L. R., Kalayjian, T., Mason, A. E., Westman, E. C., & Dalai, S. S. (2020). Treating binge eating and food addiction symptoms with low-carbohydrate ketogenic clients: A case series. *Journal of Eating Disorders, 8,* 1–7. https://doi.org/10.186/s40337-020-0278-7

Carr, M. M., Catak, P. D., Pejsa-Reitz, M. C., Saules, K. K., & Gearhardt, A. N. (2017). Measurement invariance of the Yale Food Addiction Scale 2.0 across gender and racial groups. *Psychological Assessment, 29,* 1044–1052. https://doi.org/10.1037/pas00000403

Coker Ross, C. (2017). *The food addiction recovery workbook: How to manage cravings, reduce stress, and stop hating your body.* New Harbinger Publications, Inc.

Costin, C. (2007). *The eating disorder sourcebook: A comprehensive guide to the causes, treatments, and prevention of eating disorders* (3rd ed.). McGraw-Hill

Felitti, V. J., Anda, R. F., Nordenberg, D., Williamson, D. F., Spitz, A. M., Edwards, V., Koss, M. P., & Marks, J. S. (1998). Relationship of childhood abuse and household dysfunction to many of the leading causes of death in adults: The adverse childhood experiences (ACE) study. *American Journal of Preventive Medicine, 14,* 245–258. https://doi.org/10.1016/s0749-3797(98)00017-8

Food Addicts in Recovery Anonymous. (2015). *Food addicts in recovery anonymous.* Author.

Gearhardt, A. N., & Corbin, W. R. (2012). Food addiction and diagnostic criteria for dependence. In K. D. Brownell & M. S. Gold (Eds.), *Food and addiction: A comprehensive handbook* (pp. 167–171). Oxford University Press.

Gearhardt, A. N., Corbin, W. R., & Brownell, K. D. (2009). Preliminary validation of the Yale food addiction scale. *Appetite, 52,* 430–436. https://doi.org/10.1016/j.appet.2008.12.03

Gearhardt, A. N., Corbin, W. R., & Brownell, K. D. (2016). Development of the Yale Food Addiction Scale version 2.0. *Psychology of Addictive Behaviors, 30,* 113–121. https://doi.org/10.1037/adb0000136

Gluck, M. E., Geliebter, A., Hung, J., & Yahav, E. (2004). Cortisol, hunger, and desire to binge eat following a cold stress test in obese women with binge eating disorder. *Psychosomatic Medicine, 66,* 876–881. https://doi.org/10.1097/01.psy.0000143637.63508.47

Hales, C. M., Carroll, M. D., Fryar, C. D., & Ogden, C. L. (2017). *Prevalence of obesity among adults and youth: United States 2015–2016.* National Center for Health Statistics.

Hales, C. M., Carroll, M. D., Fryar, C. D., & Ogden, C. L. (2020). *Prevalence of obesity and severe obesity among adults: United States, 2017–2018.* National Center for Health Statistics.

Hauck, C., Cook, B., & Ellrott, T. (2020). Food addiction, eating addiction and eating disorders. *Proceedings of the Nutrition Society, 79,* 103–112. https://doi.org/10.1017/S0029665119001162

Hauck, C., Weiß, A., Schulte, E. M., Meule, A., & Ellrott, T. (2017). Prevalence of 'food addiction' as measured with the Yale Food Addiction Scale 2.0 in a representative German sample and its association with sex, age and weight categories. *Obesity Facts, 10,* 12–24. https://doi.org/10.1159/000456013

Hilbert, A., Petroff, D., Herpertz, S., Pietrowsky, R., Tuschen-Caffier, B., Vocks, S., & Schmidt, R. (2019). Meta-analysis of the efficacy of psychological and mental treatments for binge-eating disorder. *Journal of Consulting and Clinical Psychology, 87,* 91–105. https://doi.org/10.037/ccp0000358

Imperatori, C., Innamorati, M., Lamis, D. A., Farina, B., Pompili, M., Contardi, A., & Fabbricatore, M. (2016). Childhood trauma in obese and overweight women with food addiction and clinical-level of binge eating. *Child Abuse and Neglect, 58,* 180–190. https://doi.org/10.1016/j.chiabu.2016.06.023

Jimenez-Murcia, S., Agura, Z., Paslakis, G., Munguia, L., Granero, R., Sanchez-Gonzalez J., Sánchez, I., Riesco, N., Gearhardt, A. N., Dieguez, C., Fazia, G., Segura-García, C., Baenas, I., Menchón, J. M., & Fernandez-Aranda, F. (2019). Food addiction in eating disorders and obesity: Analysis of clusters and implications for treatment. *Nutrients, 11,* 2633. https://doi.org/10.3390/nu11112633

Kabat-Zinn, J. (2003). Mindfulness-based interventions in context: Past, present, and future. *Clinical Psychology: Science and Practice, 10,* 144–156. https://doi.org/10.1093/clipsy/bpg016

Kristeller, J. L., & Wolever, R. Q. (2014). Mindfulness-based eating awareness training: Treatment of overeating and obesity. In R. A. Baer (Ed.), *Mindfulness-based treatment approaches: Clinican's guide to evidence base and applications* (2nd ed., pp. 121–139). Elsevier.

Leigh, S. J., & Morris, M. J. (2018). The role of reward circuitry and food addiction in the obesity epidemic: An update. *Biological Psychiatry, 131,* 31–42. https://doi.org/10.1016/j.biopsycho.2016.12.013

Lerma-Cabrera, J. M., Carvajal, F., & Lopez-Legarrea, P. (2016). Food addiction as a new piece of the obesity framework. *Nutrition Journal, 15,* 1–5. https://doi.org/10.1186/s12937-016-0124-6

Lopez-Aguilar, I., Ibarra-Reynoso, L. D. R., & Malacara, J. M. (2018). Association of Nesfatin-1, acylated Ghrelin and cortisol with scores of compulsion, food addiction, and binge eating in adults with normal weight and with obesity. *Annals of Nutrition and Metabolism, 73,* 54–61. https://doi.org/10.1159/000490357

Meule, A. (2019). A critical examination of the practical implication derived from the food addiction concept. *Current Obesity Reports, 8,* 11–17. https://doi.org/10.1007/s13679-019-0326-2

Mitchell, J. E., Devlin, M. J., de Zwaan, M., Crow, S. J., & Peterson, C. B. (2008). *Binge-eating disorders: Clinical foundations and treatment.* Guilford Press.

National Heart, Lung, and Blood Institute. (1998). *Clinical guidelines on the identification, evaluation, and treatment of overweight and obesity in adults: The evidence report.* https://www.ncbi.nlm.nih.gov/books/NBK2003

Nolan, L. J., & Jenkins, S. M. (2019). Food addiction is associated with irrational beliefs via trait anxiety and emotional eating. *Nutrients, 11,* 1711. https://doi.org/10.3390/nu11081711

Onaolapo, A. Y., & Onaolapo, O. J. (2018). Food additives, food and the concept of 'food addiction': Is stimulation of the brain reward circuit by food sufficient to trigger addiction? *Pathophysiology, 25,* 263–276. https://doi.org/10.1016/j.pathophys.2018.04.002

O'Reilly, G. A., Cook, L., Spruijt-Metz, D., & Black, D. S (2014). Mindfulness-based interventions for obesity-related eating behaviors: A literature review. *Obesity Reviews, 15,* 453–461. https://doi.org/10.1111/obr.12156

Ouellette, A. S., Rodrigue, C., Lemieux, S., Tchernof, A., Biertno, L., & Begin, C. (2018). Establishing a food addiction diagnosis using the Yale Food Addiction Scale: A closer look at the clinically significant distress/functional impairment criterion. *Appetite, 129,* 55–61. https://doi.org/10.1016/j.appt.2018.06.031

Penzenstadler, L., Soares, C., Karila, L., & Khazaal, Y. (2019). Systematic review of food addiction as measured with the Yale Food Addiction Scale: Implications for the food addiction construct. *Current Neuropharmacology, 17,* 526–538. https://doi.org/10.2174/1570159x16666181108093520

Rainey, J. C., Furman, C. R., & Gearhardt, A. N. (2018). Food addiction among sexual minorities. *Appetite, 120,* 16–22. https://doi.org/10.1016/j.appet.2-17.08.019

Ruddock, H. K., Christiansen, P., Halford, J. C. G., & Hardman, C. A. (2017). The development and validation of the Addiction-like Eating Behaviour Scale. *International Journal of Obesity, 41,* 1710–1717. https://doi.org/10.1038/ijo.2017.158

Salamone, J. D., & Correa, M. (2013). Dopamine and food addiction: Lexicon badly needed. *Biological Psychiatry, 73,* e15–e25. https://doi.org/10.1016/j.biopsych.2012.09.027

Sanlier, N., Turkozu, D., & Toka, O. (2016). Body image, food addiction, depression, and body mass index in university students. *Ecology of Food and Nutrition, 55,* 491–507. https://doi.org/10.1080/03670244.2016.1219951

Schulte, E. M., & Gearhardt, A. N. (2017). Development of the modified Yale food addiction scale version 2.0. *European Eating Disorders Review, 25,* 302–308. https://doi.org/10.1002/erv.2515

Smith, D. G., & Robbins, T. W. (2013). The neurobiological underpinnings of obesity and binge eating: A rationale for adopting the food addiction model. *Biological Psychiatry, 73,* 804–810. https://doi.org/10.1016/j.biopsych.2012.08.026

Stojek, M. M., Maples-Keller, J. L., Dixon, H. D., Umpierrez, G. E., Gillespie, C. F., & Michopoulos, V. (2019). Associations of childhood trauma with food addiction and insulin resistance in African American women with diabetes mellitus. *Appetite, 141,* 104317. https://doi.org/10.1016/j.appet.2019.104317

Tarman, V. & Werdell, P. (2014). *Food junkies: The truth about food addiction.* Dundurn.

Wang, G. J., Volkow, N. D., & Fowler, J. S. (2012). Dopamine deficiency, eating, and body weight. In K. D. Brownell & M. S. Gold (Eds.), *Food and addiction: A comprehensive handbook* (pp. 185–193). Oxford University Press.

Windle, M., Haardorfer, R., Getachew, B., Shah, J., Payne, J., Pillai, D., & Berg, C. J. (2018). A multivariate analysis of adverse childhood experiences and health behaviors and outcomes among college students. *Journal of American College Health, 66,* 246–251. https://doi.org/10.1080/07448481.2018.1431892

Wise, R. A. (2013). Dual roles of dopamine in food and drug-seeking: The drive-reward paradox. *Biological Psychiatry, 73,* 819–826. https://doi.org/10.1016/j.biopsych.2012.09.001

World Health Organization. (2018). *International statistical classification of diseases and related health problems* (11th Rev.). https://icd.who.int/browse11/l-m/en

Yu, Z. Indelicato, N. A., Fuglestad, P., Tan, M., Bane, L., & Stice, C. (2018). Sex differences in disordered eating and food addiction among college students. *Appetite, 129,* 12–18. https://doi.org/10.1016/j.appet.2018.06.028

11

Exercise Addiction

HOW DO I CONCEPTUALIZE IT?

Physical activity refers to moving one's body in a way that expends energy above baseline levels (U.S. Department of Health and Human Services [HHS], 2018). Thus, physical activity can include walking up a flight of stairs, vacuuming the carpet, mowing the lawn, or carrying an infant while grocery shopping. *Exercise* is a specific type of physical activity that is "planned, structured, repetitive, and performed with the goal of improving health or fitness" (HHS, 2018, p. 29). Hence, exercise includes activities such as cycling, swimming, running, weight lifting, practicing martial arts, and brisk walking. There are a myriad of known physical and psychological benefits of regular exercise. Research indicates that consistent exercise among healthy adults can improve bone health, sleep patterns, and cognitive functioning while also decreasing anxiety, depression, weight gain, and lowering the risk of hypertension, type 2 diabetes, cardiovascular disease, cancer, and dementia (HHS, 2018). According to the HHS (2018), American adults should exercise at a moderate intensity for 30 minutes, 5 days per week, or at a vigorous intensity for 20 minutes, 3 days per week. In addition to aerobic (i.e., cardio) exercise, experts also recommend at least 2 days per week of strength training and muscular endurance activities (HHS, 2018). For the majority of individuals, regular exercise is healthy and beneficial. However, for a small portion of exercisers, the behavior can become problematic and potentially, an addiction.

The concept of exercise addiction can be perplexing. For many people, exercise does not feel as rewarding or pleasurable as other potentially addictive behaviors (e.g., eating, gaming, drug use). How then, does it provide the positive reinforcement (i.e., positive consequences that increase the likelihood of repeating the behavior) indicative of addiction? Additionally, given expert recommendations for regular exercise, one must question how and when this repetitive behavior is deemed compulsive. Finally, even if a person seems dependent on exercise, is that necessarily detrimental? Could it be a positive addiction?

To help address these questions, Schreiber and Hausenblas (2015) provided a useful definition of exercise addiction. Specifically, they described the condition as:

> A pattern of physical activity that exceeds what most fitness and medical professionals consider "normal," causes immense psychological anguish (either during, following, or anticipation of exercise), engulfs an exercise addict's personal, professional, and social life, and is experienced by the addict as difficult to control or reduce in frequency—even in the face of illness or injury (p. 3).

Additionally, decades ago, Morgan (1979) identified three symptoms of exercise addiction: (a) daily exercise is needed to cope (along with the belief that an individual cannot miss a day of exercise), (b) withdrawal symptoms occur if the individual is unable to exercise (e.g., irritability, depression, anger, insomnia, restlessness, interpersonal conflict), and (c) exercise is continued even when contraindicated (e.g., physical injury, social conflicts, time necessary to invest in other life commitments).

Thus, like other behavioral addictions, exercise addiction is marked by the loss of control over exercise behaviors, engaging in exercise compulsively, continuing to exercise despite negative consequences (e.g., illness, injury), and craving or mental preoccupation with exercise. As the addiction progresses, exercise becomes paramount in the individual's life to the detriment of other responsibilities, opportunities, and relationships, and is the source of psychological distress. For example, although injuries are upsetting for anyone, Lichtenstein et al. (2018) found more emotional distress among injured exercisers with exercise addiction than injured exercisers without exercise addiction. Specifically, among injured exercisers with exercise addiction, 26% reported depressive symptomology and 23% reported having the thought that life was not worth living (Lichtenstein et al., 2018). Additionally, although psychiatrist William Glasser (1976, 1977) posited the idea that some compulsive behaviors (e.g., running, meditation, playing an instrument) could be considered *positive addictions*, this notion has been heavily contested by scholars and clinicians (Berczik et al., 2012). Specifically, it is argued that engagement in repetitive behaviors that are adaptive and life-enhancing is best conceptualized as passionate, committed, or highly enthusiastic engagement, rather than an addiction (Hausenblas et al., 2017; Szabo, 2010). Furthermore, addictive behaviors are defined by negative consequences, conflict, a loss of control, withdrawal symptoms, and cravings, and thus, by definition, cannot be positive (Berczik et al., 2012; Griffiths, 2005). Therefore, the concept of exercise addiction differs substantially from highly committed exercise and is marked by significant distress, negative consequences, and functional impairment.

AN INTERACTION MODEL OF EXERCISE ADDICTION

Several models exist to explain the emergence and course of exercise addiction. One of the newer, more comprehensive models is Egorov and Szabo's (2013) *interaction model*. This model encompasses personal, situational, and motivational factors to explain the development of exercise addiction among certain individuals. Although there are numerous ways for people to regulate their emotions (e.g., substance use, sexual activity, spiritual practices, social interactions, nonsuicidal self-injury), the interaction model provides context for why some individuals rely on exercise as their primary (and often, only) coping strategy.

According to the interaction model, exercise addiction is the result of the combined effects of both personal and situational factors. *Personal factors* include an individual's personality (e.g., perfectionism, neuroticism), values (e.g., health, thinness), goals (e.g., success, social praise), and past experiences with exercise (previous positive outcomes). *Situational factors* entail accessibility (exercise is almost always accessible), cost (exercise can be free), and social aspects (general acceptance and societal praise for exercising) of the behavior. Together, these personal and situational factors interact to create an individual's unique *motivation* for exercise (Egorov & Szabo, 2013).

Egorov and Szabo (2013) proposed that individuals can be motivated to exercise for several reasons including: (a) social purposes, (b) physical health purposes, (c) performance-based purposes, and (d) psychological health purposes. These four types of motivation can have therapeutic orientations (to influence one's mental state) or mastery orientations (to perform better or reach fitness goals). For those who engage in exercise for its therapeutic function, such as escaping psychological pain, exercise addiction is more likely to develop. Indeed, being motivated by negative reinforcement (i.e., decreasing something undesirable and thus increasing the likelihood that the behavior will be repeated) is characteristic of those with exercise addiction (Szabo, 2010). For example, consider a woman who makes an error at work and subsequently feels embarrassment and self-loathing. She believes that the only way to escape her negative emotions is to go for a run, despite the inclement weather, late hour, and her current ankle pain. Although regular exercise can be a useful and healthy means of mood modification, if the behavior is the *only* means of emotion regulation and motivated solely by therapeutic orientations, it carries the risk of becoming an addictive behavior.

The interaction model encourages clinicians to consider a variety of client factors (both internal and external) in the development of exercise addiction. Indeed, researchers have found empirical support for the relationship between specific personality traits and exercise addiction including perfectionism (Downs et al., 2004) and psychological inflexibility (Alcaraz-Ibanez et al., 2018). Additionally, the social approval of exercise in many societies may make it a more appealing (and often easier to hide) addictive behavior than activities such as using drugs, engaging in nonsuicidal self-injury, or gambling. Therefore, using the interaction model, counselors can assess clients' unique motivations for exercise and identify personal and social factors that contribute to the function of exercise in their lives.

PRIMARY AND SECONDARY EXERCISE ADDICTION

Exercise addiction can fall into one of two categories distinguished by the purpose of the behavior (Cunningham et al., 2016; Veal, 1987). *Primary exercise addiction* exists when an individual seeks to avoid negative mood states and experience positive feelings through compulsive exercise. In this condition, the experience of exercise is the goal in and of itself (e.g., consider a body builder who craves exercise and feels relief and pleasure when he lifts weights and exerts physical strength). *Secondary exercise addiction*, on the other hand, exists when the individual is seeking to expend calories and lose weight through exercise in the presence of an eating disorder (Berczik et al., 2012; Veal, 1987). Among those with secondary exercise addiction, weight loss, muscle tone, and calorie burn are the desired outcomes (rather than the experience of exercising). Thus, clinicians should be careful to distinguish between primary and secondary exercise addiction by assessing whether an eating disorder exists (which is indicative of secondary exercise addiction).

There is some research supporting the notion that secondary exercise addiction is more prevalent than primary exercise addiction (Cunningham et al., 2016; Trott et al., 2021). Indeed, in the study of U.S. adults (with specific recruitment of athletes and those who may have an eating disorder), researchers found that 12.02% of the sample met criteria for pathological exercise, and 77.78% of those with pathological exercise also had an eating disorder (Cunningham et al., 2016). Cunningham et al. (2016) also noted that primary exercise addiction may be more reflective of an addictive behavior while secondary exercise addiction may be more reflective of a compulsive behavior. Additionally, Trott et al. (2021) conducted a meta-analysis and found that individuals with eating disorders were over 3.5 times more likely than those without eating disorders to have exercise addiction. Thus, although similarities exist between the presentation of the two types of exercise addiction, treatment will vary depending on whether the client has a comorbid eating disorder.

EXERCISE ADDICTION AND ANOREXIA NERVOSA

Exercise addiction can exist with any eating disorder. Indeed, in the study of 1,522 women and 61 men with eating disorders, Monell et al. (2018) found that 55.1% women and 55.5% men with eating disorder not otherwise specified, 51.1% women and 45.1% men with bulimia nervosa (BN), and 40.3% of women and 36.1% men with anorexia nervosa (AN) met criteria for compulsive exercise. Additionally, Cunningham et al. (2016) found that among clients with pathological exercise, 62.2% had an unspecified feeding or eating disorder (UFED), 9.4% had binge eating disorder (BED), 5.0% had BN, and 1.1% had AN. Furthermore, researchers confirm that addressing compulsive exercise is an important component of treatment for all eating disorders (Danielsen et al., 2016). Despite the potential to co-occur with any type of disordered eating, the *Diagnostic and Statistical Manual of Mental Disorders* (5th ed.; *DSM-5*; American Psychiatric Association [APA], 2013) specifically identified excessive exercise as characteristic of a subgroup of individuals with AN. Thus the relationship between AN and exercise addiction will be considered in this chapter (for information related to BN and BED, readers are encouraged to consult Chapter 10).

The diagnostic criteria for AN include: (a) the act of food restriction leading to less than minimally healthy body weight (i.e., a body mass index less than 18.5), (b) a persistent and powerful fear of weight gain, and (c) extreme influence of one's body shape and weight on evaluation of the self (APA, 2013). AN can be categorized as the restricting type (no episodes of bingeing or purging in previous 3 months) or binge eating/purging type (episodes of bingeing or purging occurred within the previous 3 months). Individuals with AN may engage in a variety of strategies to maintain less than minimally healthy weight including compulsive exercise (APA, 2013). The prevalence of exercise addiction among those with AN has been supported by research. Specifically, among 21 women in inpatient treatment for AN, 48% met criteria for exercise dependence (Klein et al., 2004). Additionally, Keyes et al. (2015) examined psychological and physical variables among female participants with a diagnosis of AN, participants with moderate anxiety (without eating disorders), and healthy controls. The results indicated that participants with AN had a higher drive to exercise (reflecting scores on exercise addiction and obligatory exercise assessments) compared to those in the anxiety group and healthy controls (Keyes et al., 2015). Thus, although clinicians working with clients with any eating disorder should assess for exercise addiction, it may be particularly important among clients with AN.

EXERCISE ADDICTION AND BODY DYSMORPHIC DISORDER

When working with clients with exercise addiction, it is important for clinicians to be familiar with and able to recognize the signs of *body dysmorphic disorder* (APA, 2013). Classified as an obsessive-compulsive disorder (OCD), body dysmorphic disorder is characterized by a preoccupation with a perceived physical flaw (e.g., acne, wrinkles, thinning hair, the size or shape of one's facial features) and subsequent compulsive, repetitive actions in response to the perceived flaw (e.g., mirror checking, grooming, tanning, comparing themselves to others, excessive exercise). To be diagnosed with body dysmorphic disorder, preoccupation with the perceived physical defect must cause impairment and distress and should not be better accounted for by weight concerns accompanying eating disorders. Additionally, to warrant the diagnosis, the physical flaw should only be perceived, meaning that it is unobservable to others or nonexistent. Therefore, an extreme emotional response to an actual physical abnormality would not be considered body dysmorphic disorder (APA, 2013).

When diagnosing body dysmorphic disorder, clinicians can specify whether *muscle dysmorphia* is present, which entails a mental obsession centered upon the insufficiency of one's size or muscle mass. Muscle dysmorphia often is accompanied by excessive weight lifting and bodybuilding efforts coupled with high-protein diets, protein powders, and the potential use of anabolic-androgenic steroids (Specter & Wiss, 2014). Individuals with muscle dysmorphia (more frequently males; APA, 2013) are distressingly preoccupied with the belief that they are not muscular enough and therefore compulsively engage in strength training activities (often in spite of injury or other commitments) to become larger in size (Specter & Wiss, 2014). Indeed, in the study of 1,711 exercising adults from four different countries, researchers found that 38.5% were at risk for body dysmorphic disorder and 11.7% met criteria for exercise addiction (Corazza et al., 2019). The researchers also assessed for the use of fitness enhancing products (e.g., protein supplements, vitamins, steroids, caffeine) and found that participants who reported using fitness supplements were at higher risk for exercise addiction. Additionally, over 8% of the sample reported the use of anabolic-androgenic steroids or amphetamine-like fitness supplements (Corazza et al., 2019). Therefore, when counselors become aware of compulsive or addictive exercise, it is important to assess whether clients meet criteria for body dysmorphic disorder (specifically with muscle dysmorphia) and also if fitness enhancing products (e.g., steroids, stimulants) are being used.

CLINICAL NOTE 11.1

Take a moment to consider how current gender norms, body image ideals, and sexual objectification can impact eating disorders, body dysmorphic disorder, and exercise addiction among men and women.

PREVALENCE OF EXERCISE ADDICTION

Prevalence rates of exercise addiction are difficult to ascertain due to the lack of uniform diagnostic criteria and varying samples (e.g., exercisers versus the general population). For example, in a national sample of Hungarian adults, researchers found between .3% and .5% of the total sample (including regular exercisers and nonexercisers) met criteria for exercise addiction (Monok et al., 2012). Among a national sample of American adults, however, 6.4% were classified as engaging in pathological exercise (Cunningham et al., 2016). Additionally, in a community sample of almost 900 women, researchers found exercise addiction among 3.34% (Quesnel et al., 2018). As expected, prevalence rates of exercise addiction are higher among samples of regular exercisers (e.g., 8% of male recreational exercisers; Alcaraz-Ibanez et al., 2018), and even higher among those with eating disorders (e.g., 48.2% of women and 45.5% of men in eating disorder treatment; Monell et al., 2018). Moreover, some researchers have found higher prevalence rates of exercise addiction among those who practice particular forms of exercise such as running, cycling, and bodybuilding (Juwono & Szabo, 2020).

With regard to gender, Dumitru et al. (2018) reviewed 26 articles related to exercise addiction and found higher prevalence rates among men compared to women, yet other researchers did not find gender differences (Corazza et al., 2019; Fattore et al., 2014). Some scholars have posited that primary exercise addiction is more prevalent among men while secondary exercise addiction is more prevalent among women due to the high incidence of eating disorders among women (Cunningham et al., 2016; Hausenblas et al., 2017).

CLINICAL NOTE 11.2

Some support exists for the consideration of specific athletic activities in the investigation of exercise addiction. For example, among 179 cyclists, researchers found that 8.8% were at risk for primary exercise dependence and 1.18% were at risk for secondary exercise dependence (Cook & Luke, 2017). Additionally, among a sample of triathletes, 19.9% were found to be at high risk for exercise addiction (Youngman & Simpson, 2014).

NEUROSCIENCE RELATED TO EXERCISE ADDICTION

Goodman (2001) noted that individuals are motivated to engage in addictive behaviors by both *positive reinforcement* and *negative reinforcement*. For example, consider alcohol consumption: Individuals drink alcohol because of its euphoric, pleasing effects produced by the activation of reward circuitry in the brain (i.e., positive reinforcement). Alcohol also provides an escape from unwanted feelings or physiological states such as social anxiety, depression, or withdrawal symptoms (i.e., negative reinforcement). Thus, alcohol use, at least initially, is both positively and negatively reinforcing (over time, however, among those with addiction, alcohol use becomes motivated, primarily, by reducing withdrawal symptomology; thus negative reinforcement becomes more prominent in later stages of addiction).

Although rewarding effects are easy to identify with regard to alcohol and other drug use, questions have emerged related to the degree of positive reinforcement associated with exercise (which many individuals find difficult or unenjoyable). However, many scholars agree that exercise does, in fact, produce pleasurable or desirable outcomes, constituting positive reinforcement (Schreiber & Hausenblas, 2015; A. Weinstein & Y. Weinstein, 2014; Williams & Marcus, 2012). Specifically, in the study of females with exercise addiction and regular exercisers (nonaddicted), researchers found differences in asymmetric frontal brain activity (Gapiri et al., 2009). Those participants with exercise addiction had greater activity in the left prefrontal cortex, which is associated with positive affect, as opposed to right frontal activity, which is associated with negative affect (Gapiri et al., 2009), Thus, the research findings support an association between exercise and positive emotions. Furthermore, researchers examined differences among three groups of adult men: (a) those with exercise addiction, (b) regular nonaddicted exercisers, and (c) nonregular, nonaddicted exercisers (Huang et al., 2019). Using a variety of experimental tasks, the researchers concluded that those with exercise addiction had less inhibition (i.e., more impulsivity) and more activation of the reward system in response to exercise-related stimuli than other groups (Huang et al., 2019). Finally, exercise often is a component of treatment for mood disorders, such as depression, due to its mood-enhancing qualities (Goodwin et al., 2012). Therefore, it appears that exercise can be rewarding and reinforcing for certain individuals, yet the mechanisms responsible for these positive effects remain unclear.

There is a long-standing belief, especially among the general public, that the positive reinforcement of exercise is based on endogenous endorphin release, which often is referred to as a "runner's high." Although the notion is popular, research related to this phenomenon in inconclusive (Berczik et al., 2012). Exercise causes natural endorphin release into the bloodstream, yet these endogenous opioids cannot penetrate the blood–brain barrier, calling into question the immediate effects on mood (Weinstein & Weinstein, 2014; Williams & Marcus, 2012; Veal, 1987). Alternative hypotheses for the positive feelings associated with exercise attribute the reinforcement to factors such as an increase in body temperature (inducing warmth and relaxation), activation of the dopaminergic system (implicated in reward), anti-inflammatory cytokine (protein) release, and stimulation of endocannabinoids (naturally sedating neurotransmitters; Klein et al., 2004; Schreiber & Hausenblas, 2015; Weinstein & Weinstein, 2014; Williams & Marcus, 2012). Therefore, although the "runner's high" hypothesis lacks strong empirical support, there may be other neurobiological factors that cause the positive effects experienced by exercisers.

In addition to neurobiological reward, exercise can be positively reinforced by praise from others (social reinforcement), a personal sense of mastery, accomplishment, control, and even reinforcement from technology. Indeed, the rise of *wearable technology* to monitor one's step count, heart rate, and distance may increase the addictive nature of exercise by providing immediate positive reinforcement (Alter, 2017). For example, when an exerciser obtains a certain number of steps or burns a specific number of calories, a fitness device worn on the wrist, arm, or chest can provide reinforcing sounds and graphics, and keeps a record of achieved fitness goals. For those with exercise addiction, these devices may perpetuate compulsive exercise as the individual focuses on numbers rather than being mindful of their physical sensations (e.g., fatigue, pain, exhaustion; Alter, 2017). Thus, counselors working with clients with exercise addiction should assess the use, purpose, and effects of wearable technology.

In sum, although more conclusive research is needed, it is clear that exercise can be positively reinforcing for some individuals via reward circuitry activation, social accolades, or technological reinforcement. Exercise also is known to be negatively reinforcing by providing an escape from dysphoric mood and unpleasant physical states (e.g., depression, restlessness, lethargy; Szabo, 2010). Moreover, for those with exercise addiction, a period without exercise may induce cravings and withdrawal symptoms (e.g., irritability, agitation), which are reduced when exercise commences. Therefore, in light of the positive and negative reinforcement associated with the behavior, some individuals may be susceptible to developing exercise addiction.

HOW DO I IDENTIFY IT?

In a society in which the word "addiction" is used quite loosely, how does one decipher between a strong commitment to exercise and an exercise addiction? The answer lies in individuals' motivations for exercising, their response to being unable to exercise, and the consequences of exercise in their lives. Szabo (2010) noted that those who are highly committed to exercise, yet nonaddicted, are able to control the frequency and intensity of the behavior. Although they strongly desire to exercise, they do not *need* to exercise to feel okay. These exercisers typically are motivated to exercise in order to reach particular goals (e.g., health improvement, weight loss or maintenance, stress relief) and do not experience negative consequences as a result of their exercise patterns (Egorov & Szabo, 2013; Szabo, 2010). Those with exercise addiction, on the other hand, feel as though they *must* exercise to feel okay, and their next run or workout session becomes the anchor around which their lives revolve. These individuals use exercise as their sole coping mechanism and primary form of emotion regulation, and feel extreme discomfort, irritation, and depression if they are unable to work out as planned (Egorov & Szabo, 2013). Moreover, these individuals may experience a host of negative consequences resulting from their rigid, intense workout regimen such as physical injuries, relational conflicts, financial difficulties, and the neglect of other important responsibilities in order to exercise (Schreiber & Hausenblas, 2015; Szabo, 2010).

Therefore, counselors should carefully assess their clients' motivation for exercise, patterns of exercise over time (e.g., taking an exercise history), emotional experience when they are unable to exercise, effects of exercise on other facets of life, and negative consequences resulting from workout patterns (Hausenblas et al., 2017). High frequency or intensity of exercise alone is an insufficient indicator of exercise addiction (consider triathletes, marathon runners, and professional athletes who train regularly, yet have not lost control over their exercise or experience negative consequences). Instead, exercise addiction is marked by compulsive engagement in exercise (e.g., exercising in inconvenient or inappropriate times), a loss of control over exercise (e.g., failed attempts to cut back), experience of withdrawal when unable to exercise (e.g., irritability, discomfort, depression, anger), continuing to exercise despite negative consequences (e.g., injury, relational conflict, detrimental effects on other important responsibilities), and craving to exercise (e.g., mentally obsessing over next workout, inability to be in the present moment due to thoughts of exercise, strong urges to exercise; Fattore et al., 2014).

PROPOSED CRITERIA FOR COMPULSIVE EXERCISE

Although criteria for exercise addiction are not included in the *DSM-5* (APA, 2013) or the *International Classification of Diseases*, 11th Revision (*ICD-11*; World Health Organization [WHO], 2018), Dittmer et al. (2018a) proposed criteria for compulsive exercise among individuals with eating disorders. These criteria include: (a) engagement in exercise that is excessive and driven by rigid rules or mental obsession, (b) motivated to exercise as a means of preventing feared consequences or to reduce distress (stemming from distorted or maladaptive beliefs pertaining to exercise), and (c) time-consuming exercise (lasting more than 60 minutes per day) that interferes with other personal or professional responsibilities, relationships, functioning, or continues despite illness, injury, or unenjoyment. Another optional criterion is personal insight into the unreasonableness or excessive nature of the exercise behavior. The authors identified subtypes of compulsive exercise that may co-occur: (a) vigorous exercise (i.e., strenuous activity), (b) marked increases in daily movement (i.e., intentional decisions to increase physical activity throughout the day such as walking rather than driving), and (c) motor restlessness (e.g., fidgeting, repetitive movements, inability to be still; Dittmer et al., 2018a). Thus, although not formally adopted by the *DSM* or *ICD*, these criteria may be useful for clinicians as they seek to identify exercise addiction among clients.

> **CLINICAL NOTE 11.3**
>
> In addition to scholarly resources, nonacademic evidence suggests that the recognition of exercise addiction may be growing in the general public. Using an Internet search engine, researchers were able to find 100 cases of exercise addiction in articles posted on nonacademic websites (Juwono & Szabo, 2020). To be included, the articles had to describe at least one symptom of the components model of addiction (i.e., salience, withdrawal, tolerance, mood modification, conflict, relapse; Griffiths, 2005) as well as at least one negative consequence of exercise addiction (i.e., psychological, social, physical). The researchers concluded that nonacademic evidence suggests a notable incidence of exercise addiction in the general public (Juwono & Szabo, 2020).

HOW DO I ASSESS IT?

Formal assessments have been developed to help counselors screen for exercise addiction. The following are descriptions of two instruments that you may consider utilizing in your practice.

EXERCISE ADDICTION INVENTORY

Terry et al. (2004) developed a brief screening tool for exercise addiction, the Exercise Addiction Inventory (EAI), composed of six items. Each item on the EAI corresponds with a component of addiction proposed by Brown (1993) and Griffiths (1996, 2005): salience, mood modification, tolerance, withdrawal symptoms, conflict, and relapse. Respondents select responses to each EAI item using five-point Likert-type scales ranging from *strongly disagree* (1) to *strongly agree* (5). Example items on the EAI include: *Exercise is the most important thing in my life* and *If I have to miss an exercise session, I feel moody and irritable*. A score of 24 or higher is indicative of exercise addiction. The EAI was normed on undergraduate exercisers and demonstrated acceptable internal reliability (Cronbach's alpha = .84) and concurrent validity with two other exercise addiction measures (Terry et al., 2004). The six items of the EAI are listed in the appendix of the original Terry et al. (2004) article.

EXERCISE DEPENDENCE SCALE-REVISED

The Exercise Dependence Scale (EDS; Hausenblas & Downs, 2002) was developed using the criteria for substance dependence in the *Diagnostic and Statistical Manual of Mental Disorders* (4th ed.; *DSM-IV*; APA, 1994). The scale originally consisted of seven subscales (tolerance, withdrawal, continuance, lack of control, reduction of other activities, time, and intention effects) and assessed respondents' exercise behaviors and beliefs within the past 3 months. The original EDS has been revised (EDS-R; Downs et al., 2004) to 21 items, with three items corresponding to each of the original seven subscales. Respondents answer items by selecting a response on a six-point Likert-type scale ranging from *never* (1) to *always* (6). Example EDS items include: *I think about exercise when I should be concentrating on school/work* and *I exercise longer than I intend*. Item scores are summed to calculate a total score, with higher scores indicating more exercise dependence. Along with a summed score, respondents can be categorized as at risk for exercise dependence, nondependent-symptomatic, and nondependent-asymptomatic. Respondents who score 5 or 6 on items of three or more subscales are at risk, those who score 3 or 4 on items of three or more subscales are nondependent-symptomatic, and respondents who score 1 or 2 on items of three or more subscales are nondependent-asymptomatic. Among undergraduate students in fitness classes, the EDS-R demonstrated convergent validity and strong internal consistency (Cronbach's alpha scores ranging from .75 to .90 for seven subscales; Downs et al., 2004). The items on the EDS-R can be found within the Downs et al. (2004) article.

HOW DO I TREAT IT?

The means by which counselors address exercise addiction will be dependent on a number of important factors. For example, whether or not exercise addiction is comorbid with an eating disorder (AN, BN, BED, or UFED) will directly affect treatment protocols. If an eating disorder is present, counselors should ensure they have the proper training and competence to effectively work with the client (American Counseling Association, 2014, C.2.a), or consider referring the client to a trained eating disorder specialist. Additionally, the presence of a co-occurring mental illness (e.g., body dysmorphic disorder, OCD, substance use disorder) also will affect the course of treatment. Despite these distinctions, it is likely that all clinical strategies with clients with exercise addiction will include emotion regulation enhancement. Indeed, in the study of over 1,500 adolescents, researchers found that emotion regulation strategies and a drive for thinness were both significant predictors of exercise addiction (Goodwin et al., 2012). Therefore, given that exercise may be clients' primary means of mood modification, counselors and clients may need to work on identifying, labeling, and expressing emotions, increasing distress tolerance, and developing alternative, effective ways to manage negative emotions and induce positive emotions.

Although complete abstinence from all exercise is not the long-term goal, some clients may benefit from a period of abstaining from exercise (Schreiber & Hausenblas, 2015). Other clients may benefit from temporarily abstaining from their compulsive exercise behavior (e.g., running, weight lifting, cycling) while replacing it with another form of exercise or movement (e.g., dancing, group sports, yoga). A long-term goal of treatment is for clients to maintain healthy and helpful exercise patterns while abstaining from or reducing obligatory or compulsive exercise (which may take time to correctly identify and put into practice). The aim is to help clients reconnect with their bodies, become aware of and respond appropriately to physical cues and sensations (e.g., fatigue, pain, overexertion, hunger), and create a new relationship with physical activity, movement, and exercise. The development of an appropriate fitness plan can be made in conjunction with a sports therapist, a nutritionist, and/or a primary care physician.

VOICES FROM THE FIELD: Clinical Work With Exercise Addiction

Successful treatment of exercise addiction includes exploring and challenging clients' exercise-related cognitions (e.g., "exercise only counts if I sweat" or "I can only eat ____ if I exercise"). It also involves helping clients learn skills for tolerating distress and uncomfortable emotions and making behavioral changes around exercise. Typically, the two main goals for helping those struggling with exercise compulsion are to stop cold turkey (complete abstinence) or a more graduated approach (incrementally cutting down exercise). A period of total rest from exercise is recommended when helping someone to heal their relationship to exercise; however, some clients prefer a more gradual approach of challenging exercise rules. The latter might look like taking the first step of shaving off 5 minutes from their regular exercise routine.

As an eating disorder clinician and someone who previously struggled with an exercise compulsion myself, I love working with clients who are currently battling exercise addiction. One challenge for recovery is that exercise is so praised in our culture so that it may be difficult for people to identify that they have a problem. Additionally, unlike other addictions, one does not typically earn social praise by cutting down exercise. However, through the recovery process, individuals can learn how to let go of compulsive exercise and to explore forms of joyful movement that are varied, flexible, and fun.

Jennifer Rollin, MSW, LCSW-C, Therapist and Founder of The Eating Disorder Center

HEALTHY EXERCISE BEHAVIOR

When working with clients diagnosed with an eating disorder comorbid with exercise addiction, counselors should consider an integrated approach. Researchers have examined the efficacy of an intervention specifically designed for addressing compulsive exercise within standard eating disorder treatment and found promising results. Dittmer et al. (2018b) developed a manualized intervention for compulsive exercise among clients with AN entitled, *healthy exercise behavior* (HEB). Dittmer et al. (2020) conducted a randomized controlled trial to assess the effects of HEB integrated with treatment as usual, compared to treatment as usual only among female clients with both AN and compulsive exercise. The researchers found stronger reductions in the severity of compulsive exercise among clients in the HEB group (Dittmer et al., 2020).

The HEB intervention is a group therapy model that encompasses features of both cognitive behavioral therapy and exercise-based therapy. Specifically, the intervention spans eight sessions (100 minutes each) and involves emotion regulation strategies, cognitive restructuring, and the discontinuation and replacement of compulsive behaviors (Dittmer et al., 2018b). The exercise components of HEB include experimenting with various forms of movement such as yoga, partnered walking, social physical activities, playful (noncompetitive) physical activities, short intense physical activities for stress relief, and joyful, cooperative physical activity. In conjunction with these exercise-based elements, group counselors also help clients differentiate between healthy and compulsive exercise, identify risky situations that trigger urges for compulsive exercise, develop alternative coping strategies, identify and express emotions, and implement new HEB plans (Dittmer et al., 2018b). Interested readers are encouraged to consult Dittmer et al. (2018b; 2020) for more details regarding HEB.

EXPOSURE AND RESPONSE (RITUAL) PREVENTION

Counselors may also find it useful to draw from exposure and response (ritual) prevention (ERP) when working with clients with exercise addiction. Specifically, ERP is a cognitive behavioral based model used to treat clients with OCD (Foa et al., 2012). Given the potential for overlapping features between exercise addiction and OCD (e.g., mental preoccupation with exercise, compulsive need to exercise), ERP may be a helpful counseling strategy. The process of ERP includes three components: (a) expose clients to obsessive-inducing cues or triggers, (b) prevent ritual engagement, and (c) process the outcome. It is important for counselors and clients to first identify the specific stimuli that trigger the urge to engage in the ritual. Counselors and clients typically conduct a hierarchy of anxiety-producing stimuli from least to most distressing (Foa et al., 2012). For example, a female client with exercise addiction may identify the following triggers for compulsive exercise: experiencing a disappointment at work, interpersonal conflict, observing thin women in the media, and eating a high-calorie food item. The client may identify that these events stimulate emotional distress (e.g., shame, depression) as well as thoughts such as, "I am inadequate," "Being thin is my most important quality," and "I am going to get fat if I don't exercise." In response to these thoughts, the client may typically engage in 2 hours of running or fitness training to ease her distressing emotions and combat her critical thoughts.

Once triggering stimuli are identified, counselors and clients engage in exposure experiences, beginning with the least distressing trigger (Foa et al., 2012). Exposure to the cues may occur in real life (in vivo) or via the client's imagination. Importantly, prior to engaging in the in vivo or imaginary exposure to the distressing cues, counselors should have a clear understanding of the client's unique fear that prompts the obsessions and rituals. For example, with regard to exercise addiction, is the client's fear related to not being in control? Not being attractive? Succumbing to an illness? Dying? Not being accepted by others? Once the fear is understood, clients and counselors have a clearer understanding of the function of the ritual. Next, clients can practice exposure to a trigger (e.g., drinking a sugary soda, imagining being rejected by a potential romantic partner), while abstaining from engaging in the ritual (i.e., compulsive exercise). Ritual prevention is a key component of ERP and helps clients gain several important insights: (a) anxiety and fear will decrease even if they do not engage in the ritual, (b) the feared consequence rarely (if ever) occurs, and (c) clients can tolerate more distress than they previously imagined (Foa et al., 2012).

Following ritual prevention, counselors and clients process the experience to stimulate and solidify insight. Clients realize that their fears and anxieties associated with triggers are hypotheses to be tested, not undeniable conclusions. When feared outcomes do not occur in the absence of the ritual, clients disconfirm their previously held hypotheses and replace them with more accurate beliefs (e.g., "I can eat a hamburger for dinner without becoming obese overnight" or "Feelings of melancholy will eventually shift and dissipate, even if I do not go for a 10-mile jog each time I feel sad").

Another unique aspect of ERP is home visits. Counselors may visit clients in their home environment to gain more information about their obsessions and rituals or to help clients transfer what they learned in counseling to their living space (Foa et al., 2012). For example, when working with a client with exercise addiction, a home visit can help the client identify specific triggers in her living space (e.g., seeing thin women on television) and the counselor and client may engage in ritual prevention to ensure that what the client is learning in counseling can be applied at home. ERP typically includes both in-session and out-of-session exercises and should be facilitated by counselors trained in the approach. See Foa et al. (2012) for a detailed treatment manual related to ERP for OCDs.

DIAGNOSTIC CONSIDERATIONS

Exercise addiction is not included in the *DSM-5* (APA, 2013) or *ICD-11* (WHO, 2018). However, the condition frequently co-occurs with other mental health diagnoses such as body dysmorphic disorder, eating disorders, and anxiety disorders; thus, clinicians often diagnose the comorbid condition when applicable. In the case of primary exercise addiction in which an eating disorder is not present, clinicians can assess whether the client meets criteria for OCD or unspecified obsessive-compulsive and related disorders.

HOW CAN I LEARN MORE?

If you are working with clients with exercise addiction or would like to learn more about the condition, consider the following resources.

BOOKS

- Brewerton, T. D., & Dennis, A. B. (Eds.). *Eating disorders, addiction and substance use disorders: Research, clinical, and treatment perspectives* (pp. 439–457). Springer Publishing Company.
- Schreiber, K., & Hausenblas, H. A. (2015). *The truth about exercise addiction: Understanding the dark side of thinspiration.* Rowan & Littlefield.
- Szabo, A. (2010). *Addiction to exercise: A symptom or a disorder?* Nova Science Publishers.

PEER-REVIEWED ARTICLES

- Berczik, K., Szabo, A., Griffths, M. D., Kurimay, T., Kun, B., Urban, R., & Demetrovics, Z. (2012). Exercise addiction: Symptoms, diagnosis, epidemiology, and etiology. *Substance Use and Misuse, 47,* 403–417. https://doi.org/10.3109/10826084.2011.639120
- Hausenblas, H. A., Schreiber, K., & Smoliga, J. M. (2017). Addiction to exercise. *British Medical Journal, 357,* j1745. https://doi.org/10.1136/bmj.j1745
- Weinstein, A., & Weinstein, Y. (2014). Exercise addiction - diagnosis, biopsychological mechanisms and treatment issues. *Current Pharmaceutical Design, 20,* 4062–4069.

WEBSITES

- American College of Sports Medicine: www.acsm.org

- Body dysmorphic disorder foundation: bddfoundation.org
- U.S. Department of Health and Human Services Physical Activity Guidelines: health.gov/our-work/physical-activity/current-guidelines

REFERENCES

Alcaraz-Ibanez, M., Aguilar-Parra, J. M., & Alvarez-Hernandez, J. F. (2018). Exercise addiction: Preliminary evidence on the role of psychological inflexibility. *International Journal of Mental Health and Addiction, 16,* 199–206. https://doi.org/10.1007/s11469-018-9875-y

Alter, A. (2017). *Irresistible: The rise of addictive technology and the business of keeping us hooked.* Penguin Books.

American Counseling Association. (2014). *ACA code of ethics.* http://www.counseling.org/knowledge-center/ethics

American Psychiatric Association. (2013). *Diagnostic and statistical manual of mental disorders* (5th ed.). Author.

Berczik, K., Szabo, A., Griffths, M. D., Kurimay, T., Kun, B., Urban, R., & Demetrovics, Z. (2012). Exercise addiction: Symptoms, diagnosis, epidemiology, and etiology. *Substance Use and Misuse, 47,* 403–417. https://doi.org/10.3109/10826084.2011.639120

Brown, R. I. F. (1993). Some contributions of the study of gambling to the study of other addictions. In W. R. Eadington & J. A. Cornelius (Eds.), *Gambling behaviour and problem gambling* (pp. 341–272). University of Nevada Press.

Cook, B., & Luke, R. (2017). Primary and secondary exercise dependence in a sample of cyclists. *International Journal of Mental Health and Addiction, 15,* 444–451. https://doi.org/10.1007/s11469-017-9745-z

Corazza, O., Simonato, P., Demetrovics, Z., Mooney, R., van de Ven, K., Roman-Urrestarazu, A., Rácmolnár, L., De Luca, I., Cinosi, E., Santacroce, R., Marini, M., Wellsted, D., Sullivan, K., Bersani, G., & Martinotti, G. (2019). The emergence of exercise addiction, body dysmorphic disorder, and other image-related psychopathological correlates in fitness settings: A cross sectional study. *PLoS One, 14,* e0213060. https://doi.org/10.1371/journal.pone.0213060

Cunningham, H. E., Pearman, S., & Brewerton, T. D. (2016). Conceptualizing primary and secondary pathological exercise using available measures of excessive exercise. *The International Journal of Eating Disorders, 49,* 778–792. https://doi.org/10.1002/eat.22551

Danielsen, M., Ro, O., Romild, U., & Bjornelv, S. (2016). Impact of female adult eating disorder inpatients' attitudes to compulsive exercise on outcome at discharge and follow-up. *Journal of Eating Disorders, 4,* 7. https://doi.org/10.1186/s40337-016-0096-0

Dittmer, N., Jacobi, C., & Voderholzer, U. (2018a). Compulsive exercise in eating disorders: Proposal for a definition and a clinical assessment. *Journal of Eating Disorders, 6,* 42. https://doi.org/10.1186/s40337-018-0219-x

Dittmer, N., Vonderholzer, U., Monon, C., Cuntz, U., Jacobi, C., & Schlegl, S. (2020). Efficacy of a specialized group intervention for compulsive exercise in inpatients with anorexia nervosa: A randomized controlled trial. *Psychotherapy and Psychosomatics, 89,* 161–173. https://doi.org/10.1159/000504583

Dittmer, N., Voderholzer, U., von der Muhlen, M., Marwitz, M., Fumi, M., Monchi, C., Alexandridis, K., Cuntz, U., Jacobi, C., & Schlegl, S. (2018b). Specialized group intervention for compulsive exercise in inpatients with eating disorders:

Feasibility and preliminary outcomes. *Journal of Eating Disorders, 6,* 27, https://doi.org/10.1186/s40337-018-0200-8

Downs, D. S., Hausenblas, H. A., & Nigg, C. R. (2004). Factorial validity and psychometric examination of the Exercise Dependence Scale-Revised. *Measurement in Physical Education and Exercise Science, 8,* 183–201. https://doi.org/10.1207/s15327841mpee0804_1

Dumitru, D. C., Dumitru, T., & Maher, A. J. (2018). A systematic review of exercise addiction: Examining gender differences. *Journal of Physical Education and Sport, 18,* 1738–1748. https://doi.org/10.7752/jpes.2018.03253

Egorov, A. Y., & Szabo, A. (2013). The exercise paradox: An interaction model for a clearer conceptualization of exercise addiction. *Journal of Behavioral Addictions, 2,* 199–208. https://doi.org/10.556/JBA.2.2013.4.2

Fattore, L., Melis, M., Fadda, P., & Fratta, W. (2014). Sex differences in addictive disorders. *Frontiers in Neuroendocrinology, 35,* 272–284. https://doi.org/10.1016/j.yfrne.2014.04.003

Foa, E. B., Yadin, E., & Lichner, T. K. (2012). *Exposure and response (ritual) prevention for obsessive-compulsive disorder: Therapist guide* (2nd ed.). Oxford.

Gapiri, J., Etnier, J. L., & Tucker, D. (2009). The relationship between frontal brain asymmetry and exercise addiction. *Journal of Psychophysiology, 23,* 135–142. https://doi.org/10.1027/0269-8803.23.3.135

Glasser, W. (1976). *Positive addiction.* Harper and Row.

Glasser, W. (1977). Promoting client strength through positive addiction. *Canadian Counsellor, 11,* 173–175.

Goodman, A. (2001). What's in a name? Terminology for designing a syndrome of driven sexual behavior. *Sexual Addiction and Compulsivity, 8,* 191–213. https://doi.org/10.1080/107201601753459919

Goodwin, H., Haycraft, E., & Meyer, C. (2012). The relationship between compulsive exercise and emotion regulation in adolescents. *British Journal of Health Psychology, 17,* 699–710. https://doi.org/10.1111/j.2044-8287.2012.02066.x

Griffiths, M. D. (1996). Behavioural addiction: An issue for everybody? *Journal of Workplace Learning, 8,* 19–25. https://doi.org/10.1108/13665629610116872

Griffiths, M. (2005). A 'components' model of addiction within a biopsychosocial framework. *Journal of Substance Use, 10,* 191–197. https://doi.org/10.1080/14659890500114359

Hausenblas, H. A., & Downs, D. S. (2002). How much is too much? The development and validation of the Exercise Dependence Scale. *Psychology and Health, 17,* 387–404. https://doi.org/10.1080/0887044022000004894

Hausenblas, H. A., Schreiber, K., & Smoliga, J. M. (2017). Addiction to exercise. *British Medical Journal, 357,* j1745. https://doi.org/10.1136/bmj.j1745

Huang, Q., Huang, J., Chen, Y., Lin, D., Xu, S., Wei, J., Qi, C., & Xu, X. (2019). Overactivation of the reward system and efficient inhibition in exercise addiction. *Medicine and Science in Sports and Exercise, 51,* 1918–1927. https://doi.org/10.1249/mss.0000000000001988

Juwono, I. G., & Szabo, A. (2020). 100 cases of exercise addiction: More evidence for a widely researched but rarely identified dysfunction. *International Journal of Mental Health and Addiction.* https://doi.org/10.1007/s11469-020-00264-6

Keyes, A., Woerwag-Mehta, S., Bartholdy, S., Koskina, A., Middleton, B., Connan, F., Webster, P., Schmidt, U., & Campbell, I. C. (2015). Physical activity and the drive to exercise in anorexia nervosa. *International Journal of Eating Disorders, 48,* 46–54. https://doi.org/10.1002/eat.22354

Klein, D. A., Bennett, A. S., Schebendach, J., Foltin, R. W., Devlin, M. J., & Walsh, B. T. (2004). Exercise "addiction" in anorexia nervosa: Model development and pilot data. *International Journal of Neuropsychiatric Medicine, 9*, 531–537. https://doi.org/10.1017/s1092852900009627

Lichtenstein, M. B., Nielsen, R. O., Gudex, C., Hinze, C. J., & Jorgensen, U. (2018). Exercise addiction is associated with emotional distress in injured and non-injured regular exercisers. *Addictive Behaviors Reports, 8*, 33–39. https://doi.org/10.1016/j.abrep.2018.06.001

Morgan, W. P. (1979). Negative addiction in runners. *The Physician and Sports Medicine, 7*, 55–77. https://doi.org/10.1080/00913847.1979.11948436

Monell, E., Levallius, J., Forsen, M. E., & Birgegard, A. (2018). Running on empty- a nationwide large-scale examination of compulsive exercise in eating disorders. *Journal of Eating Disorders, 6*, 11. https://doi.org/10.1186/s40337-018-0197-z

Monok, K., Berczik, K., Urban, R., Szabo, A., Griffiths, M. D. Farkas, J., Magi, A., Eisinger, A., Kurimay, T., Kökönyei, G., Kun, B., Paksi, B., & Demetrovics, Z. (2012). Psychometric properties and concurrent validity of two exercise addiction measures: A population wide study. *Psychology of Sport and Exercise, 13*, 739–746. https://doi.org/10.1016/j.psychsport.2012.06.003

Quesnel, D. A., Cook, B., Murray, K., & Zamudio, J. (2018). Inspiration or thinspiration: The association among problematic internet use, exercise dependence, and eating disorder risk. *International Journal of Mental Health and Addiction, 16*, 1113–1124. https://doi.org/10.1007/s11469-017-9834-z

Schreiber, K., & Hausenblas, H. A. (2015). *The truth about exercise addiction: Understanding the dark side of thinspiration*. Rowan & Littlefield.

Specter, S. E., & Wiss, D. A. (2014). Muscular dysmorphia: Where body image, obsession, compulsive exercise, disordered eating, and substance abuse intersect in susceptible males. In T. D. Brewerton & A. B. Dennis (Eds.), *Eating disorders, addiction and substance use disorders: Research, clinical, and treatment perspectives* (pp. 439–457). Springer Publishing.

Szabo, A. (2010). *Addiction to exercise: A symptom or a disorder?* Nova Science Publishers.

Terry, A., Szabo, A., & Griffiths, M. (2004). The Exercise Addiction Inventory: A new brief screening tool. *Addiction Research and Theory, 12*, 489–499. https://doi.org/10.1080/16066350310001637363

Trott, M., Jackson, S. E., Firth, J., Jacob, L., Grabovac, I., Mistry, A., Stubbs, B., & Smith, L. (2021). A comparative meta-analysis of the prevalence of exercise addiction in adults with and without indicated eating disorders. *Eating and Weight Disorders, 26*, 37–46. https://doi.org/10.1007/s40519-019-00842-1

U.S. Department of Health and Human Services. (2018). *Physical activity guidelines for Americans* (2nd ed.). Author. https://health.gov/sites/default/files/2019-09/Physical_Activity_Guidelines_2nd_edition.pdf

Veal, D. M. W. (1987). Exercise dependence. *British Journal of Addiction, 82*, 735–740. https://doi.org/10.1111/j.1360-0443.1987.tb01539.x

Weinstein, A., & Weinstein, Y. (2014). Exercise addiction- diagnosis, bio-psychological mechanisms and treatment issues. *Current Pharmaceutical Design, 20*, 4062–4069. https://doi.org/10.2174/13816128113199990614

Williams, D. M., & Marcus, B. H. (2012). Exercise addiction and aversion: Implications for eating and obesity. In K. D. Brownell & M. S. Gold (Eds.). *Food and addiction: A comprehensive handbook* (pp. 336–341). Oxford University Press.

World Health Organization. (2018). *International statistical classification of diseases and related health problems* (11th Rev.). https://icd.who.int/browse11/l-m/en

Youngman, J., & Simpson, D. (2014). Risk for exercise addiction: A comparison of triathletes training for sprint-, Olympic-, half-ironman-, and ironman-distance triathlons. *Journal of Clinical Sport Psychology, 8,* 19–37. https://doi.org/10.1123/jcsp.2014-0010

12

Work Addiction

HOW DO I CONCEPTUALIZE IT?

According to the U.S. Bureau of Labor Statistics (2018), full-time employed workers in America work an average of 8.50 hours on weekdays and 5.39 hours on weekend days. Part-time employed workers in America work an average of 5.17 hours on weekdays and 4.81 hours on weekend days (U.S. Bureau of Labor Statistics, 2018). Thus, many Americans spend a considerable amount of their lifetimes at work—an activity that is necessary for financial security and survival. Most employees are able to disengage from work after completing their required hours and focus on other aspects of their lives. However, for a small segment of the population, work can become compulsive and lead to negative physical, psychological, and relational consequences. For these individuals, working becomes the primary means of regulating emotions. They are driven by an internal *need* to work that surpasses their desire to invest in other facets of life (e.g., personal responsibilities, friendships, romantic partners, family, leisure activities, self-care; Fassel, 1990; Robinson, 2014). Those with work addiction may persist in their rigid, unyielding work patterns despite detrimental physical and psychological consequences (e.g., stress, fatigue, anxiety, exhaustion, physical ailments). Additionally, with the advent of smartphones, video conferencing, and electronic file sharing, those with work addiction can engage in work-related activities from any location at any time. These individuals may rarely be completely disconnected from work and continuously fail to control the amount of time and energy they devote to work behaviors, despite making promises to do so. Counselors can best serve these individuals by recognizing the signs of work addiction and helping clients restore balance in their lives.

The construct of work addiction is conceptualized as having two components: a behavioral component (e.g., constant engagement in work, working beyond set hours, working on weekends and vacations) and a cognitive component (e.g., preoccupied with work, thinking about work when doing other activities, difficulty attending to the present moment due to thoughts about work; Schaufeli et al., 2008). Indeed, Atroszko et al. (2019) described work addiction as "a compulsion to work and preoccupation with work activities leading to significant harm and distress of a functionally impairing nature to the individual and/or other significantly relevant relationships (friends and family)" (p. 9). Work addiction reflects a compulsive desire to work at the expense of other responsibilities, roles, and activities. Overworking may begin as a means of coping with psychological pain or chaos in other realms of life (e.g., relationships), yet over time, work becomes the sole means of managing distress, leading to a dependency on the behavior (Atroszko et al., 2020).

Like other behavioral addictions, tolerance and withdrawal are features of work addiction. Tolerance is evidenced by increased time spent engaging in work-related activities to reach the desired emotional state (Atroszko et al., 2019). In fact, researchers found that going to work when sick (known as *presenteeism*) is significantly correlated with work addiction (Mazzetti et al., 2019). Those who are addicted to work would rather risk their health and potentially, the health of others, than refrain from working. Additionally, withdraw symptomology from work is described as similar to stimulant withdrawal (Atroszko et al., 2020) or steroid withdrawal (Robinson, 2014). The term "leisure sickness" refers to feeling ill during times when one is not working, such as weekends or vacations (consider a person who works 60 hours per week for several months and then comes down with the flu a few days into their holiday break). Rather than a separate condition, it is believed that leisure sickness actually is withdrawal from work addiction (Robinson, 2014). In a Dutch sample of working men and women, researchers found that 3.7% men and 1.7% women reported experiencing leisure sickness on weekends, and 3.7% men and 2.9% women reported experiencing leisure sickness on vacations (Vingerhoets et al., 2002). Common symptoms of leisure sickness included headaches, migraines, fatigue, common cold or influenza-like symptoms, and muscular pain (Vingerhoets et al., 2002). Although more research is needed, leisure sickness may, in fact, be the body's withdrawal response from elevated adrenaline and stress hormones (see the following for more information about the effects of adrenaline and stress).

INDIVIDUAL AND ENVIRONMENTAL PREDICTORS OF WORK ADDICTION

Work addiction is a multifaceted condition influenced by both individual and environmental components. Researchers have identified several individual characteristics that correlate with work addiction including perfectionism and achievement motivation (Mazzetti et al., 2014), neuroticism (Balducci et al., 2016), high motivation from external rewards (Spurk et al., 2016), type A personality (Clark et al., 2014), and obsessive-compulsive and/or controlling personality traits (Aziz & Uhrich, 2014). Thus, there are some personality characteristics that seem to increase one's risk of developing an addiction to work, including those related to perfectionism and a strong desire for control and achievement. Along with these individual traits, however, researchers also have identified environmental factors that contribute to the development of work addiction including, an overwork climate (in which employees perceive the need to work extended hours and on weekends/holidays; Mazzetti et al., 2014), low managerial support (Mazzetti et al., 2019), and high job demands (Andreassen et al., 2019; Balducci et al., 2016). Therefore, particular professions and working conditions may perpetuate the development of work addiction among vulnerable employees. Moreover, the behavioral manifestations of work addiction (overworking, working on evenings and weekends, constant availability) often can be praised in particular cultures, serving to reinforce the behavior (much like exercise addiction; Griffiths et al., 2018; Holland, 2008; see Chapter 11). Thus, counselors should consider both clients' individual personality traits (e.g., rigid perfectionism) and environmental conditions (e.g., high job demands) when conceptualizing work addiction (Atroszko et al., 2020).

WORK ADDICTION AND STUDY ADDICTION

Given that most individuals do not begin employment until late adolescence or early adulthood, it is important to consider whether signs of work addiction exist among younger populations. Some scholars have posited that work addiction may manifest as *study addiction* among children and teenagers (Atroszko et al., 2015; Griffiths et al., 2018). Study addiction is defined as, "being overly concerned with studying, to be driven by an uncontrollable studying motivation, and to put so much energy and effort into studying that it impairs private relationships, spare-time activities, and/or health" (Atroszko et al., 2015, p. 75). Some empirical support exists linking study addiction to work addiction. In a longitudinal study of Norwegian and Polish student samples, researchers found that study addiction at the first timepoint was a significant predictor of work addiction at the second timepoint (albeit among the Polish sample only; Atroszko et al., 2016). Moreover, study addiction has been linked to negative consequences that are similar to those associated with work addiction. For example, among college students, study addiction significantly predicted more perceived stress, lower quality of life, poorer general health, and poorer sleep quality (Atroszko et al., 2015). Therefore, the compulsive drive to engage in work may exist in childhood in the form of excessive studying and evolve into overworking in adulthood.

> **CLINICAL NOTE 12.1**
>
> It is important for counselors to consider cultural norms related to studying and educational attainment in their work with clients. For example, in South Korea (and among some Korean Americans), it is common for students to receive tutoring and take private classes after school (called *hagwon*; Yi, 2013). Between school and hagwon, Korean students could spend between 12 and 16 hours per day in educational pursuits (Mani & Trines, 2018). How might you assess and identify study addiction while considering differences in educational cultural norms?

PREVALENCE OF WORK ADDICTION

The lack of official diagnostic criteria for work addiction, coupled with difficulty distinguishing between work addiction and high work engagement, makes prevalence rates difficult to accrue. However, several researchers across the globe have provided preliminary data regarding the incidence of work addiction. A study among 1,608 working adults in Norway revealed that 7.3% met criteria for work addiction (Andreassen et al., 2019). Moreover, among a Hungarian adult sample, researchers found that 9.3% were at high risk for work addiction (Urban et al., 2019). Another Norwegian study revealed that 7.8% of a large national sample had work addiction (Andreassen et al., 2016). Finally, among a Danish sample, researchers found that 6.6% were at high risk for work addiction (Lichtenstein et al., 2019). More research is needed to investigate the prevalence of work addiction in the United States, although Sussman et al. (2011) tentatively proposed a rate of 10% among U.S. adults. With regard to gender, several researchers have noted that work addiction does not significantly differ among men and women (Andreassen et al., 2016; Clark et al., 2014; Lichtenstein et al., 2019). Some researchers, however, have posited that items on work addiction instruments may function differently among male and female participants. Thus gender bias is an important consideration in the assessment of work addiction (Beiler-May et al., 2017).

> **CLINICAL NOTE 12.2**
>
> In the study of 207 female academics in Turkey, researchers found that work addiction scores significantly predicted both work–family life conflict scores and burnout scores (Ercan Demirel & Erdirencelebi, 2019). Specifically, work–family life conflict significantly mediated the relationship between workaholism and burnout among participants. Thus, conflict between occupational and familial roles may be a significant aspect of work addiction among female professionals.

NEUROSCIENCE RELATED TO WORK ADDICTION

When considering work as a potential addiction, the reinforcing properties of the behavior must be considered. Scholars posit that hard work triggers the release of specific hormones and neurotransmitters that lead to states of high energy and alertness. Specifically, Schabracq et al. (1996) wrote, "such a state [hard work] is, at least by some people, highly valued: one feels good, there is a general feeling of control, and intrusions of unwanted thoughts are reduced to a minimum" (p. 14). Sussman (2018) noted that those with work addiction experience a type of pleasurable "high" by working and fulfilling an appetitive need, which is common among all addictions. Researchers propose that those with work addiction may become dependent on the adrenaline rush that accompanies the urgency and pressures of work (Aziz & Uhrich, 2014; Holland, 2008; Robinson, 2014). Indeed, stress from overworking activates the hypothalamic–pituitary–adrenal axis, triggering *adrenaline* and *cortisol* release, among other stress hormones (Herr et al., 2018). The hormone adrenaline (which also acts as a neurotransmitter) creates a surge of energy by increasing one's heart rate, blood pressure, blood flow to the muscles, airflow through the lungs, and glucose in the blood, therefore preparing the body for action. Robinson (2014) wrote, "Adrenaline addiction, in effect, creates addictions to crises that lead the body to produce the hormone and give workaholics their drug. On the job, workaholics routinely create and douse crises that require the body's adrenaline flow" (p. 18). These crises might include procrastinating until just before a deadline, creating large problems out of fairly minimal issues, and seeking perfection in all work projects (Holland, 2008). Indeed, members of the 12-step program Workaholics Anonymous (WA) refer to this behavior as *adrenalizing* (Workaholics Anonymous World Service Organization, 2015). Specifically, according to WA literature, work addiction is both a substance addiction (dependency on adrenaline) and a process addiction (dependency on overworking and excessive activity; Workaholics Anonymous World Service Organization, 2015).

Thus, it appears that the rush of adrenaline and other stress hormones can be rewarding among certain individuals, leading to addictive work behaviors. Genetic predispositions may make some individuals more susceptible to the rewarding properties of adrenaline than others, yet more research is needed to investigate neurobiological vulnerabilities related to work addiction. Currently, the theories related to the reinforcing, potentially addictive properties of adrenaline are based largely on clinical experiences and personal reports. Neuroscience research is needed to confirm and expand upon these theories and hypotheses.

HOW DO I IDENTIFY IT?

Consider a police officer who is "married to the job" or a surgeon who, at times, works 24-hour shifts. Are these individuals addicted to work? Maybe, or maybe not. Work addiction is distinct from high work engagement or enthusiastic investment in one's job. The number of hours spent working is not a sufficient criterion for assessing work addiction. Instead, motives for work behaviors and the effects of work-related activities on an individual's life must be explored to accurately identify work addiction. Highly committed or engaged workers often find joy and meaning in their jobs, yet also are able to disengage from work in order to invest to other realms of life (e.g., friendships, spirituality, self-care, family, leisure activities). Those with work addiction, however, feel internally compelled to work, as it is the only mechanism by which they can regulate emotions and/or achieve a sense of self-worth. In fact, Holland (2008) wrote that among those with work addiction, "work is the 'drug' of choice used to mediate emotional pain, control life and anesthetize unpleasant feelings" (p. 2). Therefore, one of the primary distinguishing factors between work addiction and high work engagement is the function of the behavior. Those who work compulsively to avoid psychological pain and escape negative mood states are more likely to have work addiction than those who are highly involved in work due to a sense of meaning and enjoyment found in their occupation.

To complicate the identification of work addiction further, manifestations of work addiction are not homogeneous. Fassel (1990) described four types of individuals with work addiction: (a) the compulsive worker (individuals who are driven to work constantly), (b) the binge worker (individuals with seemingly normal work patterns until they engage in a work binge in which they work without stopping or sleeping for days), (c) the closet worker (individuals who hide their compulsive working from others), and (d) the work anorexic (similar to those with sexual anorexia [see Chapter 5], these individuals have a compulsive aversion to work). Therefore, counselors should be aware that work addiction can take many forms. Clinicians working with clients who may be addicted to work should assess not only their motivation for work, but also explore their work history and current work patterns and behaviors.

WARNING SIGNS OF WORK ADDICTION

Although diagnostic criteria for work addiction have not been officially or uniformly endorsed by the *Diagnostic and Statistical Manual of Mental Disorders* (5th ed.; *DSM-5*; American Psychiatric Association [APA], 2013) or the *International Classification of Diseases*, 11th Revision (*ICD-11*; World Health Organization [WHO], 2018), Robinson (2014) proposed 10 warning signs to help identify work addiction. These signs include: (a) rushing and hyperbusyness (engaging in multiple tasks simultaneously), (b) the need to control (aversion to delegating tasks or asking for help), (c) perfectionism (setting unattainable standards for oneself and others), (d) difficulty with intimacy and relationships (focusing on work rather than others, missing important family events to work, avoiding emotional closeness with others), (e) work binges (working nonstop for a set period of time), (f) restlessness and the inability to relax (feelings of guilt or irritability when not working), (g) work trances (preoccupation with work at the expense of present-moment conversations or activities), (h) impatience and irritability (frustration with waiting and any perceived waste of time), (i) self-inadequacy (evaluating self-worth in light of work performance), and (j) self-neglect (little attention paid to self-care, nutrition, or personal health). If clients exhibit several of these warning signs, counselors may choose to utilize a formal measure of work addiction (described later in the chapter).

CHILDHOOD EXPERIENCES OF THOSE WITH WORK ADDICTION

Another important aspect of identifying work addiction is to explore clients' childhood experiences. Oftentimes, those with work addiction had chaotic or traumatic childhoods (e.g., parent(s) in active addiction, parent(s) with mental illness, inconsistent caregivers or living situations, abuse, neglect). Some of these children may have found that immersing themselves in chores or academic work provided a sense of security and predictability (Aziz & Uhrich, 2014; Robinson, 2014). In addition, children in chaotic households may have had chronically elevated adrenaline and stress hormone levels, thus building tolerance and a dependency on the natural chemicals (Workaholics Anonymous World Service Organization, 2015). It also is common for those with work addiction to be *parentified* as children, meaning they took on responsibilities and roles that surpassed their developmental stage (such as caring for younger siblings or a parent; Earley & Cushway, 2002). Parentified children often learn at an early age that succeeding, performing, and achieving are linked to gaining approval from others and serve to keep the chaos of the household at bay. Thus, parentified children may be at higher risk of developing study addiction in adolescence and work addiction in adulthood (Robinson, 2014).

On the other hand, children in family environments marked by rigidly high expectations, overly critical caregivers, and unachievable standards also are at risk for developing work addiction (Holland, 2008). These children may internalize the belief that their worth is directly contingent upon their performance (in school, extracurricular activities, or household responsibilities). In adulthood, these individuals may work compulsively in an attempt to meet the impossible, rigid expectations of their childhood caregivers or important early attachment figures, thus contributing to the development of work addiction. Counselors working with clients with work addiction should assess the clients' family history, early childhood experiences, and the role the clients played in their families of origin.

NEGATIVE CONSEQUENCES OF WORK ADDICTION

The relationship between overworking and physical harm is recognized worldwide. In fact, the Japanese word *karoshi* means sudden death due to overworking (occurring most often due to heart failure or stroke; Herbig & Palumbo, 1994; Ke, 2012). Research indicates that work addiction exposes individuals to chronic stress accompanied by low-grade inflammation (Girardi et al., 2019). Specifically, Girardi et al. (2019) found a positive relationship between work addiction and a proinflammatory cytokine (IL-17), which is a biomarker of inflammation. Chronic stress and inflammation caused by work addiction can lead to a variety of negative health consequences such as high blood pressure (Balducci et al., 2016; Sussman, 2012), poor sleep patterns (Salanova et al., 2016), fatigue (Atroszko et al., 2019), and cardiovascular risk (Griffiths et al., 2018). Indeed, in the study of over 500 hospital employees in Spain, researchers found that those with work addiction had higher risk of cardiovascular problems than other workers (Salanova et al., 2016). Additionally, these employees consumed more caffeine and more alcohol during the week than nonaddicted workers (Salanova et al., 2016). Taken together, these factors indicate an increased risk of physical harm among those with work addiction.

Along with the risk of physical negative consequences, work addiction also has been linked to mental health disorders including attention deficit hyperactivity disorder (ADHD), obsessive-compulsive disorder, anxiety, and depression (Andreassen et al., 2016). In a longitudinal study in Italy, researchers found that work addiction at the first timepoint significantly predicted mental distress at the second timepoint (Balducci et al., 2016). Additionally, work addiction has negative effects on individuals' relationships, including friendships, romantic partners/spouses, children, and other family members (Robinson, 2014). Given the compulsive nature of work addiction, individuals may engage in work-related activities in lieu of other obligations (thereby missing important family/social events), during time spent with others (e.g., at mealtime, on road trips, on vacation), or they may be mentally preoccupied with work, thus failing to be present and attentive. Empirical support exists for the correlation between work addiction and lower levels of friendship and relationship quality (Hancock et al., 2019), higher levels of family conflict (Sussman, 2012), and poorer family functioning (Clark et al., 2014). Thus, like other addictions, negative consequences related to work addiction impact both the individual (physically and psychologically) and those in relationship with the individual.

HOW DO I ASSESS IT?

In addition to informal assessment strategies, formal measures may be useful in your clinical work with clients reporting signs of work addiction. The following are two instruments that you may find helpful in your practice.

> **CLINICAL NOTE 12.3**
>
> In many societies, overworking is rewarded or expected; thus clients may find it difficult to recognize work addiction. Exploring negative consequences of a client's work behaviors can be a helpful way for counselors to highlight discrepancies between the client's personal values (e.g., strong family bonds, physical health, friendship, life balance) and their actions (e.g., working long hours, prioritizing work activities over family activities, working to the point of physical exhaustion, neglecting self-care). Even clients with personal values of success and achievement can examine how overworking can compromise their physical and psychological health, which can negatively affect their occupational goals.

WORK ADDICTION RISK TEST

The Work Addiction Risk Test (WART; Robinson, 1999) is a 25-item self-report measure assessing symptoms of work addiction as identified by experienced clinicians. When completing the WART, respondents consider the extent to which each item reflects their work habits/patterns and respond on a four-point Likert-type scale ranging from *never true* (1) to *always true* (4). Example items include: *I feel guilty when I am not working on something* and *I put myself under pressure with self-imposed deadlines when I work*. WART scores are derived from summing the client's responses to the 25 items. Higher scores indicate more risk of work addiction. Scores on the WART demonstrated acceptable reliability among a sample of college students (Cronbach's alpha = .88) as well as concurrent validity with measures of anxiety and type A personality traits (Robinson, 1999). All items of the WART can be found in Robinson's (1999) original article.

BERGEN WORK ADDICTION SCALE

Researchers crafted the Bergen Work Addiction Scale (BWAS; Andreassen et al., 2012) based on Brown (1993) and Griffiths's (1996, 2005) components of addiction (salience, tolerance, mood modification, relapse, withdrawal, conflict, resulting problems). Each component is represented with one item on the BWAS, totaling seven items. Respondents consider their experience with work over the previous year and respond to each item using a five-point Likert-type scale ranging from *never* (1) to *always* (5). Example items on the BWAS include: *How often during the past year have you worked in order to reduce feelings of guilt, anxiety, helplessness and depression* and *How often during the past* year have you become stressed if you have been prohibited from working. If respondents select a 4 or 5 (thus endorsing the item) on at least four of the seven items, they are classified as having work addiction. Alternatively, clinicians and researchers can sum the scores on the seven items for a total continuous BWAS score. Among a large sample of adults, scores on the BWAS demonstrated acceptable reliability (Cronbach's alpha = .84) as well as convergent and discriminant validity (Andreassen et al., 2012). The BWAS is printed in the original Andreassen et al. (2012) article.

HOW DO I TREAT IT?

Clients who present with work addiction will have varying levels of awareness and acceptance of their addictive behavior. Some clients may defend their work habits by recounting their accomplishments, while others may willingly acknowledge that their work patterns have become problematic. It may be helpful for counselors to provide psychoeducation regarding the nature of work addiction, including the role of adrenaline and potential long-term effects of elevated cortisol and other stress hormones on the body. Clients may benefit from learning that those with work addiction often use work as a means of regulating their emotions; specifically, working provides a rewarding rush of energy (i.e., positive reinforcement) as well as an escape from problems or emotional pain (i.e., negative reinforcement). Additionally, counselors can describe how some individuals use work as a means of avoiding relational intimacy or as a way to feel worthwhile. Through treatment, counselors can help clients identify the function of work in their lives and assess the effects of compulsive working. In an accepting, nonjudgmental environment, counselors can help clients identify and give voice to the negative consequences stemming from their addictive work behavior (e.g., falling asleep while driving after a work binge, missing important experiences or information due to a mental preoccupation with work, experiencing conflicts with relationship partners or family members about work, and/or lying to others about the extent of their work behaviors).

Counselors also may choose to explore the extent to which clients with work addiction use substances such as caffeine or alcohol (Salanova et al., 2016). In light of the energy needed to maintain demanding work schedules, clients may consume a large amount of caffeine or misuse prescription stimulant medications (e.g., Adderall) to stay energized. Subsequently, these clients may consume alcohol or use marijuana in order to "come down," relax, and sleep before beginning another high-energy day. Counselors should be prepared to work with comorbid substance use disorders among some clients with work addiction.

Once work addiction is acknowledged, the goal of counseling is to help clients abstain from compulsive work–related behavior and achieve a sustainable balance among life roles and activities. Like food and sex addiction, the goal of recovery is not the complete absence of the behavior (i.e., work); instead, clients identify and abstain from the compulsive aspects of work. For example, a client with work addiction may determine that recovery includes abstaining from: (a) working after set work hours (e.g., after 7 p.m. or on vacations, weekends, or holidays), (b) volunteering for more work responsibilities before current work is completed, (c) checking work email during the night when trying to sleep, and (d) lying to others about when and how much they are working. In addition to identifying compulsive behaviors from which to abstain, counselors also help clients identify replacement behaviors to cultivate more life balance. Clients may determine that overworking has substantially detracted from their social lives, family relationships, spiritual practices, or self-care activities (e.g., exercise, leisure activities, healthy eating patterns). Counselors can help clients identify ways to strengthen these areas and address the underlying thoughts and feelings that accompany engagement in nonwork-related activities (e.g., feelings of fear and vulnerability, feelings of guilt, the belief that the client may be rejected if they try to develop relationships with others). Thus, treatment for work addiction includes both the elimination of compulsive work behaviors and the installation of activities and behaviors that support life balance.

VOICES FROM THE FIELD: Clinical Work With Work Addiction

Sadly, too many in America do not see work addiction as a valid, harmful addiction that can cause substantial damage to individuals, spouses, and children. Workaholism is similar to other forms of addiction in that the individual uses work as a way to regulate their emotions and deal with their anxiety or psychological pain through performance and achievement. There is a high that comes from the adrenaline and cortisol rush of working urgently to meet deadlines and achieve the next goal. Short deadlines trigger the sympathetic nervous system, which makes the individual alert, energized, and hypervigilant. Like other addictive behaviors, those with work addiction feel compelled or driven to work to satisfy an inner urge or craving. They often lie to others about how much they are working, persist in spite of negative consequences (e.g., health problems, failing relationships), and are unable to control how much they work.

Treating work addiction involves several components—one being cognitive. Like other addictions, those with work addiction develop "stinkin thinkin," in which they endorse dichotomies ("I am the best, or I am a failure") and the belief that they *must* work. Cognitive approaches can help clients identify and adjust their maladaptive beliefs to support life balance. In fact, clients can develop work moderation plans with their counselors to find balance among four specific areas: play, work, self, and relationships. A second component of treating work addiction is mindfulness. Those with work addiction are typically living in the future, rather than the present. Mindfulness meditation can be a powerful therapeutic tool to help clients experience the present moment and pause long enough to examine the mechanisms driving their work addiction. For those with work addiction, simply finding a hobby is not enough. Recovery takes time, self-exploration, and the development of new life patterns to find balance and worth outside of overworking.

Bryan E. Robinson, PhD

MEDITATION AWARENESS TRAINING

With regard to the treatment of work addiction, scholars have examined the effects of mindfulness-based approaches. Specifically, Van Gordon et al. (2017) explored the impact of an 8-week Meditation Awareness Training (MAT) on a sample of employees with work addiction. MAT is a group intervention in which participants engage in meditation practices stemming from Buddhist traditions to increases awareness and acceptance of the present moment (Van Gordon, Shonin, Dunn, et al., 2017; Van Gordon, Shonin, Sumich, et al., 2014). The MAT intervention consists of eight, 2-hour group sessions along with two individual support sessions. Topics of the group sessions include: an introduction to meditation and mindfulness, impermanence and emptiness, cultivating joy, generosity, ethical awareness, loving-kindness, compassion, equanimity, and letting go. The group sessions begin with a presentation of information (45 minutes), followed by group discussion related to session content (35 minutes), and concludes with a guided meditative exercise (30 minutes; Van Gordon et al., 2017). It is recommended that the facilitator of the MAT groups should have at least 3 years of personal meditation experience. Along with weekly group sessions, participants engage in their own daily meditative practice (Van Gordon et al., 2014).

In their study, Van Gordon et al. (2017) divided participants into an experimental group (MAT intervention) and control group (waitlist for MAT intervention). The researchers found evidence of decreased workaholism symptoms and psychological distress among those who completed the MAT intervention. Additionally, MAT group members demonstrated increased job satisfaction and work engagement at the end of the intervention. The improvements made among members of the MAT intervention group were sustained at a 3-month follow-up (Van Gordon et al., 2017). Therefore, some empirical evidence exists to support the use of mindfulness-based interventions, specifically meditation awareness, in the treatment of work addiction.

RATIONAL EMOTIVE BEHAVIORAL THERAPY

Scholars also have proposed the use of Rational Emotive Behavioral Therapy (REBT) when working with clients with work addiction (Burwell & Chen, 2002). The goal of REBT is to replace clients' irrational beliefs (in the form of rigid, dogmatic demands such as "should," "must," and "ought-to" statements) with rational beliefs (in the form of preferential and flexible statements; Ellis, 2001). Although REBT focuses on cognitions, it proposes that thoughts, feelings, and behaviors are always interacting with one another; therefore, altering irrational beliefs also will affect an individual's emotions and actions (Ellis, 2001). With regard to work addiction, irrational, absolutistic beliefs may entail: "I must be the best employee at my job," "I should not have to delegate or ask for help," or "I must work constantly to be valuable." Counselors using REBT help clients identify irrational beliefs and replace them with more rational preferences. For example, rational beliefs related to work may entail: "I want to do well at my job, yet if I make a mistake, I can learn from it," "There are times when delegating tasks and asking for help will make me a better employee," and "My work performance is not what defines me as a person." REBT counselors help clients move from conditional self-acceptance ("I am worthwhile if I am the best employee at my job") to unconditional self-acceptance ("I am worthwhile because I am a human being"; Ellis, 2001).

A key aspect of REBT is the ABC model in which activating events (or adversities; A) trigger beliefs (B), which lead to emotional and behavioral consequences (C; Ellis, 2001; Ellis & Dryden, 1997). Using this model, REBT counselors teach clients that activating events (A) do not in and of themselves cause emotional and behavioral consequences (C). Instead, the client's beliefs (B) about the activating event cause consequences (C). Therefore, according to the ABC model, activating events generate beliefs (which can be rational or irrational), which lead to emotional states and subsequent behaviors. The aim of REBT counseling is to help clients become aware of their irrational beliefs ("I should be working, even on weekends"), engage in a technique called *disputing* to logically challenge the belief ("What would happen if you didn't work on a weekend? Could you handle the outcome?" or "Is it really true that all good employees must work beyond set hours?"), and replace the irrational belief with a rational belief ("There may be times when I have to work on the weekends, but this should be the exception, not the rule. Along with my role as an employee, my role as a parent is important to me too."). Using cognitive techniques (disputing), emotive techniques (rational emotive imagery), and behavioral techniques (shame-attacking exercises), counselors can help clients learn the tenets of REBT and replace dogmatic demands with flexible preferences (Ellis, 2001; Ellis & Dryden, 1997). For those who want to learn more about REBT training, visit the Albert Ellis Institute at albertellis.org.

12-STEP SUPPORT

WA began in the early 1980s as a fellowship for those who had lost control over their work behaviors. Like Alcoholics Anonymous, WA consists of in-person meetings, a recovery book, sponsorship, reliance on a Higher Power, and working the 12 steps (the first of which is, "we admitted we were powerless over work—that our lives had become unmanageable" [Workaholics Anonymous World Service Organization, 2015, p. 25]). WA offers a list of 20 questions to help individuals determine whether they have work addiction. Example questions include: *Are you more drawn to your work or activity than close relationships, rest, etc.* and *Do you immerse yourself in activities to change how you feel or avoid grief, anxiety, and shame.* According to WA, answering three or more of the 20 questions in the affirmative is indicative of work addiction. WA promotes the practices of doing one thing at a time (as opposed to multi-tasking), underscheduling (to create margin for unexpected tasks or events), consistently making time for play and recreation, and creating boundaries around work activities (rather than allowing them to spill over into other facets of life; Workaholics Anonymous World Service Organization, 2015).

In WA, individuals work with their sponsors to create *bottom lines* and *top lines* to define recovery. Bottom lines describe the compulsive, out-of-control activities and behaviors from which the WA member is committed to abstaining (e.g., working more than 40 hours per week, checking work emails while driving, lying about work). Along with bottom lines, WA members also create top lines, which are goals, hopes, and aspirations for recovery. Top lines may include designating time each day in which all electronic devices are turned off, engaging in a daily spiritual practice, attending WA meetings each week, and taking at least one day off from work on the weekend (Workaholics Anonymous World Service Organization, 2015). As a free program with meetings available across the country, WA may be a helpful supplemental resource for clients with work addiction. To learn more about WA, visit their website at www.workaholics-anonymous.org.

DIAGNOSTIC CONSIDERATIONS

Currently, a diagnosis for work addiction does not exist in the *DSM-5* (APA, 2013) or *ICD-11* (WHO, 2018). Given that work addiction often simultaneously exists with other mental health concerns (e.g., anxiety, depression, ADHD, substance use disorder), counselors may choose to diagnose the co-occurring disorder, if appropriate. If a co-occurring disorder is not present, clients may meet criteria for adjustment disorder (if there is an identifiable stressor) or obsessive-compulsive personality disorder (OCPD; which should not be confused with obsessive-compulsive disorder; APA, 2013). Scholars have noted several similarities between work addiction and OCPD; thus counselors should carefully assess the symptoms and criteria to determine the appropriate diagnosis (Atroszko et al., 2020). Importantly, counselors should consider that "other comorbid or underlying psychological problems should not be viewed as exclusion criteria for work addiction" (Atroszko et al., 2019, p. 10). Therefore, clients may have two primary disorders—work addiction and another mental health concern.

HOW CAN I LEARN MORE?

If you are working with clients with work addiction or would like to learn more about the condition, consider the following resources.

BOOKS

- Fassel, D. (1990). *Working ourselves to death: The high cost of workaholism, the rewards of recovery*. HarperCollins Publishers.
- Robinson, B. E. (2014). *Chained to the desk: A guidebook for workaholics, their partners and children, and the clinicians who treat them* (3rd ed.). New York University Press.
- Workaholics Anonymous World Service Organization. (2015). *The workaholics anonymous book of recovery* (2nd ed.). Author.

PEER-REVIEWED ARTICLES

- Atroszko, P. A., Demetrovics, Z., & Griffiths, M. D. (2019). Beyond the myths about work addiction: Toward consensus on definition and trajectories for future studies on problematic overworking. *Journal of Behavioral Addictions, 8*, 7–15. https://doi.org/10.1556/2006.8.2019.11
- Clark, M. A., Michel, J. S., Zhdanova, L., Pui, S. Y., & Baltes, B. B. (2014). All work and no play? A meta-analytic examination of the correlates and outcomes of workaholism. *Journal of Management, 42*, 1836–1873. https://doi.org/10.1177/0149206314522301
- Griffiths, M. D., Demetrovics, Z., & Atroszko, P. A. (2018). Ten myths about work addiction. *Journal of Behavioral Addictions, 7*, 845–857. https://doi.org/10.1556/2006.7.2018.05

WEBSITES

- Bryan Robinson, Are you a Workaholic?: www.bryanrobinsononline.com/are-you-a-workaholic
- Mindfulness-Based Professional Training Institute: mbpti.org
- Workaholics Anonymous: www.workaholics-anonymous.org

REFERENCES

American Psychiatric Association. (2013). *Diagnostic and statistical manual of mental disorders* (5th ed.). Author.

Andreassen, C. S., Griffiths, M. D., Hetland, J., & Pallesen, S. (2012). Development of a work addiction scale. *Scandinavian Journal of Psychology, 53,* 265–272. https://doi.org/10.1111/j.1467-9450.2012.00947

Andreassen, C. S., Griffiths, M. D., Sinha, R., Hetland, J., & Pallesen, S. (2016). The relationship between workaholism and symptoms of psychiatric disorders: A large-scale cross sectional study. *PLoS One, 11,* e0152978. https://doi.org/10.1371/journal.pone.0152978

Andreassen, C. S., Nielsen, M. B., Pallesen, S., & Gjerstad, J. (2019). The relationship between psychosocial work variables and workaholism: Findings from a nationally representative survey. *International Journal of Stress Management, 26,* 1–10. https://doi.org/10.1037/str0000073

Atroszko, P. A., Andreassen, C. S., Griffiths, M. D., & Pallensen, S. (2015). Study addiction—A new area of psychological study: Conceptualization, assessmen, and preliminary empirical findings. *Journal of Behavioral Addictions, 4,* 75–84. https://doi.org/10.1556/2006.4.2015.007

Atroszko, P. A., Andreassen, C. S., Griffiths, M. D., & Pallensen, S. (2016). The relationship between study addiction and work addiction: A cross-cultural longitudinal study. *Journal of Behavioral Addictions, 5,* 708–714. https://doi.org/10.1556/2006.5.2016.076

Atroszko, P. A., Demetrovics, Z., & Griffiths, M. D. (2019). Beyond the myths about work addiction: Toward consensus on definition and trajectories for future studies on problematic overworking. *Journal of Behavioral Addictions, 8,* 7–15. https://doi.org/10.1556/2006.8.2019.11

Atroszko, P. A., Demetrovics, Z., & Griffiths, M. D. (2020). Work addiction, obsessive-compulsive personality disorder, burn-out, and global burden of disease: Implications from the ICD-11. *International Journal of Environmental Research and Public Health, 17,* 660. https://doi.org/10.3390/ijerph17020660

Aziz, S., & Uhrich, B. (2014). The causes and consequences of workaholism. In R. J. Burke & D. A. Major (Eds.), *Gender in organizations: Are men allies or adversaries to women's career development?* Edwards Elgar Publishing.

Balducci, C., Avanzi, L., & Fraccaroli, F. (2016). The individual "costs" of workaholism: An analysis based on multisource and prospective data. *Journal of Management, 44,* 2961–2986. https://doi.org/10.1177/0149206316658348

Beiler-May, A., Williamson, R. L., Clark, M. A., & Carter, N. T. (2017). Gender bias in the measurement of workaholism. *Journal of Personality Assessment, 99,* 104–110. https://doi.org/10.1080/00223891.2016.1198795

Brown, R. I. F. (1993). Some contributions of the study of gambling to the study of other addictions. In W. R. Eadington & J. A. Cornelius (Eds.), *Gambling behaviour and problem gambling* (pp. 341–272). University of Nevada Press.

Burwell, R., & Chen, C. P. (2002). Applying REBT to workaholic clients. *Counseling Psychology Quarterly, 15,* 219–228. https://doi.org/10.1080/09515070210143507

Clark, M. A., Michel, J. S., Zhdanova, L., Pui, S. Y., & Baltes, B. B. (2014). All work and no play? A meta-analytic examination of the correlates and outcomes of workaholism. *Journal of Management, 42,* 1836–1873. https://doi.org/10.1177/0149206314522301

Earley, L., & Cushway, D. (2002). The parentified child. *Clinical Child Psychology and Psychiatry, 7,* 163–178. https://doi.org/10.1177/1359104502007002005

Ellis, A. (2001). *Overcoming destructive beliefs, feelings, and behaviors: New directions for rational emotive behavioral therapy.* Prometheus Books.

Ellis, A. & Dryden, W. (1997). *The practice of rational emotive behavior therapy* (2nd ed.). Springer Publishing.

Ercan Demirel, E., & Erdirencelebi, M. (2019). The relationship of burnout with workaholism mediated by work-family life conflict: A study on family academicians. *Journal of Language and Linguistic Studies, 15,* 1300–1316. https://doi.org/10.17263/jlls.668436

Fassel, D. (1990). *Working ourselves to death: The high cost of workaholism, the rewards of recovery.* HarperCollins Publishers.

Girardi, D., De Carlo, A., Dal Corso, L., Andreassen, C. S., & Falco, A. (2019). Is workaholism associated with inflammatory response? The moderating role of work engagement. *Testing, Psychometrics, Methodology in Applied Psychology, 26,* 305–322. https://doi.org/10.4473/TPM26.2.9

Griffiths, M. D. (1996). Behavioural addiction: An issue for everybody? *Journal of Workplace Learning, 8,* 19–25. https://doi.org/10.1108/13665629610116872

Griffiths, M. (2005). A 'components' model of addiction within a biopsychosocial framework. *Journal of Substance Use, 10,* 191–197. https://doi.org/10.1080/14659890500114359

Griffiths, M. D., Demetrovics, Z., & Atroszko, P. A. (2018). Ten myths about work addiction. *Journal of Behavioral Addictions, 7,* 845–857. https://doi.org/10.1556/2006.7.2018.05

Hancock, M. G., Balkin, R. S., Reiner, S. M., Williams, S., Hunter, Q., Powell, B., & Juhnke, G. A. (2019). Life balance and work addiction among NCAA administrators and coaches. *Career Development Quarterly, 67,* 264–270. https://doi.org/10.1002/cdq.12195

Herbig, P. A., & Palumbo, F. A. (1994). Karoshi: Salaryman sudden death syndrome. *Journal of Managerial Psychology, 9,* 11–16. https://doi.org/10.1108/02683949410075831

Herr, R. M., Almer, C., Loerbroks, A., Barrech, A., Elfantel, I., Siegrist, J., Gundel, H., Angerer, P., & Li, J. (2018). Association of work stress with hair cortisol concentrations-Initial findings from a perspective study. *Psychoneuroendocrinology, 89,* 134–137. https://doi.org/10.1016/j.psyneuen.2018.01.011

Holland, D. W. (2008). Work addiction: Costs and solutions for individuals, relationships and organizations. *Journal of Workplace Behavioral Health, 22,* 1–15. https://doi.org/10.1080/15555240802156934

Ke, D. S. (2012). Overwork, stroke, and Karoshi-death from overwork. *Acta Neurologica Taiwanica, 21,* 54–59.

Lichtenstein, M. B., Malkenes, M., Sibbersen, C., & Hinze, C. J. (2019). Work addiction is associated with increased stress and reduced quality of life: Validation of the Bergen work addiction scale in Danish. *Scandinavian Journal of Psychology, 60,* 145–151. https://doi.org/10.1111/sjop.12506

Mani, D., & Trines, S. (2018). *Education in South Korea.* https://wenr.wes.org/2018/10/education-in-south-korea

Mazzetti, G., Schaufeli, W. B., & Guglielmi, D. (2014). Are workaholics born or made? Relations of workaholism with person characteristics and overwork climate. *International Journal of Stress Management, 21,* 227–254. https://doi.org/10.1037/a0035700

Mazzetti, G., Vignoli, M., Guglielmi, D., & Schaufeli, W. B. (2019). Work addiction and presenteeism: The buffering role of managerial support. *International Journal of Psychology, 54*, 174–179. https://doi.org/10.1002/ijop.12449

Robinson, B. E. (1999). The Work Addiction Risk Test: Development of a tentative measure of workaholism. *Perceptual & Motor Skills, 88*, 199–210. https://doi.org/10.2466/PMS.88.1.199-210

Robinson, B. E. (2014). *Chained to the desk: A guidebook for workaholics, their partners and children, and the clinicians who treat them* (3rd ed). New York University Press.

Salanova, M., Lopez-Gonzalez, A. A., Llorens, S., del Libano, M., Vincente-Herrero, M. T., & Tomas-Salva, M. (2016). Your work may be killing you: Workaholism, sleep problems, and cardiovascular risk. *Work and Stress, 30*, 228–242. https://doi.org/10.1080/02678373.2016.1203373

Schabracq, M. J., Cooper, C. L., & Winnubst, J. A. M. (1996). Work and health psychology: Towards a theoretical framework. In M. J. Schabracq, J. A. M. Winnubst, & C. L. Cooper (Eds.), *Handbook of work and health psychology* (pp. 3–32). Wiley and Sons.

Schaufeli, W. B., Taris, T. W., & Rhenen, W. V. (2008). Workaholism, burnout, and work engagement: Three of a kind or three different kinds of employee well-being? *Applied Psychology: An International Review, 57*, 173–203. https://doi.org/10.111/j.1464-0597.2007.00285.x

Spurk, D., Hirschi, A., & Kauffeld, S. (2016). A new perspective on the etiology of workaholism. *Journal of Career Assessment, 24*, 747–764. https://doi.org/10.1177/1069072715616127

Sussman, S., Lisha, N., & Griffiths, M. (2011). Prevalence of the addictions: A problem of the majority or the minority. *Evaluation and the Health Professions, 34*, 3–56. https://doi.org/10.1177/0163278710380124

Sussman, S. (2012). Workaholism: A review. *Journal of Addiction Research and Therapy, Suppl. 6*(1), 4120. https://doi.org/10.4172/2155-6105.s6-001

Sussman, S. (2018). Ten myths (or facts?) about workaholism: An appetitive motivation framework. *Journal of Behavioral Addictions, 7*, 884–887. https://doi.org/10.1556/2006.7.2018.120

Urban, R., Kun, B., Mozes, T., Soltesz, P., Paksi, B., Farkas, J., Kökönyei, G., Orosz, G., Maráz, A., Felvinczi, K., Griffiths, M. D., & Demetrovics, Z. (2019). A four-factor model of work addiction: The development of the work addiction risk test revised. *European Addiction Research, 25*, 145–160. https://doi.org/10.1159/000499672

U.S. Bureau of Labor Statistics. (2018). *Average hours employed people spent working on days worked by day of the week*. https://www.bls.gov/charts/american-time-use/emp-by-ftpt-job-edu-h.htm

Van Gordon, W., Shonin, E., Dunn, T. J., Garcia-Campayo, J., Demarzo, M. M. P., & Griffiths, M. D. (2017). Meditation awareness training for the treatment of workaholism: A controlled trial. *Journal of Behavioral Addictions, 6*, 212–220. https://doi.org/10.1556/2006.6.2017.021

Van Gordon, W., Shonin, E., Sumich, A., Sundin, E. C., & Griffiths, M. D. (2014). Meditation Awareness Training (MAT) for psychological well-being in a sub-clinical sample of university students: A controlled pilot study. *Mindfulness, 5*, 381–391. https://doi.org/10.1007/s12671-012-0191-5

Vingerhoets, A. J. J. M., van Huijgevoort, M., & van Heck, G. L. (2002). Leisure sickness: A pilot study on its prevalence, phenomenology, and background. *Psychotherapy and Psychosomatics, 71*, 311–317. https://doi.org/10.1159/000065992

Workaholics Anonymous World Service Organization. (2015). *The workaholics anonymous book of recovery* (2nd ed.). Author.
World Health Organization. (2018). *International statistical classification of diseases and related health problems* (11th Rev.). https://icd.who.int/browse11/l-m/en
Yi, J. (2013). Tiger moms and liberal elephants: Private, supplemental education among Korean-Americans. *Society, 50,* 190–195. https://doi.org/10.1007/s12115-013-9638-0

13

Shopping Addiction

HOW DO I CONCEPTUALIZE IT?

Shopping and spending are key aspects of life in the United States, and the accumulation of debt is common. According to the Federal Reserve Bank of New York (2020), total household debt in the first quarter of 2020 reached 14.30 trillion dollars. Credit card debt contributed a substantial portion of that number (.89 trillion dollars), following auto loans (1.35 trillion), student loans (1.53 trillion), and housing debt (10.10 trillion; Federal Reserve Bank of New York, 2020). The extent of debt in the United States is reflective of the prevalence and priority of shopping, even when individuals do not currently have the money to pay for their desired items.

In today's society, there are numerous ways that people can shop, from outlet stores and shopping malls to television shopping networks and e-commerce platforms. Additionally, product advertisements and marketing strategies have become ubiquitous (e.g., television, radio, billboards, catalogs, magazines, online pop-up ads). Despite the unprecedented ease of shopping and quantity of daily advertisements, many individuals are able to spend money, manage debt, and engage in shopping behaviors without incurring problems. However, for a small portion of the population, buying and spending becomes a compulsive behavior that is continued despite an array of negative consequences (e.g., financial problems, relational conflict, psychological distress). These individuals lose control over their shopping behaviors and crave shopping or are preoccupied with thoughts of shopping when they are not making purchases. It is likely that these individuals have shopping addiction.

Like other addictive behaviors, shopping can become a primary means of regulating emotions for some people. Marketing campaigns and advertisements suggest that shopping is the antidote for emotional pain by associating products (e.g., new car) with positive feelings (e.g., confidence; Benson, 2008). Known colloquially as "retail therapy," shopping to enhance one's mood is a widely accepted and encouraged behavior. Indeed, the act of finding a good bargain, purchasing a desirable item, or acquiring the attention of store employees can temporarily induce positive feelings. Thus, when individuals feel restless, melancholy, or inadequate, they can go to a retail store or online shopping platform to reduce negative emotions. Sohn and Choi (2014) noted, "excessive and compulsive purchases are often fueled by the need to escape from an unpleasant feeling/condition" (p. 244). Therefore, shopping can be both positively reinforcing (i.e., elicit pleasurable feelings) and negatively reinforcing (i.e., diminish undesirable feelings).

It is important to note that those with shopping addiction find the *process* of shopping reinforcing, often more so than the acquisition of new items. Rose and Dhandayudham (2014) noted, "The highly experiential and sensory nature of shopping provides rewards in itself to the individual, separate from the rewards of the purchase act" (p. 83). In this way, shopping addiction is akin to gambling addiction (see Chapter 8) in which individuals become addicted to the *experience* of gambling, or being in action, rather than an addiction to the monetary payouts. In fact, there is some evidence to suggest underlying commonalities between gambling disorder and shopping addiction (Diez et al., 2018; Granero, Fernandez-Aranda, Bano, et al., 2016; Granero, Fernandez-Aranda, Mestre-Bach, et al., 2017; Guerrero-Vaca et al., 2019). In both instances, individuals find the process (i.e., shopping or gambling) rewarding, regardless of the outcome (i.e., new possession or payout). Indeed, some individuals with shopping addiction never use or wear their purchases (Benson, 2008; Muller et al., 2015), further emphasizing the rewarding nature of the process of shopping rather than the products only.

The development of shopping addiction often is a gradual process in which individuals engage in more shopping and become more preoccupied with the activity over time. Eventually, searching for bargains, buying, and spending become the most salient activities in the individual's life and they continue to engage in shopping activities despite negative consequences (e.g., indebtedness, bankruptcy, relational conflict, guilt, shame, financial problems, criminal behavior; Benson, 2008; Muller et al., 2015). Sohn and Choi (2014) interviewed nine Korean women with shopping addiction and identified five phases of the disorder: (a) retail therapy (shopping to enhance mood), (b) denial (justifying shopping endeavors and ignoring negative consequences, (c) debt-ridden (borrowing money, maxing out credit cards), (d) impulsive buying (making hasty purchasing decisions without considering repercussions), and (e) compulsive buying (unable to limit, stop, or control shopping behaviors; preoccupied with buying). Therefore, although shopping may begin as a rewarding pastime or temporary means to lift one's mood (i.e., retail therapy), for vulnerable individuals, it may develop into a compulsive behavior marked by cravings, the loss of control, and negative consequences.

ONLINE SHOPPING

With the advent of e-commerce, individuals now can shop at any time, day or night, without leaving their homes. According to the U.S. Census Bureau (2020), retail e-commerce sales exceeded 160 billion dollars in the first quarter of 2020. Online retailers provide consumers with a large variety of products at the tap of a finger or click of a mouse. The access and ease of online shopping is an important consideration of shopping addiction. Indeed, Muller et al. (2019) found that 33.6% of clients seeking treatment for compulsive buying disorder likely had an online buying disorder, specifically. Features of online retail sites and shopping apps, such as storing credit card numbers and pop-up advertisements prompted by viewing patterns, make online shopping a seamless, barrier-free process.

To help conceptualize online shopping addiction, Rose and Dhandayundham (2014) developed a model highlighting potential predictor variables. According to the model, predictors common to all addictions including low self-esteem, low self-regulation, and negative emotional states also are relevant to online shopping addiction. Additionally, predictors unique to internet shopping such as enjoyment, social anonymity, and cognitive overload can explain the development of online shopping addiction. Specifically, the level of enjoyment elicited by the process of shopping, which is contingent upon individuals' reward sensitivity, is a meaningful predictor of shopping addiction. Moreover, the anonymity of shopping online, including how often, how much, and when shopping takes place, makes e-commerce appealing for those who wish to conceal their purchasing behaviors. Finally, the cognitive overload created by e-commerce retail platforms (e.g., vivid graphics, notifications, regularly changing stimuli, special offers, coupons, pop-up advertisements) may lead to increased arousal and decreased self-control among online shoppers. The authors also purported that women may be more susceptible to online shopping addiction due to the fact that women have been socialized to assume shopping roles in the household (Rose & Dhandayudham, 2014). Thus, among susceptible individuals, these predictors can increase the risk of shopping addiction, particularly, online shopping.

Another important feature of online shopping is the means of making transactions. When shopping online, individuals use credit cards or electronic money transfers (e.g., PayPal) rather than purchasing products with cash. Researchers have found that different methods of payment have differing neurological effects on shoppers. For example, using functional magnetic resonance imaging (fMRI), researchers found that paying with cash (compared to paying with a credit card or smartphone) increases activation of the parietal cortex, insula, and posterior cingulate cortex, which are implicated in negative emotions and aversive stimuli (Ceravolo et al., 2019). Thus, when paying with cash, individuals are more likely to feel the pain associated with the loss of money than when paying with credit cards or on smartphones. For those with shopping addiction, the use of cash, rather than credit cards, may be a helpful aspect of treatment by encouraging the activation of neural regions that process loss, pain, and other negative emotions to potentially inhibit compulsive spending (Ceravolo et al., 2019). Indeed, Benson (2008) noted, "The immediacy of cash is vastly more 'real' than the very muffled impact of plastic" (p. 86). When working with clients with shopping addiction, counselors should carefully assess clients' engagement in a variety of shopping behaviors, both on- and off-line. Developing new plans for technology use may be an important component of counseling for clients who compulsively buy and shop online.

NEUROMARKETING

To aid in the conceptualization of shopping addiction, counselors should be aware of the growing field of *neuromarketing*, which merges psychology, economics, and neuroscience to understand human decision-making (Javor et al., 2013). According to the Neuromarketing Science and Business Association (NMSBA), neuromarketing "uses neuroscience (brain research) to reveal subconscious consumer decision-making processes" (NMSBA, n.d,. para. 2). Specifically, by using brain imaging and neurotechnology, the field of neuromarketing claims to help companies determine the effectiveness of their advertisements, the emotions elicited by brands and products, and the prices that provoke pain among potential buyers (NMSBA, n.d.). Rather than relying on consumer self-report, which assumes that purchasing behaviors are consciously motivated, neuromarketing seeks to utilize brain-based measurements (e.g., EEG, fMRI) and biometrics (e.g., eye tracking, facial emotional coding, galvanic skin response) to analyze unconscious decision-making processes (Karmarkar & Plassmann, 2019; Lin, 2018; Ulman et al., 2015). Thus, one of the aims of neuromarketing is to appeal to shoppers' automatic processes of their limbic systems (which are involved in emotional responses) rather than relying on the executive functioning of the prefrontal cortex (Hartson, 2012).

Neuromarketing, also known as consumer neuroscience, examines neurological reward circuitry, emotion activation, and aversion responses to assess consumers' preferred brands and the impact of promotional campaigns or marketing strategies (Javor et al., 2013). This information can assist with product packaging decisions, promotional decisions, and even item placement in stores (Karmarkar & Plassmann, 2019). The premise behind neuromarketing is that by using neural signals, researchers can better predict consumer purchasing behaviors. Karamarkar and Plassmann (2019) noted, "by measuring a distinct set of signals from consumers, neural methods offer novel dimensions of insight into consumer preferences, message receptivity, and behavior at individual and market levels" (p. 183). Despite the growing popularity of the notion of neuromarketing, more validation research is needed to assess the extent to which the employed neural strategies can effectively predict complex human behavior (Ulman et al., 2015). That said, it is important for counselors to be aware of the claims of neuromarketing and potential impact on vulnerable populations, such as those with shopping addiction.

> **CLINICAL NOTE 13.1**
>
> There are many methods of recording neural activity in neuromarketing, including EEG, PET, facial electromyography, and skin conductance (Lin, 2018). Another means of gathering data in neuromarketing is eye tracking. Specifically, eye tracking follows and records eye movements and gaze patterns among consumers to assess the stimuli to which they pay attention. Eye tracking "provides realistic evidence of what people are likely to look at, which makes it a powerful method for neuromarketers to evaluate marketing effectiveness" (Lin, 2018, p. 208).

SHOPPING ADDICTION AND HOARDING DISORDER

Although some overlap exists, clinicians should understand the distinctions between shopping addiction and *hoarding disorder*. Specifically, shopping addiction reflects an addiction to the process of buying and spending (Benson, 2008; Rose & Dhandayudham, 2014), while hoarding disorder reflects difficulty parting with possessions, even those that seem to have little value (e.g., newspapers, magazines; American Psychiatric Association [APA], 2013). According to the *Diagnostic and Statistical Manual of Mental Disorders* (5th ed.; *DSM-5*; APA, 2013), hoarding disorder is characterized by five criteria including: (a) trouble parting with belongings/possessions, (b) distress caused by the idea of discarding possessions and a fervent desire to save items (regardless of their worth), (c) substantial clutter in living spaces caused by collecting and storing items, (d) significant distress and functional impairment caused by the accumulation of items and thought of discarding the items, (e) the patterns of behavior are not caused by a medical issue, and (f) the patterns of behavior are not caused by another mental health concern. Thus, those with hoarding disorder are aversive to discarding possessions, which results in the accumulation of items and significant clutter (APA, 2013).

Importantly, those with hoarding disorder may display features of shopping addiction. Specifically, hoarding disorder has a specifier of *excessive acquisition*, in which the individual unnecessarily acquires items in addition to experiencing difficulty discarding them (APA, 2013). One form of excessive acquisition could be through compulsive shopping (along with collecting free items or stealing). One way to differentiate between shopping addiction and hoarding disorder is to assess the motivation for the behavior. Those with hoarding disorder seek to acquire items to store and keep without discarding (reflecting potential attachment issues), while those with shopping addiction seek to regulate their mood through the process of shopping (i.e., experience pleasure and avoid negative emotions). Despite potential differences in the function of the behavior, it is important to note that hoarding disorder and shopping addiction can co-occur. Indeed, in the study of 66 individuals with compulsive buying behaviors, researchers found that 62.1% also demonstrated compulsive hoarding behaviors (Mueller et al., 2007). In addition, Lawrence et al. (2014) found that hoarding significantly predicted compulsive buying among a community sample of 70 adults. Finally, using a sample from Taiwan and the United Kingdom, Lo and Harvey (2014) found that hoarding significantly predicted compulsive buying among Taiwanese participants, yet not participants from the United Kingdom. The researchers suggested that although a relationship exists between compulsive buying and hoarding, it appears that those who compulsively buy are seeking positive affect via shopping, rather than acting upon the desire to collect items, which is characteristic of hoarding (Lo & Harvey, 2014). Therefore, it is important for counselors to assess clients' shopping history, patterns, and motivation to determine whether clients have hoarding disorder, shopping addiction, or both.

PREVALENCE OF SHOPPING ADDICTION

Prevalence rates of shopping addiction are difficult to obtain given the lack of uniform diagnostic criteria for the disorder; however, some frequency reports exist in the literature. Among representative samples of adults, researchers found that 4.9% had shopping addiction, and among shopping-specific samples, the prevalence rate increased to 16.2% (Maraz et al., 2016a). Moreover, in a sample of adults in Spain, researchers found that 7.1% had shopping addiction (Otero-Lopez & Villardefrancos, 2014). Among a British and Taiwanese sample recruited from various internet forums, researchers found compulsive shopping rates of 12% and 16% respectively (Lo & Harvey, 2014). Additionally, among a sample of U.S. consumers between the ages of 18 and 45, researchers found that 20% were compulsive buyers (Mrad & Cui, 2020).

Data also suggest that the prevalence of shopping addiction is increasing, likely as a result of the growing popularity of e-commerce. In fact, consultations among individuals seeking treatment for compulsive buying disorder increased from 2.48% to 5.53% in a 10-year time span (Granero et al., 2016). Furthermore, some research suggests that shopping addiction is more prevalent among women (Andreassen et al., 2015; Otero-Lopez & Villardefrancos, 2014), while other researchers did not find gender differences in prevalence rates (Muller et al., 2014; Nicoli de Mattos et al., 2016). With regard to age of onset, researchers have found that shopping addiction began at 19.7 years (Black et al., 2012) and 21.85 years (Nicoli de Mattos et al., 2016).

NEUROSCIENCE RELATED TO SHOPPING ADDICTION

Shopping can be a highly rewarding experience. The anticipation of a good find (e.g., "thrill of the hunt" Benson, 2008, p. 140), the attention from store employees, the successful discovery of a highly desirable item, and praise from others regarding purchases can lead to reward circuitry activation in the brain. The personal experience of reward varies considerably from one person to the next depending on the sensitivity of the individual's neurological reward system (Rose & Dhandayudham, 2014). Genetic and neurological differences in reward sensitivity explain why "some behaviors, in some people, can be hyperstimulating enough to create addiction-like behaviors and brain changes" (Hartson, 2012, p. 65). In the study of compulsive buying, researchers found that participants' sensitivity to reward (measured by a self-report questionnaire examining participants' reactions to rewards) was a significant predictor of compulsive buying symptomology (Lawrence et al., 2014). Additionally, researchers have found that those with shopping addiction score higher on sensation-seeking (Maraz et al., 2015) and novelty-seeking (Black et al., 2012) than those without shopping addiction, which could be explained by low reward sensitivity. Indeed, the need for sensation and novelty may reflect low baseline dopaminergic levels (a neurotransmitter implicated in reward), necessitating engagement in rewarding behaviors (e.g., shopping) to stimulate dopamine release (Black et al., 2012).

Another variable to consider is the amount of dopaminergic stimulation triggered by shopping behaviors (recall that dopamine is the neurotransmitter implicated in the "wanting" or desire aspect of reward; Berridge & Kringelbach, 2015; Berridge & Robinson, 2016). Activities such as drug taking and sexual acts can trigger powerful surges of dopamine, among other neurotransmitters implicated in reward. Rather than a large spike in dopamine release, however, compulsive shopping (either online or in person) can lead to chronic, mild hyperstimulation of dopamine in the reward system, which also can lead to neuroadaptations (Hartson, 2012). Indeed, researchers have found that activation in the reward center of the brain differs between those with compulsive buying patterns and those without. Specifically, among 23 women with compulsive buying disorder and 26 normal shoppers (noncompulsive buyers), researchers used fMRI to determine that compulsive buyers had more activity in the nucleus accumbens (a brain structure implicated in reward circuitry) when shown a potential product to purchase compared to noncompulsive buyers (Raab et al., 2011). The significantly higher activation of the nucleus accumbens among those with compulsive buying indicates that these individuals experience more reward when viewing available products and a stronger desire to make a purchase than those without compulsive buying behavior. In addition, when these same groups of women were shown the prices for products, those with compulsive buying disorder showed significantly less insula activity, the region of the brain implicated in negative emotional processing. Therefore, nascent fMRI evidence reveals that those with shopping addiction may experience more reward from the potential of making a purchase and less inhibitory negative emotions from the cost associated with the purchase than those without shopping addiction (Raab et al., 2011).

Finally, data also reveal that some neurocognitive functioning differences may exist among those with shopping addiction and those without. Researchers tested 23 adults with shopping addiction and 23 matched controls and found that those with shopping addiction had poorer spatial working memory (associated with inhibited self-regulation, less control, and more automatic behaviors), inferior motor impulse control (indicating difficulty inhibiting behavior), and problems adapting behavior according to risk (poor risk adjustment skills) compared to nonaddicted controls (Derbyshire et al., 2014). Thus, researchers confirmed differences in cognitive strategies including impulsivity and decision-making among those with shopping addiction when compared to normal shoppers (Derbyshire et al., 2014). Taken together, this neurological evidence suggests that those with shopping addiction may have stronger reward responses to shopping cues and more difficulty employing self-regulation, decision-making, and self-control strategies when compared to those without shopping addiction.

CLINICAL NOTE 13.2

Like other addictive behaviors, those with shopping addiction experience cravings or strong urges to shop. In the study of 277 adults in Germany, researchers found subjective craving for shopping scores increased as participants were shown shopping-related cues (Trotzke et al, 2020). Additionally, there was a strong correlation between craving scores and the severity of buying–shopping disorder among participants (Trotzke et al., 2020). In light of the ubiquitous nature of product advertisements in many societies, consider how this may affect susceptible clients' cravings for shopping behaviors.

HOW DO I IDENTIFY IT?

Although diagnostic criteria for shopping addiction are not included in the *DSM-5* (APA, 2013), the coding tool of the *International Classification of Diseases* (*ICD-11*; World Health Organization [WHO], 2018) identifies compulsive buying–shopping disorder as an example of other specified impulse-control disorders (a residual category of impulse-control disorders). According to the *ICD-11*, impulse-control disorders are marked by (a) the failure to resist urges to engage in a rewarding activity, (b) persisting in the behavior despite negative consequences to the individual or others, and (c) significant distress or functional impairment resulting from the behavior. Disorders classified in the impulse-control category include pyromania, kleptomania, and compulsive sexual behavior disorder (WHO, 2018). It appears that compulsive buying–shopping disorder also is an appropriate code within this section, although specific criteria were not provided.

Despite the lack of criteria in the *DSM-5* and *ICD-11*, McElroy et al. (1994) proposed three criteria for compulsive buying based on the phenomenological study of 20 individuals with compulsive buying disorder. The resulting criteria included: (a) maladaptive buying patterns marked by irresistible preoccupations and impulses to shop/buy, and/or frequent acts of spending that exceed what can be afforded; (b) preoccupation, impulses, and behaviors related to buying that cause distress and interfere with one's functioning (e.g., debt, criminal behavior, bankruptcy); and (c) the problematic buying does not happen only in manic or hypomanic episodes. According to McElroy et al. (1994), endorsing these three criteria is indicative of compulsive buying disorder.

When identifying shopping addiction, it is important for clinicians to determine whether compulsive buying is a primary condition or a symptom of another mental health disorder. For example, impulsive spending is one of the potential criteria for borderline personality disorder (BPD; APA, 2013). Additionally, the criteria for both bipolar I and bipolar II disorders include references to buying sprees in the descriptions of manic and hypomanic episodes (APA, 2013). Therefore, compulsive, out-of-control shopping could be a symptom of BPD, a symptom of bipolar disorder, evidence of an independent, primary shopping addiction, or evidence of shopping addiction comorbid with another mental health diagnosis. Indeed, in the study of over 1,400 adult shoppers in Hungary, researchers found that 8.5% had compulsive buying disorder, 7.7% had BPD, and 2.2% had both compulsive buying disorder and BPD. Counselors are encouraged to review the diagnostic criteria for both BPD and bipolar I and II when working with clients who report overshopping and excessive spending. If co-occurring disorders exist, counselors can best serve clients by addressing both the addictive behavior and mental health concerns simultaneously.

SHOPPING ADDICTION AND MENTAL HEALTH

Those with shopping addiction are likely to have comorbid mental health concerns, either full co-occurring disorders or symptoms of mental health issues. Researchers found that those with shopping addiction have higher levels of anxiety, depression, hostility, and somatization compared to those without shopping addiction (Otero-Lopez & Villardefrancos, 2014). In Hungary, those with shopping addiction were found to have higher levels of psychological distress and lower self-esteem than those without shopping addiction (Maraz et al., 2015). Additionally, among a sample of 171 adults with shopping addiction, 95.9% had another mental health diagnosis including generalized anxiety disorder (55% men and 55.6% women), major depressive episodes (55% men and 53% women), suicide risk (45% men and 39.8% women), and panic disorder (15% men and 30% women; Nicoli de Mattos et al., 2016). Moreover, Muller et al. (2014) found that among 102 clients in treatment for shopping addiction, 65.7% also were at risk for major depressive disorder. Therefore, counselors should be prepared to assess and attend to psychological symptomology that may have preceded the shopping addiction, developed concurrently with the addiction, or developed as a consequence of compulsive shopping.

HOW DO I ASSESS IT?

Several assessment instruments exist for compulsive buying or shopping addiction. The following are descriptions of two brief screening tools that can be useful in your work with clients who show signs of shopping addiction.

COMPULSIVE BUYING SCALE

The Compulsive Buying Scale (CBS; Faber & O'Guinn, 1992) was developed as a means to screen for compulsive buying and is one of the most popular assessments in shopping addiction research (Maraz et al., 2016a). The short, seven-item scale was developed based on the study of compulsive buying, discussions with counselors, and qualitative research methods. Each CBS item corresponds with a five-point Likert-type scale ranging from *very often* (1) to *never* (5). Respondents indicate the extent to which they have experienced feelings, motives, and behaviors related to compulsive buying including: *felt anxious or nervous on days I didn't go shopping* and *bought items even though I couldn't afford them*. Lower scores are indicative of more compulsive buying symptomology. The authors of the CBS found excellent internal consistency among scale scores (Cronbach's alpha = .95), and the CBS also demonstrated construct validity (Faber & O'Guinn, 1992). The entire scale and scoring instructions can be found in the appendix of the original Faber and O'Guinn (1992) article.

BERGEN SHOPPING ADDICTION SCALE

Authors of the Bergen Shopping Addiction Scale (BSAS; Andreassen et al., 2015) sought to develop an updated, brief screening assessment for shopping addiction with language inclusive of both online and off-line shopping. Using Brown (1993) and Griffiths's (1996, 2005) components of addiction (salience, mood modification, conflict, tolerance, relapse, withdrawal, and resulting problems), Andreassen et al. (2015) developed 28 initial items. After testing the items among a large Norwegian sample, the final scale included seven items, each corresponding to one component of addiction (Brown, 1993; Griffiths, 1996, 2005). Example items include: *I shop/buy things in order to change my mood* and *I think about shopping/buying things all the time*. The BSAS items correspond with five-point Likert-type scales ranging from *completely disagree* (0) to *completely agree* (4). Total scores are obtained by summing the seven items, with higher scores indicating more symptoms of shopping addiction. BSAS scores demonstrated good reliability (Cronbach's alpha = .87) and convergent validity (Andreassen et al., 2015). The items of the BSAS are listed in Table 1 of the original Andreassen et al. (2015) article.

HOW DO I TREAT IT?

Treating shopping addiction is a multifaceted process. Along with addressing the immediate problematic behavior (i.e., compulsive shopping), counselors also must address underlying issues that prompt compulsive shopping (e.g., emotion regulation deficits, low self-esteem, unresolved trauma), as well as any co-occurring mental health concerns or addictions. A helpful starting place may be for counselors and clients to examine the function of the compulsive shopping behaviors in the client's life. Potential motives for overshopping include: to increase self-esteem, to avoid something, to hurt someone, to earn love from others, to self-soothe, to enhance self-image and appearance, to cope with trauma or loss, to establish a sense of control, and to find meaning/purpose (Benson, 2008). Once the purpose of shopping behaviors is identified, counselors can help clients address this need in more adaptive, balanced ways.

CLINICAL NOTE 13.3

Motives for compulsive shopping can vary among clients. Researchers examined compulsive buying among undergraduate students in the United States and found several significant predictors including materialism, the pain of paying, and anhedonia (Harnish et al., 2019). Specifically, participants with higher levels of materialism (placing great importance on owning material goods), less pain when spending money (can spend money easily), and more anhedonia (difficulty experiencing pleasure) were more likely to engage in compulsive buying (Harnish et al., 2019). Among other motives, counselors should assess whether clients' compulsive shopping is a means of acquiring possessions to increase social status, a means of stimulating pleasure, or fueled by a lack of consideration of the consequences of spending.

Counselors also want to help clients increase control over their shopping behaviors. Rather than acting impulsively in response to cues from the limbic system of the brain (one of the aims of neuromarketing strategies; Hartson, 2012), counselors can help clients pause long enough to enlist the decision-making strategies of the prefrontal cortex. For example, Benson (2008) suggested clients create a *Shopping Reminder Card* containing six questions for them to answer (preferably in writing) before making a purchase: (a) Why am I here?, (b) How do I feel?, (c) Do I need this?, (d) What if I wait?, (e) How will I pay for it?, and (f) Where will I put it? (Benson, 2008, p. 64). The practice of answering these questions before engaging in shopping activities can assist clients in making mindful, deliberate purchases (Benson, 2008).

With regard to specific counseling approaches, there are many ways to address shopping addiction. In a meta-analysis of treatment methods for compulsive buying, researchers found that group counseling was the most popular approach, particularly group interventions that included mindfulness and cognitive behavioral components (Goslar et al., 2020). Additionally, researchers determined that a 12-week individualized cognitive behavioral therapy intervention that emphasized psychoeducation regarding shopping addiction, stimulus control strategies, exposure with response prevention, cognitive restructuring, and skills training effectively decreased compulsive buying episodes among participants (Granero et al., 2017). Furthermore, shopping addiction has been linked to lower levels of self-esteem (Raab et al., 2011; Rodriguez-Villarino et al., 2006) and higher appearance orientation (more value placed on physical appearance; Slack et al., 2019); thus, cognitive strategies (e.g., Socratic questioning, disputing, or cognitive restructuring) related to beliefs linking self-worth to possessions may be helpful. Overall, the use of cognitive behavioral strategies as well as mindfulness exercises may be useful integrations into counselors' work with clients who shop compulsively.

As with other behavioral addictions (e.g., food addiction, work addiction, exercise addiction), the goal of shopping addiction treatment is not to completely abstain from the behavior. Instead, the aim of clinical work with clients with shopping addiction is to identify and abstain from the compulsive, out-of-control buying behaviors. To help accomplish this goal, counselors and clients can determine triggers that prompt addictive shopping and help clients respond in alternative ways (i.e., develop healthy coping strategies). Moreover, counselors and clients can ascertain whether particular forms of shopping are more problematic than others (e.g., online shopping, auctions, high-end retail stores) and create plans to abstain from these shopping methods, at least temporarily.

STOPPING OVERSHOPPING GROUP TREATMENT PROGRAM

Benson and Eisenach (2013) developed a unique group counseling approach for working with clients with shopping addiction called the *Stopping Overshopping Group Treatment Program*. In conjunction with daily reading and

> ## VOICES FROM THE FIELD: Clinical Work With Shopping Addiction
>
> In my practice, I approach working with clients with shopping addictions much like any other process or behavioral addiction. I have found that there are many commonalities among individuals with addiction, such as underlying unmet needs and trauma histories. Clients with shopping addiction do not typically identify shopping as their presenting concern. Instead, these clients often report struggling with intense relational issues.
>
> Initially, clients with shopping addiction may have limited awareness or be in denial regarding the problematic nature of their shopping behaviors. My goals for these clients are to increase their awareness, equip them with skills for tolerating distress and regulating their emotions, and address the root cause of the compulsive shopping. I have learned that every client's maladaptive behavior, including shopping addiction, is rooted in trauma. The client is shopping or compulsively spending to fill a void, numb a discomfort, or fuel intensity. It is imperative, therefore, that counselors help clients identify what drives the desire to act out their addictive behavior (compulsive shopping) and increase their ability to tolerate discomfort. Successful treatment of shopping addiction entails identifying the underlying traumas and helping clients gain skills to respond to trauma triggers in more effective and adaptive ways.
>
> I would encourage clinicians working with clients who present with shopping addiction or compulsive spending to approach their clients with an open mind. It is from a nonevaluative, curious mind-set that counselors can gain insight into the trauma histories of their clients and understand what need(s) shopping fulfills. Each client with shopping addiction will present differently; so it is important to understand the uniqueness of each client's shopping experience. For example, some clients will compulsively spend on small ticket items and some will compulsively spend on flashy, high ticket items. Regardless of the presentation of the shopping addiction, however, it is important to explore the client's experience before, during, and after shopping and uncover the ways in which the addictive behavior is linked to previous trauma.
>
> Taylor Zebrosky, MS, LPC; Owner/Therapist, Highland Village Counseling, PLLC

journaling activities from Benson's (2008) workbook, group members attend 100-minute meetings, one time per week, for 12 weeks. Group members are encouraged to interact with other group members on an online forum between group counseling sessions. The overshopping group intervention assists group members in uncovering the function of their overshopping behaviors, identifying triggers of compulsive buying, exploring values and strengths, and learning mindful shopping practices (Benson & Eisenach, 2013). Each group meeting consists of meditation practices, sharing progress of weekly goals, discussing journal/writing assignments detailed in Benson's (2008) workbook, and receiving psychoeducation. Benson et al. (2014) conducted a randomized controlled trial to test the efficacy of the Stopping Overshopping Group Treatment Program. Six women participated in the overshopping group while five women served as the control group (Benson et al., 2014). At the conclusion of the 12-week intervention, those in the Stopping Overshopping Group demonstrated significant declines in the frequency and severity of their compulsive buying behaviors (significant reductions in money spent, time spent, and frequency of compulsive buying episodes) compared to the control group. Moreover, these treatment gains were upheld at a 6-month follow-up (Benson et al., 2014). Thus, preliminary evidence exists for the efficacy of the group treatment program in decreasing addictive shopping behaviors.

DEVELOPING A PERSONAL FINANCE PLAN

Another important component of treatment for shopping addiction is related to money management. Specifically, researchers have highlighted the association between financial attitudes and shopping addiction. Among 225 adults, researchers found that less financial impulse control, less financial organization, and more anxiety about money, significantly predicted compulsive buying (Spinella et al., 2014). Additionally, compulsive buying was associated with more credit card debt and less likelihood of having a savings account among the sample (Spinella et al., 2014). Therefore, clients may benefit from psychoeducation and organizational skills related to managing finances, investing and saving, interacting with creditors, interpreting interest rates on credit cards, and augmenting credit scores. Counselors may be equipped and trained to provide this type of financial education, or may choose to consult with (or refer clients to) a credit counselor or debt management professional.

Either with or without consultation with a financial management professional, counselors and clients can work together to develop a *finance plan* to help clients restructure their relationship with money. This plan can entail behaviors in which clients will engage and behaviors from which clients will abstain. For example, it is recommended that those with shopping addiction refrain from using credit cards and develop new systems for spending that involve only the use of cash, debit cards, or checks (Benson, 2008). Clients also may identify a trusted other (e.g., family member) to manage their money for them. Another potentially helpful component of a client's finance plan is to begin tracking all income and expenses and creating a sustainable budget. Moreover, clients may choose to abstain from making purchases without spending a designated amount of time (e.g., 24 hours) in which they consider the benefits and drawbacks of the purchase. Additionally, some research exists supporting a relationship between compulsive buying and brand addiction (i.e., compulsive urge to purchase items from a favorite brand). Thus clients may determine specific brands from which they will abstain making purchases (Mrad & Cui, 2020). Furthermore, clients may plan only to shop in person rather than using online retail sites. Counselors can help clients develop this plan while enlisting the help of local financial counseling professionals, and/or directing clients to self-help books and services (e.g., Dave Ramsey at https://www.daveramsey.com/ or resources from the Federal Trade Commission at https://www.consumer.ftc.gov/articles/getting-out-debt#Self-Help).

12-STEP SUPPORT

Debtors Anonymous (DA) is a 12-step program that began in the 1970s to help those with compulsive debt. The first step of DA is, "we admitted we were powerless over debt—that our lives had become unmanageable" (DA, 2014, p. XVIII). Along with those with shopping addiction, DA can be a useful resource for anyone who has trouble with compulsive debt (e.g., those with gambling addiction, those with poor financial saving habits, those who regularly rely on borrowing money). DA provides 15 questions to help individuals assess whether the fellowship may be useful, such as: *Does the pressure of your debts cause you to have difficulty sleeping* (DA, 2014, p. XXXII) and *Have you ever developed a strict regimen for paying off your debts, only to break it under pressure* (DA, 2014, p. XXXIII). Endorsing eight or more of the 15 questions suggests that individuals may have issues with compulsive debt.

Like other 12-step fellowships, DA includes a primary text and literature, meetings, sponsorship, and spiritual components (e.g., reliance on a Higher Power). Unique to DA is the practice of recording all spending and income, and meeting with two other DA members (called a pressure relief meeting) to develop spending and action plans to help manage finances and resolve debt. According to DA, recovery from compulsive debting is solvency, or the cessation of incurring any new unsecured debt (DA, 2014). To learn more about DA, visit www.debtorsanonymous.org.

DIAGNOSTIC CONSIDERATIONS

With regard to diagnosing, counselors working with clients with shopping addiction should assess whether clients meet criteria for hoarding disorder, bipolar disorder, or BPD. If clients do not meet criteria for these disorders, counselors may choose to diagnose existing co-occurring disorders such as depression, anxiety, or panic disorder (Nicoli de Mattos et al., 2016), or coaddictions such as gambling disorder (Granero et al., 2016) or eating disorders (Slack et al., 2019). In the event that co-occurring mental disorders and coaddictions are not present, counselors can consider whether a diagnosis of other specified or unspecified obsessive-compulsive and related disorder is appropriate (APA, 2013).

HOW CAN I LEARN MORE?

If you are working with clients with shopping addiction or would like to learn more about the condition, consider the following resources.

BOOKS

- Benson, A. L. (2008). *To buy or not to buy: Why we overshop and how to stop.* Trumpeter Books.
- Cardella, A. (2010). *Spent: Memoirs of a shopping addict.* Little, Brown and Company.
- Muller, A., & Mitchell, J. E. (Eds.). (2011). *Compulsive buying: Clinical foundations and treatment.* Routledge.

PEER-REVIEWED ARTICLES

- Hartson, H. (2012). The case for compulsive shopping as an addiction. *Journal of Psychoactive Drugs, 44,* 64–67. https://doi.org/10.1080/02791072.2012.660110
- Muller, A., Mitchell, J. E., & de Zwaan, M. (2015). Compulsive buying. *The American Journal on Addictions, 24,* 132–137. https://doi.org/10.1111/ajad.12111
- Rose, S., & Dhandayudham, A. (2014). Towards an understanding of Internet-based problem shopping behavior: The concept of online shopping addiction and its proposed predictors. *Journal of Behavioral Addictions, 3,* 83–89. https://doi.org/10.1556/JBA.3.2014.003

WEBSITES

- Debtors Anonymous: debtorsanonymous.org
- Neuromarketing Science and Business Association: nmsba.com
- Stopping Overshopping: www.shopaholicnomore.com

REFERENCES

American Psychiatric Association. (2013). *Diagnostic and statistical manual of mental disorders* (5th ed.). Author.

Andreassen, C. S., Griffiths, M. D., Pallesen, S., Bilder, R. M., Torsheim, T., & Aboujaoude, E. (2015). The Bergen shopping addiction scale: Reliability and validity of a brief screening test. *Frontiers in Psychology, 6,* 1374. https://doi.org/10.3389/fpsyg.2015.01374

Benson, A. L. (2008). *To buy or not to buy: Why we overshop and how to stop.* Trumpeter Books.

Benson, A. L., & Eisenach, D. A. (2013). Stopping overshopping: An approach to the treatment of compulsive buying disorder. *Journal of Groups in Addiction and Recovery, 8,* 3–24. https://doi.org/10.1080/1556035x.2013.727724

Benson, A. L., Eisenach, D., Abrams, L., & van Stolk-Cooke, K. (2014). Stopping overshopping: A preliminary randomized controlled trial of group therapy for compulsive buying disorder. *Journal of Groups in Addiction and Recovery, 9,* 97–125. https://doi.org/10.1080/1556035x.2014.868725

Berridge, K. C., & Kringelbach, M. L. (2015). Pleasure systems in the brain. *Neuron, 86,* 646–664. https://doi.org/10.1016/j.neuron.2015.02.018

Berridge, K. C., & Robinson, T. E. (2016). Liking, wanting and the incentive-sensitization theory of addiction. *The American Psychologist, 71,* 670–679. https://doi.org/10.1037/amp0000059

Black, D. W., Shaw, M., McCormick, B., Bayless, J. D., & Allen, J. (2012). Neuropsychological performance, impulsivity, ADHD symptoms, and novelty seeking in compulsive buying disorder. *Psychiatry Research, 200,* 581–587. https://doi.org/10.1016/j.psychres.2012.06.003

Brown, R. I. F. (1993). Some contributions of the study of gambling to the study of other addictions. In W. R. Eadington & J. A. Cornelius (Eds.), *Gambling behaviour and problem gambling* (pp. 341–272). University of Nevada Press.

Ceravolo, M. G., Fabri, M., Fattobene, L., Polonara, G., & Raggetti, G. (2019). Cash, card or smartphone: The neural correlates of payment methods. *Frontiers in Neuroscience, 13,* 1188. https://doi.org/10.3389/fnins.2019.01188

Debtors Anonymous. (2014). *A currency of hope.* Debtors Anonymous General Service Board, Inc.

Derbyshire, K. L., Chamberlain, S. R., Odlaug, B. L., Schreiber, L. R. N., & Grant, J. E. (2014). Neurocognitive functioning in compulsive buying disorder. *Annals of Clinical Psychiatry, 26,* 57–63.

Diez, D., Aragay, N., Soms, M., Prat, G., Bonet, P., & Casas, M. (2018). Women with compulsive buying or gambling disorder: Similar profiles for different behavioural addictions. *Comprehensive Psychiatry, 87,* 95–99. https://doi.org/10.1016/j.comppsych.2018.09.02

Faber, R. J., & O'Guinn, T. C. (1992). A clinical screener for compulsive buying. *Journal of Consumer Research, 1,* 459–469. https://doi.org/10.1086/209315

Federal Reserve Bank of New York. (2020). *Household debt and credit report.* https://www.newyorkfed.org/microeconomics/hhdc.html

Goslar, M., Leibetseder, M., Muench, H. M., Hofmann, S. G., & Laireiter, A. R. (2020). Treatments for internet addiction, sex addiction and compulsive buying: A meta-analysis. *Journal of Behavioral Addictions, 9,* 14–43. https://doi.org/10.1556/2006.2020.005

Granero, R., Fernandez-Aranda, F., Bano, M., Steward, T., Mestre-Bach, G., del Pino-Gutierrez, A., Moragas, L., Mallorquí-Bagué, N., Aymamí, N., Goméz-Peña, M., Tárrega, S., Menchón, J. M., & Jimenez-Murcia, S. (2016). Compulsive buying disorder clustering based on sex, age, onset, and personality traits. *Comprehensive Psychiatry, 68,* 1–10. https://doi.org/10.1016/j.comppsych.2016.03.003

Granero, R., Fernandez-Aranda, F., Mestre-Bach, G., Steward, T., Bano, M., Aguera, Z., Mallorquí-Bagué, N., Aymamí, N., Gómez-Peña, M., Sancho, M., Sánchez, I., Menchón, J. M., Martín-Romera, V., & Jimenez-Murcia, S. (2017). Cognitive behavioral therapy for compulsive buying behavior: Predictors of treatment outcome. *European Psychiatry, 39,* 57–65. https://doi.org/10.1016/j.eurpsy.2016.06.004

Griffiths, M. D. (1996). Behavioural addiction: An issue for everybody? *Journal of Workplace Learning, 8,* 19–25. https://doi.org/10.1108/13665629610116872

Griffiths, M. (2005). A 'components' model of addiction within a biopsychosocial framework. *Journal of Substance Use, 10,* 191–197. https://doi.org/10.1080/14659890500114359

Guerrero-Vaca, D., Granero, R., Fernandez-Aranda, F., Gonzalez-Dona, J., Muller, A., Brand, M., Steward, T., Mestre-Bach, G., Mallorquí-Bagué, N., Aymamí, N., Gómez-Peña, M., Del Pino-Gutiérrez, A., Baño, M., Moragas, L., Martín-Romera, V., Menchón, J. M., & Jimenez-Murcia, S. (2019). Underlying mechanism of the comorbid presence of buying disorder with gambling disorder: A pathways analysis. *Journal of Gambling Studies, 35,* 261–273. https://doi.org/10.1007/s10899-018-9786-7

Harnish, R. J., Bridges, K. R., Gump, J. T., & Carson, A. E. (2019). The maladaptive pursuit of consumption: The impact of materialism, pain of paying, social anxiety, social support, and loneliness on compulsive buying. *International Journal of Mental Health and Addiction, 17,* 1401–1416. https://doi.org/10.1007/s11469-018-9883-y

Hartson, H. (2012). The case for compulsive shopping as an addiction. *Journal of Psychoactive Drugs, 44,* 64–67. https://doi.org/10.1080/02791072.2012.660110

Javor, A., Koller, M., Lee, N., Chamberlain, L., & Ransmayr, G. (2013). Neuromarketing and consumer neuroscience: Contributions to neurology. *BMC Neurology, 13,* 1–12. https://doi.org/10.1186/147-2377-13-13

Karmarkar, U. R., & Plassmann, H. (2019). Consumer neuroscience: Past, present, and future. *Organizational Research Methods, 22,* 174–195. https://doi.org/10.1177/1094428117730598

Lawrence, L. M., Ciorciari, J., & Kyrios, M. (2014). Relationships that compulsive buying has with addiction, obsessive-compulsiveness, hoarding, and depression. *Comprehensive Psychiatry, 55,* 1137–1145. https://doi.org/10.1016/j.comppsych.2014.03.005

Lin, W. M. (2018). Demystifying neuromarketing. *Journal of Business Research, 91,* 205–220. https://doi.org/10.1016/j.jbusres.2018.05.036

Lo, H. Y., & Harvey, N. (2014). Compulsive buying: Obsessive acquisition, collecting or hoarding? *International Journal of Mental Health and Addiction, 12,* 453–469. https://doi.org/10.1007/s11469-014-9477-2

Maraz, A., Griffiths, M. D., & Demetrovics, Z. (2016a). The prevalence of compulsive buying: A meta analysis. *Addiction, 111,* 408–419. https://doi.org/10.1111/add.13223

Maraz, A., Urban, R., & Demetrovics, Z. (2016b). Borderline personality disorder and compulsive buying: A multivariate etiological model. *Addictive Behaviors, 60*, 117–123. https://doi.org/10.1016/j.addbeh.2016.04.003

Maraz, A., van den Brink, W., & Demetrovics, Z. (2015). Prevalence and construct validity of compulsive buying disorder in shopping mall visitors. *Psychiatry Research, 228*, 918–924. https://doi.org/10.1016/j.psychres.2015.04.012

McElroy, S. L., Keck, P. E., Pope, H. G., Smith, J. M. R., & Strakowski, S. M. (1994). Compulsive buying: A report of 20 cases. *The Journal of Clinical Psychiatry, 55*, 242–248.

Mrad, M., & Cui, C. C. (2020). Comorbidity of compulsive buying and brand addiction: An examination of two types of addictive consumption. *Journal of Business Research, 113*, 339–408. https://doi.org/10.1016/j.jbusres.2019.09.023

Mueller, A., Mueller, U., Albert, P., Mertens, C., Silbermann, A., Mitchell, J. E., & de Zwaan, M. (2007). Hoarding in a compulsive buying sample. *Behaviour Research and Therapy, 45*, 2754–2763. https://doi.org/10.1016/j.brat.2007.07.012

Muller, A., Claes, L., Georgiadou, E., Mollenkamp, M., Voth, E. M., Faber, R. J., Mitchell, J. E., & de Zwaan, M. (2014). Is compulsive buying related to materialism, depression or temperament? Findings from a sample of treatment-seeking patients with CB. *Psychiatry Research, 216*, 103–107. https://doi.org/10.1016/j.psychres.2014.01.012

Muller, A., Mitchell, J. E., & de Zwaan, M. (2015). Compulsive buying. *The American Journal on Addictions, 24*, 132–137. https://doi.org/10.1111/ajad.12111

Muller, A., Steins-Loeber, S., Trotzke, P., Vogel, B., Georgiadou, E., & de Zwaan, M. (2019). Online shopping in treatment-seeking patients with buying-shopping disorder. *Comprehensive Psychiatry, 94*, 152120. https://doi.org/10.1016/j.comppsych.2019.152120

Neuromarketing Science and Business Association. (n.d.). *What is neuromarketing.* https://nmsba.com/neuromarketing/what-is-neuromarketing

Nicoli de Mattos, C., Kim, H. S., Requiao, M. G., Marasaldi, R. F., Filomensky, T. Z., Hodgins, D. C., & Tavares, H. (2016). Gender differences in compulsive buying disorder: Assessment of demographic and psychiatric co-morbidities. *PLoS One, 11*, 1–11. https://doi.org/10.1371/journal.pone.0167365

Otero-Lopez, J. M., & Villardefrancos, E. (2014). Prevalence, sociodemographic factors, psychological distress, and coping strategies related to compulsive buying: A cross sectional study in Galicia, Spain. *BMC Psychiatry, 14*, 101. https://doi.org/10.1186/1471-244x-14-101

Raab, G., Elgar, C. E., Neuner, M., & Weber, B. (2011). The neural basis of compulsive buying. In A. Muller & J. E. Mitchell (Eds.), *Compulsive buying: Clinical foundations and treatment* (pp. 63–86). Routledge.

Rodriguez-Villarino, R., Gonzalez-Lorenzo, M., Fernandez-Gonzalez, A., Lameiras-Fernandez, M., & Foltz, M. L. (2006). Individual factors associated with buying addiction: An empirical study. *Addiction Research and Theory, 14*, 511–525. https://doi.org/10.1080/16066350500527979

Rose, S., & Dhandayudham, A. (2014). Towards an understanding of Internet-based problem shopping behavior: The concept of online shopping addiction and its proposed predictors. *Journal of Behavioral Addictions, 3*, 83–89. https://doi.org/10.1556/JBA.3.2014.003

Slack, F. J., Rottschaefor, K. M., Harnish, R. J., Gump, J. T., & Bridges, K. R. (2019). Compulsive buying: The impact of attitudes toward body image, eating disorders, and physical appearance investment. *Psychological Reports, 122,* 1632–1650. https://doi.org/10.1177/0033294118789042

Sohn, S. H., & Choi, Y. J. (2014). Phases of shopping addiction evidenced by experiences of compulsive buyers. *International Journal of Mental Health and Addiction, 12,* 243–254. https://doi.org/10.1007/s11469-013-9449-y

Spinella, M., Lester, D., & Bijou, Y. (2014). Compulsive buying tendencies and personal finances. *Psychological Reports, 115,* 670–674. https://doi.org/10.2466/18.02.PR0.115c27z0

Trotzke, P., Muller, A., Brand, M., Starcke, K., & Steins-Loeber, S. (2020). Buying despite negative consequences: Interaction of craving, implicit cognitive processes, and inhibitory control in the context of buying-shopping disorder. *Addictive Behaviors, 110,* 106523. https://doi.org/10.1016/j.addbeh.2020.106523

U.S. Census Bureau. (2020). *Quarterly retail ecommerce sales: 1st quarter 2020.* https://www.census.gov/retail/mrts/www/data/pdf/ec_current.pdf

Ulman, Y., Cakar, T., & Yildiz, G. (2015). Ethical issues in neuromarketing: "I consume, therefore I am!". *Science and Engineering Ethics, 21,* 1271–1284. https://doi.org/10.1007/S11948-014-9581-5

World Health Organization. (2018). *International statistical classification of diseases and related health problems* (11th Rev.). https://icd.who.int/browse11/l-m/en

14

Advocating for Clients With Behavioral Addictions

WHAT IS ADVOCACY?

For many people, the word *advocacy* brings to mind images of lobbying in front of the Capitol Building or mobilizing a grassroots movement to influence public policy. Although these activities certainly are important, they represent only a fraction of what advocacy entails. At its core, advocacy is any effort to remove barriers to clients' wellness and any strategy to promote human dignity (Brubaker & Goodman, 2012; Lewis et al., 2011; Toporek & Daniels, 2018). Indeed, Lee (2012) concisely described an advocate as, "an individual who pleads for a cause" (p. 111). Advocacy efforts can span from individual client empowerment to large-scale social action (Toporek et al., 2009). Rather than something that other professionals do, advocacy is the responsibility of *all* practicing counselors (American Counseling Association [ACA], 2014). Indeed, Lewis et al. (2011) noted, "Advocacy is not an 'add-on' that is separate from the counselor's work with clients and students. Advocacy is, instead, a natural outgrowth of the counselor's empathy and experience" (p. 9). Therefore, as counselors engage with clients and become aware of systemic barriers impeding their wellness and personal goals, counselors are moved to advocate.

The ACA *Code of Ethics* (2014) defines advocacy as the "promotion of the well-being of individuals, groups, and the counseling profession within systems and organizations" and efforts to "remove barriers and obstacles that inhibit access, growth, and development" (p. 20). According to the *Code of Ethics,* counselors are charged with advocating for clients at multiple levels ranging from individual to institutional (ACA, 2014, A.7.a.). Additionally, the *Multicultural and Social Justice Counseling Competencies*

(MSJCC; Ratts et al., 2015) stress the importance of advocacy in conjunction with clinical services. The fourth domain of the MSJCC encompasses both counseling and advocacy interventions and implores counselors to intervene "with, and on behalf, of clients at the intrapersonal, interpersonal, institutional, community, public policy, and international/global levels" (Ratts et al., 2015, p. 11). Finally, the World Health Organization (WHO; 2003) also provided a guide for advocacy within the field of mental health. Specifically, advocacy in this domain serves to decrease the discrimination and stigma of those with mental health concerns and increase positive outcomes. The elements of advocacy put forth by the WHO (2003) include strategies to raise awareness, provide accurate information through education and training, and denounce myths and misrepresentations related to mental illness. Some barriers specific to those with mental health concerns are stigma, ineffective treatment services, high cost of treatment services, and the lack of prevention efforts (WHO, 2003).

Thus, in light of the many mandates and guidelines for advocacy that exist among mental health professional organizations, it is clear that all counselors and mental health professionals are, indeed, advocates. Along with providing effective intervention services related to presenting concerns, counselors are charged with removing barriers to clients' wellness and promoting the rights, dignity, and positive outcomes of those they serve. Although advocacy efforts can apply to a multitude of barriers and obstacles, this chapter specifically focuses on advocating for clients, groups, and populations with behavioral addictions.

ADDICTION ADVOCACY

To understand advocacy for behavioral addictions, it is important to examine the history and context of advocacy efforts related to chemical addiction. Addiction to substances has been conceptualized in various ways in the United States, yet a marked shift in the narrative occurred with the emergence of the "war on drugs" that began in the early 1970s (Lassiter & Spivey, 2018; Polcin, 2014). This "war" led to "tough on drugs" policies, such as mandatory minimum sentences and the mass incarceration of individuals who commit nonviolent drug crimes (Alexander, 2012; Polcin, 2014). The narrative around addiction quickly became one of fear and criminality rather than a discourse marked by compassion and treatment (Polcin, 2014). Thus, advocacy efforts over the past several decades have focused on shifting public opinion from a narrative of fear to increased understanding of the neuroscience of substance use, the disease model of addiction, and the need for rehabilitation, support, and effective treatment services (i.e., shifting the notion of substance use from a criminal justice issue to a public health issue). Despite some success, there is still a long way to go in these advocacy efforts, particularly regarding the racial bias inherent in the enforcement of drug laws (Alexander, 2012).

CLINICAL NOTE 14.1

Although data indicates that members of all racial and ethnic groups use alcohol and other drugs at similar rates, those arrested for drug-related charges are disproportionately more likely to be people of color (Alexander, 2011, 2012). Indeed, Alexander (2011) noted:

> The so-called War on Drugs has driven the quintupling of our prison population in a few short decades. The vast majority of the startling increases in incarceration in America is traceable to the arrest and imprisonment of poor people of color from nonviolent, drug-related offenses. (p. 16)

How might racial bias affect whether an individual using illicit drugs is ushered into a treatment program or ushered into the criminal justice system?

In 2001, the New Recovery Advocacy Movement (NRAM) was formed with the aim of "eliminating policy barriers to addiction recovery and promoting a policy environment in which addiction recovery can flourish" (White et al., 2012, p. 304). This movement is dedicated to removing obstacles that hinder individuals from entering and persisting in recovery. Specifically, the NRAM is a "social movement led by people in addiction recovery and their allies aimed at altering public and professional attitudes toward addiction recovery, promulgating recovery-focused policies and programs, and supporting efforts to break intergenerational cycles of addiction and related problems" (Faces and Voices of Recovery, n.d., para 1). Thus, according to the NRAM, some of the most prevalent barriers faced by individuals with addiction are stigmatization, public skepticism regarding recovery success, the lack of programs focused on recovery support, and the lack of effective prevention and intervention efforts related to intergenerational patterns of addiction. Consequently, the aims of the NRAM are to: (a) change public perception of addiction by focusing on effective solutions, (b) expose the public to individuals living in long-term recovery, (c) combat the stigmatization and dehumanization of individuals with addiction, (d) increase the efficacy and accessibility of treatment and recovery support, and (e) support policies and legislation that remove barriers to recovery (White, 2007). In alignment with the goals of the NRAM, the American Society of Addiction Medicine (ASAM, 2019) recently contributed to efforts to destigmatize addiction by providing an updated definition of addiction emphasizing the fact that it is a "chronic medical disease" (p. 2). Additionally, the definition includes a statement disputing the assumption of poor prognoses by noting that addiction treatment is just as effective as the treatment of other diseases (ASAM, 2019). By providing this new definition, the ASAM is contributing to the destigmatization of addiction.

Although many of these advocacy efforts have almost exclusively addressed chemical addiction, they have set the stage for advocating for individuals with any type of addiction (importantly, the ASAM definition refers to both chemical and behavioral addictions). Rather than reinventing the wheel, advocates of individuals with behavioral addictions can join with the already successful advocacy movement of chemical addiction to shift public opinion, increase effective and affordable treatment, and work to destigmatize behavioral addictions. For example, one strategy of the NRAM is to celebrate recovery publicly so that the general population is aware that recovery is possible and prevalent (White, 2007). From rallies and marches to public events and national recovery month (i.e., September; see recoverymonth.gov), advocates seek to make recovery known and celebrated. Along with raising awareness and publicly celebrating recovery from alcohol and other drugs, celebrating recovery from behavioral addictions such as gambling, internet gaming, sex, pornography, food, work, or nonsuicidal self-injury can be just as powerful with regard to shifting public opinion. More than simply raising awareness that behavioral addictions exist, advocacy efforts must include informing the public that people can successfully initiate and persist in recovery from addictive behaviors.

ADVOCATING FOR THOSE WITH BEHAVIORAL ADDICTIONS

Advocacy efforts for those with behavioral addictions can take many forms and occur at individual, community, or societal levels. According to the *ACA Advocacy Competencies* (Toporek & Daniels, 2018; Toporek et al., 2009), advocacy can take place across six domains spanning from micro- to macrolevels of interventions with varying amounts of client involvement. Specifically, at each of the three advocacy levels (individual, community, public), counselors can advocate on behalf of clients (i.e., counselors as the primary actors) or with clients (i.e., clients as the primary actors with counselors' support). The first advocacy domain, *client empowerment*, entails helping clients develop self-advocacy skills to address the systemic barriers to their wellness (counselor advocates with the client at individual level). The second domain, *client advocacy*, includes counselors acting on a client's behalf to dismantle or remove barriers with the client's collaboration and consent (counselor advocates on behalf of the client at the individual level). The third advocacy domain, *community collaboration*, involves partnering with a group to support them in their efforts to remove systemic barriers (counselor advocates with a group at the community level). The fourth domain, *systems advocacy*, occurs when counselors act on behalf of a group to generate positive systemic change (counselor advocates on behalf of a group at the community level). The fifth domain, *collective action*, encompasses partnering with a population to address barriers and increase public awareness (counselor advocates with a population at the public level). Finally, the sixth advocacy domain, *social/political advocacy*, consists of counselors using their interpersonal skills to cultivate systemic change on behalf of entire populations who are facing oppressive barriers (counselor advocates on behalf of a population at the public level; Toporek & Daniels, 2018; Toporek et al., 2009).

Counselors can employ advocacy interventions within each of these six domains as they advocate with and on behalf of individuals with behavioral addictions. The following are examples of advocacy efforts at each of the three levels of advocacy described within the ACA Advocacy Competencies (individual, community, public; Toporek & Daniels, 2018; Toporek et al., 2009). It is important to note that these are just a few possible ways to advocate for clients and populations with behavioral addictions. Counselors are encouraged to consider additional forms of advocacy as they become aware of barriers faced by their clients and members of their local communities with behavioral addictions.

ADVOCACY AT THE INDIVIDUAL LEVEL

One of the primary ways in which counselors can advocate with (client empowerment), and on behalf of (client advocacy), individual clients with behavioral addictions is to provide psychoeducation about the nature of addiction. Oftentimes, clients and others in clients' lives (e.g., family members, employers, supervisors, religious leaders, coworkers, friends, neighbors) have only minimal knowledge (if any) about behavioral addictions. It is possible that clients and others may not have heard of becoming addicted to a behavior and thus lack a mental category for the condition. Subsequently, clients, and those with whom clients interact, may draw erroneous conclusions about the cause, course, and treatment of behavioral addictions. Without accurate, current information regarding addictive behaviors, clients can succumb to intense amounts of shame and their loved ones can experience feelings of hopelessness.

In addition to a general lack of knowledge, opinions about behavioral addictions often are influenced by the harmful actions of those with addiction. When speaking about substance use disorders, Volkow (2020) said,

> People who are addicted to drugs sometimes lie or steal and can behave aggressively, especially when experiencing withdrawal or intoxication-triggered paranoia. These behaviors are transgressions of social norms that make it hard even for their loved ones to show them compassion (p. 1289).

Similarly, clients with behavioral addictions may break promises, keep secrets, lie, steal, betray others, and/or put themselves or others in risky situations. Thus, it is easy for friends, family members, romantic partners, and clients themselves to adopt a *moral model* of addiction, meaning they conceptualize addiction as a personal choice stemming from some sort of moral failing (Lassiter & Spivey, 2018). Specifically, Brickman et al. (1982) noted that the moral model assumes that the individual is responsible for both causing and solving the problem (i.e., addiction). From this perspective, individuals with addiction are perceived as fully responsible for becoming addicted and thus must find ways to help themselves become unaddicted. By way of psychoeducation, however, counselors can introduce clients and their loved ones to the *biopsychosocial model* of addiction, which conceptualizes addiction as a complex disorder with genetic/biologic, psychological, and social factors (Marlatt & Baer, 1988; Skewes & Gonzalez, 2013). Rather than causing their own addictions, the biopsychosocial model proposes that clients' genetic predispositions put them at higher risk for the development of addiction. These genetic predispositions coupled with psychological difficulties and societal access to drugs of abuse or addictive behaviors all contributed to the emergence of the addiction.

Thus, counselors are in prime positions to advocate for and with their clients by providing accurate information about addiction in comprehensible terms that clients and their loved ones can easily understand. To advocate in this way, counselors must have working knowledge of the nature of behavioral addictions including genetic predispositions and risk factors, relevant neuroscience, the influence of psychological trauma and other mental health concerns, and the effects of increased availability and societal norms related to the behavior. Clients can then share this information with others in their lives (self-advocacy) or collaborate with their counselor to share this information with others (counselor advocates on behalf of the client). Specifically, helping clients and those in the clients' lives gain accurate information about behavioral addictions and shift from the moral model to the biopsychosocial model can be a powerful form of advocacy.

For example, consider a client with gambling addiction who loses his family's personal savings during a weekend binge at the casino. Rather than perceiving this client as sick and in need of treatment, the client himself and members of his family conceptualize him as immoral and selfish (reflecting the moral model of addiction). Moreover, rather than conceptualizing his addiction as an illness or mental disorder, they conceptualize his behavior as a personal choice from which he could refrain if he so desired. In this case, client advocacy may involve teaching the client and his family about the etiology, progression, and treatment of gambling addiction. Specifically, the client and his family may benefit from understanding that although many people gamble, a small portion of the population has biological, psychological, and social risk factors that make them more susceptible to the development of a gambling addiction (thus reflecting the biopsychosocial model). Teaching the client and his family about the impact of naturally rewarding behaviors in the brain, the role of dopamine in reward, individual differences in reward sensitivity, and the strong effects of a variable ratio reinforcement schedule in gambling activities may help foster a more accurate perception of gambling addiction. Additionally, reading through the diagnostic criteria of gambling disorder in the *Diagnostic and Statistical Manual of Mental Disorders* (5th ed.; *DSM-5*; American Psychiatric Association [APA], 2013) with the client and his family can provide details related to common symptoms of gambling addiction and underscore the widely held acceptance of gambling disorder. Finally, counselors can discuss the elements of treatment for gambling addiction and emphasize that many individuals with gambling addiction have been able to initiate and persist in recovery. The counselor can refer the client to a local Gambler's Anonymous meeting (www.gamblersanonymous.org) and the family to a Gam-Anon meeting (a fellowship for the loved ones of those with gambling addiction; www.gam-anon.org). In this way, counselors can advocate for their clients by raising awareness related to the biopsychosocial nature of behavioral addictions, debunking myths and dispelling inaccurate information, and instilling hope related to treatment and recovery.

Of course, counselors will be unable to advocate in this manner if they themselves endorse *biases* and stereotypes regarding clients with behavioral addictions. Counselors must do the important and necessary work of inspecting their own personal beliefs and attitudes in order to identify biases regarding behavioral addictions. For example, along with the general public, counselors may question whether particular behavioral addictions are "real," assume poor prognoses among addicted clients, and/or subscribe to the moral model of addiction. Indeed, Lassiter and Spivey (2018) wrote:

> Just as racism, sexism, and homophobia are internalized in us all, the moral model is all around us and in us. Acknowledging and embracing this potential is the only way for these biases to not have undue influence on our interactions with addicted clients (p. 42).

Counselors may best address their biases by becoming more informed about the nature of behavioral addictions and learning from individuals in recovery. Specially, counselors can seek out continuing education opportunities, consume the most current research, seek supervision, consult with other mental health professionals who have experience working with behavioral addictions, and attend open 12-step support group meetings to humanize those with behavioral addictions. To be effective advocates at any level, counselors must engage in continuous self-reflection and work to dismantle their own stereotypes and biases.

CLINICAL NOTE 14.2

To identify potential biases, consider engaging in a simple mental exercise. Clear your mind, and, without censorship, ask yourself what comes up for you when you hear terms such as, "sex addiction," "food addiction," "social media addiction," "shopping addiction," "love addiction," or "nonsuicidal self-injury." Often, the thoughts, images, and knee-jerk reactions triggered by these terms reveal potential biases and areas for growth.

ADVOCACY AT THE COMMUNITY LEVEL

Beyond advocating for individual clients, counselors are well suited to advocate for groups of people with behavioral addictions in their local communities. At this level of advocacy, counselors can partner with existing groups to enhance their efforts (community collaboration) or initiate advocacy efforts on behalf of particular groups (systems advocacy). A very practical form of advocacy at the community level is to ensure that effective, *local treatment* is available for a variety of behavioral addictions. For example, with the rise of online gambling, all communities should be equipped with clinicians who have training and knowledge related to gambling addiction (e.g., International Certified Gambling Counselor), not just those communities located near casinos. In fact, the ubiquitous nature of the internet contributes to a variety of behavioral addictions including social media addiction, internet gaming addiction, shopping addiction, and cybersex addiction. It is important that clinicians in local communities are familiar with evolving technology and internet features in order to accurately assess and provide treatment for internet-based addictions. If counselors feel unqualified to address particular behavioral addictions, it is important to acquire the necessary training or ensure that there are local referral sources available for clients. For example, if a counselor becomes aware that clients with sex addiction are seeking treatment in other cities because there are no local providers who are competent in treating sex addiction (e.g., Certified Sex Addiction Therapists), there is an opportunity to advocate for these clients by ensuring that effective, local treatment opportunities are available.

If practitioners in a local community lack knowledge and skills related to a particular type of behavioral addiction, it is important to address this competency gap. Rather than working in silos, counselors, social workers, psychologists, and psychiatrists can join together to share resources and co-sponsor training events related to behavioral addictions to increase competency. The practitioners in a particular community may choose to bring in experts in specific behavioral addictions to provide large-group trainings or create additional opportunities for continuing education (e.g., host conferences or workshops). By working together, mental health providers in a community can ensure that clients with behavioral addictions have access to local and effective treatment services.

Another example of community level advocacy is to initiate *prevention efforts* for behavioral addictions in school settings (K–12). School counselors or community mental health counselors in schools are uniquely positioned to instigate prevention efforts for a variety of behavioral addictions. For instance, almost all forms of addiction are linked to issues in emotion regulation. Specifically, individuals seek to escape negative mood states or induce positive mood states by engaging in a rewarding behavior (e.g., taking a drug, using pornography, eating, checking social media, having sex, gaming). When naturally rewarding behaviors become the primary and/or sole means of emotion regulation, individuals can become dependent on the behavior to feel good (positive reinforcement) and to stop feeling bad (negative reinforcement). Opportunities for school-age children to develop effective emotion regulation skills may help students become better prepared to cope with negative emotions, find healthy ways to generate positive emotions, and engage in appropriate self-regulation. It is very possible that these skills can contribute to a decreased risk of developing behavioral addictions later in life.

Additionally, many individuals with behavioral addictions report engaging in their addictive behavior for the first time during their adolescent years. Counselors can develop programs to help students become aware of the addictive potential of particular behaviors (e.g., gaming, cybersex, gambling, social media, overexercising) and learn to engage with these activities in a healthy manner. For example, school counselors can initiate programs regarding how to cultivate healthy relationships with internet gaming. Rather than demonizing internet games, counselors can explore the potential benefits of internet gaming with students (e.g., developing community, enhancing problem-solving skills, increasing attention and focus, utilizing social skills), while also providing information about how to monitor one's relationship with gaming and recognize signs of compulsive behavior. Specifically, this prevention effort could include teaching students about the rewarding nature of internet games (i.e., age-appropriate neuroscience education), assessing motives for gaming (e.g., social connection, enjoyment, escaping problems, feel a sense of accomplishment, feel euphoria, decrease depressive or anxious symptoms), developing boundaries and limits for internet gaming, identifying risks associated with gaming addiction, recognizing negative consequences of gaming, and providing directions for what to do if students feel they have lost control of their gaming behaviors. In sum, rather than waiting for addiction to emerge and then responding with treatment, school counselors and clinical mental health counselors in schools can proactively facilitate prevention efforts to decrease the risk of behavioral addictions developing in the first place.

ADVOCACY AT THE PUBLIC LEVEL

There are many opportunities for counselors to advocate with (collective action) or on behalf of (social/political advocacy) the whole population of individuals with behavioral addictions at the public level. Counselors can work to address the *stigma* associated with behavioral addictions, which is a barrier to help-seeking behaviors. McGinty and Barry (2020) noted that stigma is "persistent, pervasive and rooted in the belief that addiction is a personal choice reflecting a lack of willpower and a moral failing" (p. 1291). Counselors can dispel these myths (and others) by publicly sharing their experience working with clients with a variety of behavioral addictions. Given that many people in the general public may not have personal relationships with individuals with behavioral addictions (to their knowledge), counselors can describe amalgams of their clinical experiences (while keeping clients' identities anonymous) to humanize those with addictive behaviors (McGinty & Barry, 2020). Indeed, by using various media outlets (e.g., internet, radio, podcasts, social media, newspapers, magazines, television) clinicians can explain that for some people, naturally rewarding behaviors can become compulsive, out of control, continue despite negative consequences, and lead to cravings or mental preoccupation. Additionally, counselors with experience working with behavioral addictions can publicly confirm that these clients *can* and *do* get better and treatment can be successful. Raising public awareness about the prevalence of behavioral addictions and the efficacy of quality treatment can help reduce the stigma and shame associated with addictive behaviors and promote help-seeking among this population.

Another way for counselors to advocate at the public level is to *conduct research* on their clinical work to determine what treatment approaches are most effective for clients with behavioral addictions. Whether clinicians work independently or partner with counselor educators or researchers, more data is needed to determine the best treatment strategies to use with clients with behavioral addictions. For example, in recent decades, addiction treatment has shifted from confrontation-based strategies (e.g., strategies to break through clients' denial) to more collaborative approaches (e.g., motivational interviewing; Miller & Rollnick, 2013). Despite these changes, however, "the conventional wisdom that addicts are incapable of change without coercion remains deeply entrenched, affecting both treatment models and the attitudes of the general public" (Lewis & Eder, 2010, p. 169). Therefore, experimental, randomized controlled trials (RCTs) are needed to identify the efficacy of various treatment approaches with behavioral addictions. RCTs, in which participants are randomly assigned to either an intervention or control group, are "the most rigorous and robust research method for determining whether a cause–effect relation exists between an intervention and an outcome" (Bhide et al., 2018, p. 386). Along with RCTs to increase the evidence base of potential treatment strategies, counselors can advocate for clients with behavioral addictions by publishing clinical manuals to guide novice counselors in their work. Treatment manuals, such as the manual describing the nine-session intervention for nonsuicidal self-injury (Treatment for Self-Injurious Behavior; Andover, Schatten, Morris, & Miller, 2015; Andover, Schatten, Morris, et al., 2017), can help counselors develop a therapeutic plan when working with behavioral addictions for the first time. Finally, clinicians and researchers can advocate at the public level by developing uniform, empirically validated diagnostic criteria for behavioral addictions to propose for inclusion in future editions of the *DSM* (APA, 2013) or *International Classification of Diseases* (World Health Organization [WHO], 2018). Universally accepted diagnostic criteria can help garner accurate prevalence-rate data and aid in the identification of behavioral addictions. Additionally, formal diagnoses can influence insurance coverage for the treatment of addictive behaviors, making services more affordable and accessible to the general public.

Finally, counselors also can become involved in influencing laws and public policy related to the regulation of behaviors that have the potential to become addictive. For example, counselors may feel passionate about influencing laws and policies that limit pornography access among young internet users, enforce internet gaming time limits or forced breaks, or regulate daily fantasy sports betting among college students. Counselors who have knowledge pertaining to the prevalence of behavioral addictions and associated negative consequences are vital to influencing public policy and legal statutes related to these activities. Clinicians can share their experiences and perspectives with lobbyists for specific causes, speak with legislators, or spearhead letter-writing campaigns to government agencies or congressional representatives.

CLINICAL NOTE 14.3

In light of the many examples of advocacy described in this chapter, is there one that you feel most passionate about? Consider specific examples of how you may be able to remove just one obstacle or barrier faced by individuals with behavioral addictions. What would be the first step?

LOOKING TO THE FUTURE

Counselors can do a lot of good by providing clinical services in their counseling offices, yet "other situations will demand that counselors work in the community in the role of advocate to address systemic issues that affect clients" (Ratts & Greenleaf, 2018, p. 84). If each counselor engages in advocacy efforts at individual, community, and public levels to remove barriers faced by clients with behavioral addictions, great change can be expected. Whether by providing accurate information regarding the neuroscience of behavioral addictions, publicly working to decrease stigmatization and discrimination of addicted clients, ensuring that all communities have access to local treatment services for clients with behavioral addictions, enhancing mental health training programs by infusing content related to behavioral addictions throughout program curriculum, or partnering with lobbyists to change laws and policies in favor of rehabilitation and affordable treatment for individuals with behavioral addictions, there are ample opportunities for counselors to advocate with and on behalf of addicted clients. Counselors have the responsibility to use their influence to advocate for positive change and remove systemic barriers that impede the growth, development, and wellness of those with behavioral addictions.

REFERENCES

Alexander, M. (2011). Cruel and unequal. *Sojourners Magazine, 40,* 16–18.

Alexander, M. (2012). *The new Jim Crow: Mass incarceration in the age of colorblindness.* The New Press.

American Counseling Association. (2014). *ACA code of ethics.* http://www.counseling.org/knowledge-center/ethics

American Psychiatric Association. (2013). *Diagnostic and statistical manual of mental disorders* (5th ed.). Author.

American Society of Addiction Medicine. (2019). *Definition of addiction.* https://www.asam.org/docs/default-source/quality-science/asam's-2019-definition-of-addiction-(1).pdf?sfvrsn=b8b64fc2_2

Andover, M. S., Schatten, H. T., Morris, B. W., Holman, C. S., & Miller, I. W. (2017). An intervention for nonsuicidal self-injury in young adults: A pilot randomized controlled trial. *Journal of Consulting and Clinical Psychology, 85,* 620–631. https://doi.org/10.1037/ccp00000206

Andover, M. S., Schatten, H. T., Morris, B. W., & Miller, I. W. (2015). Development of an intervention for non-suicidal self-injury in young adults: An open pilot trial. *Cognitive and Behavioral Practice, 4,* 491–503. https://doi.org/10.1016/j.cbpra.2014.05.003

Bhide, A., Shah, P. S., & Acharya, G. (2018). A simplified guide to randomized controlled trials. *Acta Obstetricia et Gynecologica Scandinavica, 97,* 380–387. https://doi.org/10.1111/aogs.13309

Brickman, P., Rabinowitz, V. C., Karuza, J., Coates, D., Cohn, E., & Kidder, L. (1982). Models of helping and coping. *American Psychologist, 37,* 368–384. https://doi.org/10.1037/0003-066X.37.4.368

Brubaker, M. D., & Goodman, R. D. (2012). Client advocacy: In action. In C. Y. Chang, C. A. Barrio Minton, A. L. Dixon, J. E. Myers, & T. J. Sweeney (Eds.), *Professional counseling excellence through leadership and advocacy* (pp. 141–161). Routledge.

Faces and Voices of Recovery. (n.d.). *New recovery movement basics.* https://facesandvoicesofrecovery.org/blog/2016/01/04/new-recovery-movement-basics

Lassiter, P. S., & Spivey, M. S. (2018). Historical perspectives and the moral model. In P. S. Lassiter & J. R. Culbreth (Eds.), *Theory and practice of addiction counseling* (pp. 27–46). Sage Publishing.

Lee, C. C. (2012). Social justice as the fifth force in counseling. In C. Y. Chang, C. A. Barrio Minton, A. L. Dixon, J. E. Myers, & T. J. Sweeney (Eds.), *Professional counseling excellence through leadership and advocacy* (pp. 109–120). Routledge.

Lewis, J. A., & Eder, J. (2010). Substance abuse counseling and social justice advocacy. In M. J. Ratts, R. L. Toporek, & J. A. Lewis (Eds.), *ACA advocacy competencies: A social justice framework for counselors* (pp. 161–172). American Counseling Association.

Lewis, J. A., Ratts, M. J., Paladino, D. A., & Toporek, R. L. (2011). Social justice counseling and advocacy: Developing new leadership roles and competencies. *Journal for Social Action in Counselling and Psychology, 3,* 5–16. https://doi.org/10.33043/jsacp.3.1.5-16

Marlatt, G. A., & Baer, J. S. (1988). Addictive behaviors: Etiology and treatment. *Annual Review of Psychology, 39,* 223–252. https://doi.org/10.1146/annurev.ps.39.020188.001255

McGinty, E. E., & Barry, C. L. (2020). Stigma reduction to combat the addiction crisis-developing an evidence base. *New England Journal of Medicine, 382*,1291–1292. https://doi.org/10.1056/NEJMp2000227

Miller, W. R., & Rollnick, S. (2013). *Motivational interviewing: Helping people change* (3rd ed.). Guilford Press.

Polcin, D. L. (2014). Addiction science advocacy: Mobilizing political support to influence public policy. *International Journal of Drug Policy, 25*, 329–331. https://doi.org/10.1016/j.drugpo.2013.11.002

Ratts, M. J., & Greenleaf, A. T. (2018). Counselor-advocate-scholar model: Changing the dominant discourse in counseling. *Journal of Multicultural Counseling and Development, 46*, 78–96. https://doi.org/10.1002/jmcd.12094

Ratts, M. J., Singh, A. A., Nassar-McMillan, S., Butler, S. K., & McCullough, J. R. (2015). *Multicultural and social justice counseling competencies*. https://www.counseling.org/docs/default-source/competencies/multicultural-and-social-justice-counseling-competencies.pdf?sfvrsn=20

Skewes, M. C., & Gonzalez, V. M. (2013). The biopsychosocial model of addiction. In P. M. Miller, A. W. Blume, D. J. Kavanagh, K. M. Kampman, M. E. Bates, M. E. Larimer, N. M. Petry, P. De Witte, & S. A. Ball (Eds.), *Principles of addiction: Comprehensive addictive behaviors and disorders* (Vol. 1, pp. 61–70). Academic Press.

Toporek, R. L., & Daniels, J. (2018). *2018 update: American Counseling Association advocacy competencies.* https://www.counseling.org/docs/default-source/competencies/aca-advocacy-competencies-updated-may-2020.pdf?sfvrsn=f410212c_4

Toporek, R. L., Lewis, J. A., & Crethar, H. C. (2009). Promoting systemic change through the ACA Advocacy Competencies. *Journal of Counseling and Development, 87*, 260–268. https://doi.org/10.1002/j.1556-6678.2009.tb00105.x

Volkow, N. D. (2020). Stigma and the toll of addiction. *The New England Journal of Medicine, 382*, 1289–1290. https://doi.org/10.1056/NEJMp1917360

White, W. L. (2007). The new recovery advocacy movement in America. *Addiction, 102*, 696–703. https://doi.org/10.1111/j.1360-0443.2007.01808.x

White, W. L., Kelly, J. F., & Roth, J. D. (2012). New addiction-recovery support institutions: Mobilizing support beyond professional addiction treatment and recovery mutual aid. *Journal of Groups in Addiction and Recovery, 7*, 297–317. https://doi.org/10.1080/1556035X.2012.705719

World Health Organization. (2003). *Advocacy for mental health*. https://www.who.int/mental_health/policy/services/1_advocacy_WEB_07.pdf?ua=1

World Health Organization. (2018). *International statistical classification of diseases and related health problems* (11th Rev.). https://icd.who.int/browse11/l-m/en

INDEX

ABUSI. *See* Alexian Brothers Urge to Self-Injure Scale
acceptance and commitment therapy (ACT), 112–113
ACEs. *See* adverse childhood experiences
ACT. *See* acceptance and commitment therapy
Adaptive Information Processing (AIP) model, 134
addiction
  components model, 4–5
  cycle, 8
  definition, 2–3
  vs. excessive healthy enthusiasm, 4
  genogram, 25
  and trauma, 29–31
Addiction-like Eating Behaviour Scale (AEBS), 194
adolescent
  brain development, 22–23
  nonsuicidal self-injury, 165
  pornography, 100–102
  study addiction, 227
adrenaline, 30, 229
adverse childhood experiences (ACEs), 29
  and addiction, 29–31
  childhood obesity, 191
  sex addiction, 82
advocacy
  ASAM definition, 267–268
  behavioral addictions, 268–269
  chemical addiction, 266

community level, 272–273
definition, 265
individual level, 269–271
MSJCC, 265–266
NRAM, 267
public level, 273–275
AEBS. *See* Addiction-like Eating Behaviour Scale
AGA. *See* American Gaming Association
agents, behavioral addictions, 7–8
agonists, 19
AIP model. *See* Adaptive Information Processing model
Alcoholics Anonymous, 50
Alexian Brothers Urge to Self-Injure Scale (ABUSI), 175
American Gaming Association (AGA), 143
American Society of Addiction Medicine (ASAM), 2, 17, 267–268
amygdala, 20, 22, 169
anorexia nervosa, exercise addiction, 208–209
antagonists, 19
antisocial personality, gambling, 148
anxious attachment styles, sex addiction, 84
anxious-avoidant attachment, 83
anxious-resistant attachment, 83
arousal template, continued pornography use, 105
ASAM. *See* American Society of Addiction Medicine

attachment, sex addiction, 83–84, 90–91
attraction, 121
avatar, 35
axon, 18

BBGS. *See* Brief Biosocial Gambling Screen
BED. *See* binge eating disorder
behavioral addiction, 47
  adolescent, 3
  advocacy, 268–269
  criteria, 3
  four Cs, 5–6
  genetic predisposition, 24–25
  neuroscience (*see* neuroscience)
  offline addictive behaviors, 1–2
  prevalence rates, 1
  public health model, 7–12
  rewarding behaviors, 2
behavioral conditioning, 147
Bergen Facebook Addiction Scale (BFAS), 66
Bergen Shopping Addiction Scale (BSAS), 6, 254–255
Bergen Social Media Addiction Scale (BSMAS), 66
Bergen Work Addiction Scale (BWAS), 233–234
BFAS. *See* Bergen Facebook Addiction Scale
binge eating, 187
binge eating disorder (BED), 187–188
biopsychosocial model of addiction, 8, 17, 270
BN. *See* bulimia nervosa
body dysmorphic disorder, 209–210
borderline personality disorder (BPD), 173, 253
bottom-up process, emotion regulation, 169
brain development, adolescent, 22–23
Brief Biosocial Gambling Screen (BBGS), 154–155
BSAS. *See* Bergen Shopping Addiction Scale
BSMAS. *See* Bergen Social Media Addiction Scale
bulimia nervosa (BN), 187
bupropion, internet gaming addiction, 49
BWAS. *See* Bergen Work Addiction Scale

Canadian Problem Gambling Index (CPGI), 154
Carnes's 30-task model, 89–90
CBS. *See* Compulsive Buying Scale
CBT. *See* cognitive behavioral therapy
CCS. *See* Composite Codependency Scale
Celebrate Recovery, 115
Certified Sex Addiction Therapist (CSAT), 93
CGAA. *See* Computer Gaming Addicts Anonymous
chain analysis, 178
chemical addiction, 1
chilling effect, 106
classic sex addiction, 100
client advocacy, 268
client empowerment, advocacy, 268
codependence, love addiction
  attachment issues and childhood trauma, 126
  childhood trauma, 125
  definition, 125
  difficulties, 125
  pathological love, 126
Co-Dependents Anonymous (CoDA) program, 124
cognitive behavioral therapy (CBT)
  food addiction, 198–199
  gambling addiction, 157
cognitive behavioral therapy-internet addiction (CBT-IA), 48
cognitive defusion, 112
cognitive distortions, gambling addiction, 146–147
cognitive fusion, ACT, 112
collective action, advocacy, 268
community collaboration, advocacy, 268
community level advocacy, 272–273
components model of addiction, 4–5
Composite Codependency Scale (CCS), 132
compulsive buying, 246
Compulsive Buying Scale (CBS), 254
compulsive overeating, 188
compulsive sexual behavior, 77, 81, 84
Computer Gaming Addicts Anonymous (CGAA), 50
consumer neuroscience, 248–249
contemporary sex addiction, 100

cortisol, 30, 229
Council for Accreditation of Counseling and Related Educational Programs (CACREP), 3
CPGI. *See* Canadian Problem Gambling Index
CSAT. *See* Certified Sex Addiction Therapist
cyberbullying
  offline bullying, 62–63
  perpetration, 63
  social media addiction, 62–63
  victimization, 63
cyberloafing, 64
cybersex addiction. *See also* pornography and cybersex addiction
  at-risk users, 103
  categories, 99
  gender, 103
  recreational users, 103
  sexually addicted users, 103
cybersquatting, 101
cyclical limerence, 124

DA. *See* Debtors Anonymous
daily fantasy sports (DFS), 150
Debtors Anonymous (DA), 259
Deliberate Self-Harm Inventory (DSHI), 174
dendrites, 18
DFS. *See* daily fantasy sports
Diagnostic and Statistical Manual of Mental Disorders 5th ed (DSM-5), 2, 42, 71
  anorexia nervosa, 209
  binge eating disorder, 187
  body dysmorphic disorder, 210
  borderline personality disorder, 253
  bulimia nervosa, 187
  hoarding disorder, 249
  internet gaming addiction, 44
  nomophobia, 56
  nonsuicidal self-injury, 171
  social media addiction, 71
dialectical behavior therapy (DBT), 177–178
dissociative symptoms, nonsuicidal self-injury, 167
dopamine release, 20
  food addiction, 190

love addiction, 127–128
repeated pornography use, 105
shopping addiction, 251
social media addiction, 60–61
DSHI. *See* Deliberate Self-Harm Inventory
DSM-5. *See* Diagnostic and Statistical Manual of Mental Disorders 5th ed
dysregulated stress response system, 30–31

EAI. *See* Exercise Addiction Inventory
eating addiction, 187
eating disorders, food addiction, 1871–88
EDS. *See* Exercise Dependence Scale
EGMs. *See* electronic gambling machines
electronic gambling machines (EGMs), 143, 145
EMDR. *See* eye movement desensitization and reprocessing
emotion regulation, 8
  exercise addiction
  food addiction, 185–186, 194–195
  gambling addiction, 144, 157
  internet gaming, 48
  love addiction, 127
  nonsuicidal self-injury, 166, 167, 169, 176
  pornography, 108
  prevention efforts, 272–273
  sex addiction, 90–91
endogenous chemical release, 19
environment, behavioral addiction specificity, 9–10
epigenetics, 29
ERP. *See* exposure and response (ritual) prevention
eSports, 41
exercise addiction
  activities, 205
  anorexia nervosa, 208–209
  assessment instruments, 215–216
  body dysmorphic disorder, 209–210
  clinical work, 217
  compulsive behaviors, 206
  definition, 206
  diagnostic considerations, 220
  emotional distress, 206
  interaction model, 207–208

exercise addiction (cont.)
  motivation, 207
  neuroscience, 211–213
  prevalence, 210–211
  primary, 208
  proposed criteria, 213–214
  resources, 220–221
  secondary, 208
  symptoms, 206
  treatment, 216–219
Exercise Addiction Inventory (EAI), 215
Exercise Dependence Scale (EDS), 216
exogenous chemicals, 19
experiential avoidance, ACT, 112
exposure and response (ritual) prevention (ERP), 218–219
eye movement desensitization and reprocessing (EMDR), 134–135

Facebook
  addiction, 57–58
  motives, 57
Fantasy Sports and Gaming Association (FSGA), 150
fear of missing out (FoMO), 61–62
fixed ratio reinforcement schedules, 147
FoMO. *See* fear of missing out
food addiction
  assessment instruments, 193–194
  clinical work, 195–196
  cognitive behavioral therapy, 198–199
  controversy, 186–187
  diagnostic considerations, 199–200
  vs. eating disorder, 195
  eating disorders, 187–188
  hedonic eating, 192
  mental health, 192–193
  mindfulness-based interventions, 196–198
  neuroscience, 189–191
  overweight/obese individuals, 186
  prevalence, 189
  resources, 200–201
  symptoms, 10–11
  and trauma, 191
  treatment, 194–200
  12-step support, 199
Food Addicts in Recovery Anonymous (FA), 195

FSGA. *See* Fantasy Sports and Gaming Association
functional magnetic resonance imaging (fMRI)
  love addiction, 127
  online shopping addiction, 247

GA. *See* Gamblers Anonymous
Gamblers Anonymous (GA), 153, 159
gambler's fallacy, 146
gamblification, 149
gambling, 36, 60
gambling addiction
  activities, 144–145
  assessment and screening tools, 153–155
  clinical work, 156–157
  cognitive behavioral therapy, 157
  cognitive distortions, 146–147
  and criminal behavior, 152–153
  diagnostic criteria, 151
  electronic gambling machines, 145
  gambling forms, 143
  internet gambling, 144–145
  motivational interviewing, 158–159
  negative consequences, 42–43
  neuroscience, 147–149
  prevalence, 145–146
  resources, 160
  risk factors, 152
  self-exclusion, 159
  sports betting and daily fantasy sports, 149–150
  stock market investments, 145
  and suicide, 153
  treatment, 155–160
  12-step support, 159–160
Gaming Disorder Test (GDT), 45
gaming genres, 37, 38
genetic predisposition, behavioral addiction, 24–25
genogram, 25
group-based positive psychology interventions, 69
group counseling
  food addiction, 196–198
  sex addiction, 90–91
  shopping addiction, 255–256
  social media addiction, 70

harm reduction therapy, internet gaming, 48
HBI. *See* Hypersexual Behavior Inventory
healthy exercise behavior (HEB), 218
HEB. *See* healthy exercise behavior
hedonic eating, 192
hoarding disorder, 249–250
host, behavioral addiction, 8–9
hyperphagia, 186
Hypersexual Behavior Inventory (HBI), 87
hypersexual disorder, 84, 85
hypersexuality, sex addiction, 79
hypothalamic–pituitary–adrenal (HPA) axis, 30

ICD-11. *See* International Classification of Diseases, 11th Revision
IGDS9-SF. *See* Internet Gaming Disorder Scale-Short Form
individual level advocacy, 269–271
inflexible attention, ACT, 112
insecure attachment styles, sex addiction, 83
interaction model of exercise addiction, 207–208
internal family systems (IFS) therapy, 113–114
International Classification of Diseases, 11th Revision (ICD-11), 2, 42, 50, 71
  exercise addiction, 214
  food addiction, 200
  gambling disorder, 151
  pornography and cybersex addiction, 107, 115
  sex addiction, 84
  shopping addiction, 252
  work addiction, 230
internet addiction, 36–37
  diagnostic criteria, 63
  positive psychology intervention, 69
Internet Addiction Test (IAT), 36, 66
Internet and Technology Addicts Anonymous (ITAA), 71
internet gaming addiction, 144–145
  assessment, 44–46
  cognitive behavioral therapy-internet addiction, 48
  diagnosis, 42
  diagnostic considerations, 50
  eSports, 41
  gaming nature, 37–38
  vs. internet addiction, 36–37
  massively multiplayer online, 35
  mental health, 43–44
  motives, 39
  neuroscience, 39–41
  prevalence, 38
  resources, 51
  seven-step treatment approach, 49
  treatment strategies, 46–50
  12-step support programs, 50
internet gaming disorder (IGD), 41
Internet Gaming Disorder Scale-Short Form (IGDS9-SF), 44–45
ITAA. *See* Internet and Technology Addicts Anonymous

Jessica Logan Act, 102

LAI. *See* Love Addiction Inventory
LAI-SF. *See* Love Addiction Inventory Short Form
learning, 21–22
leisure sickness, 226
limerence, 123–124
limerent object, 123
loot boxes, 40
love addiction
  assessment instruments, 131–132
  characteristics, 129–130
  clinical work, 133–134
  codependence, 124–126
  diagnostic considerations, 137
  EMDR, 134–135
  limerence, 123–124
  negative consequences, 130
  neuroscience, 126–128
  prevalence, 126
  proposed criteria, 129
  psychodrama therapy, 135
  resources, 137–138
  vs. sex addiction, 122–123
  treatment, 132–137
  12-step support, 136
Love Addiction Inventory (LAI), 131
Love Addiction Inventory Short Form (LAI-SF), 131

massively multiplayer online (MMO) games, 35
MAT. *See* Meditation Awareness Training
MB-EAT. *See* Mindfulness-Based Eating Awareness Training
MBIs. *See* mindfulness-based interventions
MDMA. *See* methylenedioxymethamphetamine
Meditation Awareness Training (MAT), 236
mesolimbic dopamine system pathway, 20–21
methylenedioxymethamphetamine (MDMA), 128
Mindfulness-Based Eating Awareness Training (MB-EAT), 197
mindfulness-based interventions (MBIs), 196–198
MOGQ. *See* Motives for Online Gaming Questionnaire
moral model of addiction, 269–270
motivational interviewing, gambling addiction, 158–159
Motives for Online Gaming Questionnaire (MOGQ), 45–46
MSJCC. *See* Multicultural and Social Justice Counseling Competencies
MUDs. *See* Multi-User Dungeons
Multicultural and Social Justice Counseling Competencies (MSJCC), 11, 265–266
Multi-User Dungeons (MUDs), 35
Murphy vs. National Collegiate Athletic Association, 149
muscle dysmorphia, 210
myelination, 23

neuroadaptations
  abuse and rewarding activities, 26
  addiction cycle, 27
  chemical addiction, 26
  dopaminergic system downregulation, 26–27
  novel stimuli, 26–27
  supernormal stimuli, 26
neuromarketing, 248–249
Neuromarketing Science and Business Association (NMSBA), 248

neurons, 18
neuroplasticity, 19, 105
neuroscience
  brain circuity, 17
  exercise addiction, 211–213
  food addiction, 189–191
  gambling addiction, 147–149
  genetic and environmental factors interaction, 28–31
  genetic predisposition, 24–25
  internet gaming addiction, 39–41
  love addiction, 126–128
  neuroadaptations, 26–28
  neurotransmission, 18–19
  nonsuicidal self-injury, 168–170
  pornography, 104–106
  reward circuitry, 19–22
  sex addiction, 81–83
  shopping addiction, 251–252
  social media addiction, 59–61
  work addiction, 229
neurotransmission, 18–19
neurotransmitters, 18, 21
New Recovery Advocacy Movement (NRAM), 267–268
nomophobia, 56
nonsuicidal self-injury (NSSI)
  assessment measures, 174–175
  behaviors, 165
  clinical work, 176–177
  diagnostic considerations, 179
  dialectical behavior therapy, 177–178
  functional behavioral analysis, 176
  gender differences, 168
  motives, 166–167
  neuroscience, 168–170
  prevalence rates, 167–168
  proposed criteria, 171–172
  resources, 180
  social contagion, 170–171
  vs. suicide attempt, 172–173
  TF-CBT, 179
  treatment, 175–179, 178
  types, 166
  with and without borderline personality disorder, 173
Non-Suicidal Self-Injury Disorder Scale (NSSIDS), 174–175
novel stimuli, 26–27

NRAM. *See* New Recovery Advocacy Movement
NSSI. *See* nonsuicidal self-injury
NSSIDS. *See* Non-Suicidal Self-Injury Disorder Scale

obesity, food addiction, 186
obsessive-compulsive disorder (OCD), 209
  diagnostic considerations, 220
  exposure and response (ritual) prevention, 218–219
online sexual behavior, 99, 107
online shopping addiction, 247–248
operant conditioning, 59
opioids, 169
other specified feeding or eating disorder (OSFED), 200
overworking, 226
oxytocin release, love addiction, 128

PACE. *See* pragmatics, attraction, communication, expectations
pain pathway, 168
pathological exercise, 208. *See also* exercise addiction
pathological gambling, 36. *See also* gambling addiction
pathological love, 126. *See also* love addiction
PCES-SF. *See* Pornography Consumption Effects Scale-Short Form
PCQ. *See* Pornography Craving Questionnaire
PED scale. *See* Positive Effects Dimension scale
personal finance plan, 258–259
physical activity, 205
pornography and cybersex addiction
  acceptance and commitment therapy, 112–113
  adolescent, 100–102
  assessment instruments, 108–110
  clinical work, 111–112
  diagnostic considerations, 115
  ethical considerations, 106
  internal family systems therapy, 113–114
  negative consequences, 108
  neuroscience, 104–106
  prevalence, 103
  proposed criteria, 107–108
  resources, 115–116
  and sexting, 100–102
  treatment, 110–115
  12-step support groups, 114–115
  virtual reality (VR), 100
Pornography Consumption Effects Scale-Short Form (PCES-SF), 109
Pornography Craving Questionnaire (PCQ), 110
positive addictions, 206
positive psychology intervention, social media addiction, 69
PPUS. *See* Problematic Pornography Use Scale
pragmatics, attraction, communication, expectations (PACE), 9–10
primary exercise addiction, 208
Problematic Pornography Use Scale (PPUS), 109
Problematic Social Networking Services Use Scale (PSUS), 66–67
proinflammatory cytokine (IL-17), 232
PSUS. *See* Problematic Social Networking Services Use Scale
psychodrama therapy, love addiction, 135
psychoeducation
  behavioral addiction, 269
  food addiction, 195
  internet gaming addiction, 49
  social media addiction, 61
public health model, behavioral addictions, 13
  agents, 7–8
  environment, 9–11
  epidemiologic triad, 7
  host, 8–9
  vector, 11–12

racial discrimination, 10
randomized controlled trials (RCTs), 274
Rational Emotive Behavioral Therapy (REBT), 237
RCTs. *See* randomized controlled trials
REBT. *See* Rational Emotive Behavioral Therapy

retail therapy, 246
reward circuitry
  adolescent brain development, 22–23
  dopamine, 20–21
  mesolimbic dopaminergic pathway, 20–21
  rewards and learning, 21–22
  wanting and liking, 20
reward deficiency syndrome (RDS), 24–25, 190
rewards and learning, 21–22
reward system, 19, 81
romantic love, 121

SAA. *See* Sex Addicts Anonymous
SAST-R. *See* Sexual Addiction Screening Test-Revised
SCS. *See* Sexual Compulsivity Scale
secondary exercise addiction, 208
secure attachment, sex addiction, 83
self-as-context, ACT, 112
self-directed emotions, sex addiction, 79
self-esteem, social media addiction, 65
self-exclusion, gambling addiction, 159
self-expanding activities, love addiction, 133
self-injury, *See* nonsuicidal self-injury
self-punishment, nonsuicidal self-injury, 167
sex addiction
  assessment instruments, 86–87
  and attachment, 83–84
  attachment and emotion regulation, 90–91
  clinical work, 88–89
  compulsive sexual behavior, 77
  diagnostic considerations, 92
  emotion regulation, 77
  four-part cycle, 78–79
  vs. love addiction, 122–123
  mood modification, 78
  negative consequences, 85
  neuroscience, 81–83
  obsession and rituals, 77
  prevalence, 80–81
  proposed criteria, 84–85
  resources, 93
  vs. sexual offending, 79–80
  treatment, 87–92
  12-step support, 91–92

Sex Addicts Anonymous (SAA), 77, 91–92
Sexaholics Anonymous, 115
Sex and Love Addicts Anonymous (SLAA), 136
sexting and pornography
  definition, 101
  policies and regulations, 101
  school counselors, 102
Sexual Addiction Screening Test-Revised (SAST-R), 86
sexual anorexia, 77
Sexual Compulsives Anonymous, 115
Sexual Compulsivity Scale (SCS), 86–87
sexually addicted sex offender, 80
sexually concerned, 80
sexual maps, 106
sexual offending, 79–80
shame, sex addiction, 79
shopping addiction
  assessment instruments, 254–255
  clinical work, 257
  counseling approaches, 256
  diagnostic considerations, 259–260
  group counseling approach, 256–258
  hoarding disorder, 249–250
  marketing campaigns and advertisements, 245
  mental health, 253–254
  neuromarketing, 248–249
  neuroscience, 251–252
  online shopping, 247–248
  overshopping motives, 255
  personal finance plan, 258–259
  phases, 246
  prevalence rates, 250–251
  proposed criteria, 252–253
  resources, 260
  treatment, 255–259
  12-step support, 259
Shopping Reminder Card, 256
SLAA. *See* Sex and Love Addicts Anonymous
sleep disturbance, social media addiction, 64–65
smartphone addiction, 10
  proposed criteria, 63–64
  vs. social media addiction, 56–57
SMAS. *See* Social Media Addiction Scale
social contagion, 170–171
social media addiction

assessment tools, 65–67
clinical work, 68
cyberbullying, 62–63
diagnostic considerations, 71
fear of missing out, 61–62
feedback features, 55
Instagram, 55
mood modification, 58
motives, 57–58
negative consequences, 64–65
neuroscience, 59–61
positive psychology intervention, 69
prevalence, 58–59
proposed criteria, 63
resources, 72
vs. smartphone addiction, 56–57
social networking, 55
technology plan, 69–70
treatment, 67–71
12-step support program, 71
Social Media Addiction Scale (SMAS), 66
social networking, 55
social/political advocacy, 269
SOGS. *See* South Oaks Gambling Screen
South Oaks Gambling Screen (SOGS), 154
sports betting and daily fantasy sports, 149–150
stalking behaviors, love addiction, 130
Stopping Overshopping Group Treatment Program, 256–258
stress response system, 29–30
    food addiction, 191
    sex addiction, 82
suicide
    assessment, internet gaming addiction, 46
    gambling addiction, 153
    nonsuicidal self-injury, 172–173
supernormal stimuli, 26, 104, 190
synapses, 18
systems advocacy, 268

teleology, 39
TF-CBT. *See* trauma-focused cognitive behavioral therapy
Three Circles technique, 92
top-down process, emotion regulation, 169
toxic stress, 30, 82
trauma

adverse childhood experiences, 29
food addiction, 191
love addiction, 175, 179
nonsuicidal self-injury, 166–167, 179
pornography and cybersex addiction, 99–100
sex addiction, 81–83
shopping addiction, 255–256
stress response system, 29–30
systemic oppression, 10
work addiction, 231
trauma-focused cognitive behavioral therapy (TF-CBT)
    components of, 179
    nonsuicidal self-injury (NSSI), 179
Treatment for Self-Injurious Behavior (T-SIB), 178
T-SIB. *See* Treatment for Self-Injurious Behavior
12-step support program
    food addiction, 199
    gambling addiction, 159–160
    internet gaming addiction, 50
    love addiction, 136
    pornography and cybersex addiction, 114–115
    sex addiction, 91–92
    shopping addiction, 259
    social media addiction, 71
    work addiction, 238

UFED. *See* unspecified feeding or eating disorder
unspecified feeding or eating disorder (UFED), 209

variable ratio reinforcement schedules, 40, 60, 147
vasopressin release, love addiction, 128
vector, behavioral addiction, 11–12

War on Drugs, 267
WART. *See* Work Addiction Risk Test
wearable technology, 212
work addiction
    assessment strategies, 232–234
    childhood experiences, 231
    clinical work, 235–236
    cultural norms, 228
    identification, 229–230

work addiction (*cont.*)
  individual and environmental predictors, 226–227
  leisure sickness, 226
  negative consequences, 232
  neuroscience, 229
  overworking, 226
  prevalence, 228
  resources, 239
  study addiction, 227
  treatment, 234–238
  12-step support, 238
  warning signs, 230–231
Work Addiction Risk Test (WART), 233
Workaholics Anonymous, 238
work anorexic, 230
work-family life conflict, 228

Yale Food Addiction Scale (YFAS), 192, 193
YFAS. *See* Yale Food Addiction Scale

www.ingramcontent.com/pod-product-compliance
Ingram Content Group UK Ltd.
Pitfield, Milton Keynes, MK11 3LW, UK
UKHW021833140426
5217IPUK00021B/1419